NANOMEDICINE AND CANCER THERAPIES

Advances in Nanoscience and Nanotechnology
Volume 2

NANOMEDICINE AND CANCER THERAPIES

Edited By
**Mathew Sebastian, MD, Neethu Ninan,
and Eldho Elias**

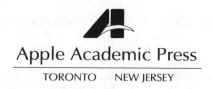

Apple Academic Press

TORONTO   NEW JERSEY

© 2013 by
Apple Academic Press Inc.
3333 Mistwell Crescent
Oakville, ON L6L 0A2
Canada

Apple Academic Press Inc.
1613 Beaver Dam Road, Suite # 104
Point Pleasant, NJ 08742
USA

First issued in paperback 2021

Exclusive worldwide distribution by CRC Press, a Taylor & Francis Group

ISBN 13: 978-1-77463-237-6 (pbk)
ISBN 13: 978-1-926895-18-5 (hbk)

Library of Congress Control Number: 2012935668

Library and Archives Canada Cataloguing in Publication

Nanomedicine and cancer therapies / edited by Mathew Sebastian, Neethu Ninan and Eldho Elias.
(Recent advances in nanoscience and nanotechnology; v.2)

Includes bibliographical references and index.
ISBN 978-1-926895-18-5
1. Nanomedicine. 2. Cancer–Treatment. 3. Cancer–Diagnosis.
4. Nanotechnology. I. Sebastian, Mathew II. Ninan, Neethu
III. Elias, Eldho IV. Series: Recent advances in nanoscience and nanotechnology; v.2

R857.N34N36 2012   610.28   C2011-908742-1

Apple Academic Press also publishes its books in a variety of electronic formats. Some content that appears in print may not be available in electronic format. For information about Apple Academic Press products, visit our website at **www.appleacademicpress.com**

Advances in Nanoscience and Nanotechnology

Series Editors-in-Chief

Sabu Thomas, PhD

Dr. Sabu Thomas is the Director of the School of Chemical Sciences, Mahatma Gandhi University, Kottayam, India. He is also a full professor of polymer science and engineering and Director of the Centre for nanoscience and nanotechnology of the same university. He is a fellow of many professional bodies. Professor Thomas has authored or co-authored many papers in international peer-reviewed journals in the area of polymer processing. He has organized several international conferences and has more than 420 publications, 11 books and two patents to his credit. He has been involved in a number of books both as author and editor. He is a reviewer to many international journals and has received many awards for his excellent work in polymer processing. His h Index is 42. Professor Thomas is listed as the 5th position in the list of Most Productive Researchers in India, in 2008.

Mathew Sebastian, MD

Dr. Mathew Sebastian has a degree in surgery (1976) with specialization in Ayurveda. He holds several diplomas in acupuncture, neural therapy (pain therapy), manual therapy and vascular diseases. He was a missionary doctor in Mugana Hospital, Bukoba in Tansania, Africa (1976-1978) and underwent surgical training in different hospitals in Austria, Germany, and India for more than 10 years. Since 2000 he is the doctor in charge of the Ayurveda and Vein Clinic in Klagenfurt, Austria. At present he is a Consultant Surgeon at Privatclinic Maria Hilf, Klagenfurt. He is a member of the scientific advisory committee of the European Academy for Ayurveda, Birstein, Germany, and the TAM advisory committee (Traditional Asian Medicine, Sector Ayurveda) of the Austrian Ministry for Health, Vienna. He conducted an International Ayurveda Congress in Klagenfurt, Austria, in 2010. He has several publications to his name.

Anne George, MD

Anne George, MD, is the Director of the Institute for Holistic Medical Sciences, Kottayam, Kerala, India. She did her MBBS (Bachelor of Medicine, Bachelor of Surgery) at Trivandrum Medical College, University of Kerala, India. She acquired a DGO (Diploma in Obstetrics and Gynaecology) from the University of Vienna, Austria; Diploma Acupuncture from the University of Vienna; and an MD from Kottayam Medical College, Mahatma Gandhi University, Kerala, India. She has organized several international conferences, is a fellow of the American Medical Society, and is a member of many international organizations. She has five publications to her name and has presented 25 papers.

Dr. Yang Weimin

Dr. Yang Weimin is the Taishan Scholar Professor of Quingdao University of Science and Technology in China. He is a full professor at the Beijing University of Chemical Technology and a fellow of many professional organizations. Professor Weimin has authored many papers in international peer-reviewed journals in the area of polymer processing. He has been contributed to a number of books as author and editor and acts as a reviewer to many international journals. In addition, he is a consultant to many polymer equipment manufacturers. He has also received numerous award for his work in polymer processing.

Contents

List of Contributors .... *ix*

List of Abbreviations .... *xiii*

Preface .... *xvii*

1. **Nanotechnological Based Systems for Cancer** 1

   Jagat R. Kanwar, Ganesh Mahidhara, and Rupinder K. Kanwar

2. ***In vivo* Spectroscopy for Detection and Treatment of GBM with NPt Implantation** 19

   José de la Rosa, Diego Adrián Fabila, Luis Felipe Hernández, Edgard Moreno, Suren Stolik, Gabriela de la Rosa, Mayra Álvarez, Alfonso Arellano, Tessy López, R. Mercado, J. L. Soto, L. Arredondo, J. Bustos, A. Mosqueda, and I. Rivero

3. **Nanobiotechnology for Antibacterial Therapy and Diagnosis** 31

   Jagat R. Kanwar, Kislay Roy, and Rupinder K. Kanwar

4. **Chitosan Nanoparticles** 41

   Divyen Shah, Vaishali Londhe, and Rima Shah

5. **Synthesis and Biomedical Application of Silver Nanoparticles** 55

   M. Saravanan and V. Anil Kumar

6. **Recent Advances in Cancer Therapy Using Phytochemicals** 69

   Hullathy Subban Ganapathy, Rajakani Senthil Nagarajan, and Hirotaka Ihara

7. **Mitochondrial Dysfunction and Cancer: Modulation by Palladium α-Lipoic Acid Complex** 75

   C. V. Krishnan, M. Garnett, and F. Antonawich

8. **Unity of Mind and Body: The Concept of Life Purpose Dominant** 131

   Bukhtoyarov Oleg Viktorovich and Samarin Denis Mikhaylovich

9. ***Thuja occidentalis* and Breast Cancer Chemoprevention** 143

   B. K. Ojeswi, M. Khoobchandani, S. Medhe, D. K. Hazra, and M. M. Srivastava

10. **Antioxidants and Combinatorial Therapies in Cancer Treatment** 157

    Arpita Saxena

11. ***Eruca sativa* Inhibits Melanoma Growth: A Scientific Evidence** 163

    M. Khoobchandani, N. Ganesh, L. Valgimigli, and M. M. Srivastava

12. **Optical and Mechanical Investigations of Nanostructures for Biomolecular Detection** 173

    G. Malegori, D. Nardi, F. Banfi, C. Giannetti, and G. Ferrini

13. Suffering and Comfort in Portuguese Cancer Patients **189**

João Luís Alves Apóstolo, Rita Susana Soares Capela, and Inês Barata Sá Castro

References **199**
Index **245**

List of Contributors

Mayra Álvarez
Laboratorio de Nanotecnología, Instituto Nacional de Neurología y Neurocirugía "MVS", Insurgentes Sur 3877, La Fama, CP-14269, D.F., México.

F. Antonawich
Garnett McKeen Laboratory, Inc, Bohemia, New York-11716–1735, USA

João Luís Alves Apóstolo
RN, PhD, Health Sciences Research Unit: Nursing, Coimbra Nursing School, Avenida Bissaya Barreto—Apartado-7001, 3046 851 Coimbra Portugal

Alfonso Arellano
Laboratorio de Nanotecnología, Instituto Nacional de Neurología y Neurocirugía "MVS", Insurgentes Sur 3877, La Fama, CP-14269, D.F., México.

L. Arredondo
Hospital Civil de Guadalajara, Salvador de Quevedo y Zubieta No. 750 Esq. Sierra Nevada, Independencia, CP-44340, Guadalajara, Jal., México.

F. Banfi
Dipartimento di Matematica e Fisica, Università Cattolica, I-25121 Brescia, Italy,

J. Bustos
Departamento de Atención a la Salud, Universidad Autónoma Metropolitana Xochimilco, Calzada del Hueso 1100, Villa Quietud, CP-04960, D.F., México.

Rita Susana Soares Capela
RN, Master in Palliative Care, Oncology/Haematology Unit of the Portuguese Institute of Oncology of Porto, Portugal, Rua Dr. António Bernardino de Almeida

Inês Barata Sá Castro
Grant holder, Health Sciences Research Unit: Nursing, Coimbra Nursing School, Avenida Bissaya Barreto—Apartado-7001, 3046-851 Coimbra–Portugal

Diego Adrián Fabila
Instituto Politécnico Nacional, Unidad Profesional "Adolfo López Mateos", SEPI-ESIME ZAC., Lindavista, CP-07738, D.F., México.

G. Ferrini
Dipartimento di Matematica e Fisica, Università Cattolica, I-25121 Brescia, Italy.

Hullathy Subban Ganapathy
Priority Organization for Innovation and Excellence, Kumamoto University, 2-39-1 Kurokami, Kumamoto-860–8555, Japan

N. Ganesh
Jawaharlal Nehru Cancer Hospital and Research Centre, Bhopal-422001, India

M. Garnett
Garnett McKeen Laboratory, Inc, Bohemia, New York 11716-1735, USA

C. Giannetti
Dipartimento di Matematica e Fisica, Università Cattolica, I-25121 Brescia, Italy.

D. K. Hazra
S.N Medical College, Agra, India-282002.

Luis Felipe Hernández
Instituto Politécnico Nacional, Unidad Profesional "Adolfo López Mateos", SEPI-ESIME ZAC., Lindavista, CP-07738, D.F., México.

Hirotaka Ihara
Department of Applied Chemistry and Biochemistry, Faculty of Engineering, Kumamoto University, 2-39-1 Kurokami, Kumamoto-860–8555, Japan

Jagat R. Kanwar
Laboratory of Immunology and Molecular Biomedical Research (LIMBR), Centre for Biotechnology and Interdisciplinary Biosciences (BioDeakin), Institute for Technology and Research Innovation (ITRI), Geelong Technology Precinct (GTP), Deakin University, Pigdons Road, Waurn Ponds, Geelong, Victoria-3217, Australia.

Rupinder K. Kanwar
Laboratory of Immunology and Molecular Biomedical Research (LIMBR), Centre for Biotechnology and Interdisciplinary Biosciences (BioDeakin), Institute for Technology and Research Innovation (ITRI), Geelong Technology Precinct (GTP), Deakin University, Pigdons Road, Waurn Ponds, Geelong, Victoria-3217, Australia.

M. Khoobchandani
Department of Chemistry, Faculty of Science, Dayalbagh Educational Institute, Agra, India-282110.

C. V. Krishnan
Garnett McKeen Laboratory, Inc, Bohemia, New York-11716–1735, USA.
Department of Chemistry, Stony Brook University, New York-11794–3400, USA.

Anil Kumar V.
Department of Biotechnology, Faculty of Science and Humanities, SRM University, SRM Nagar, Kattankulathur, Chennai, Tamilnadu-603203, India.

Vaishali Londhe
School of Pharmacy & Technology Management, SVKM's NMIMS, Mumbai, Maharashtra-400057, India.

Tessy López
Laboratorio de Nanotecnología, Instituto Nacional de Neurología y Neurocirugía "MVS", Insurgentes Sur 3877, La Fama, CP-14269, D.F., México.
Departamento de Atención a la Salud, Universidad Autónoma Metropolitana Xochimilco, Calzada del Hueso 1100, Villa Quietud, CP-04960, D.F., México.
Department of Chemical Engineering, Tulane University, New Orleans, LA-70118.

Ganesh Mahidhara
Laboratory of Immunology and Molecular Biomedical Research (LIMBR), Centre for Biotechnology and Interdisciplinary Biosciences (BioDeakin), Institute for Technology Research and Innovation (ITRI), Deakin University, Waurn Ponds, Victoria-3217, Australia.

G. Malegori
Dipartimento di Matematica e Fisica, Università Cattolica, I-25121 Brescia, Italy.

S. Medhe
Department of Chemistry, Faculty of Science, Dayalbagh Educational Institute, Agra, India-282110.

R. Mercado
Hospital Civil de Guadalajara, Salvador de Quevedo y Zubieta No. 750 Esq. Sierra Nevada, Independencia, CP-44340, Guadalajara, Jal., México.

Samarin Denis Mikhaylovich
Center for Medical and Social Rehabilitation UFSIN Russia of Kaliningrad region 10–103, ul. V. Gakuna-236009, Kaliningrad, Russian Federation.

Edgard Moreno
Instituto Politécnico Nacional, Unidad Profesional "Adolfo López Mateos", SEPI-ESIME ZAC., Lindavista, CP-07738, D.F., México.

A. Mosqueda
Departamento de Atención a la Salud, Universidad Autónoma Metropolitana Xochimilco, Calzada del Hueso 1100, Villa Quietud, CP-04960, D.F., México.

Rajakani Senthil Nagarajan
Priority Organization for Innovation and Excellence, Kumamoto University, 2-39-1 Kurokami, Kumamoto-860–8555, Japan.

D. Nardi
Dipartimento di Matematica e Fisica, Università Cattolica, I-25121 Brescia, Italy.

B. K. Ojeswi
Department of Chemistry, Faculty of Science, Dayalbagh Educational Institute, Agra, India-282110.

I. Rivero
Instituto Nacional de Investigaciones Nucleares, Carretera México-Toluca S/N, La Marquesa, CP 52750, Ocoyoacac, México, México.

Gabriela de la Rosa
Laboratorio de Nanotecnología, Instituto Nacional de Neurología y Neurocirugía "MVS", insurgentes Sur 3877, La Fama, CP-14269, D.F., México.

José de la Rosa
Instituto Politécnico Nacional, Unidad Profesional "Adolfo López Mateos", SEPI-ESIME ZAC., Lindavista, CP-07738, D.F., México.

Kislay Roy
Laboratory of Immunology and Molecular Biomedical Research (LIMBR), Centre for Biotechnology and Interdisciplinary Biosciences (BioDeakin), Institute for Technology and Research Innovation (ITRI), Geelong Technology Precinct (GTP), Deakin University, Pigdons Road, Waurn Ponds, Geelong, Victoria-3217, Australia.

M. Saravanan
Department of Biotechnology, Faculty of Science and Humanities, SRM University, SRM Nagar, Kattankulathur, Chennai, Tamilnadu-603203, India.

Arpita Saxena
Division of Cancer Pharmacology, Indian Institute of Integrative Medicine (CSIR), Canal Road, Jammu Tawi-180001, India.

Divyen Shah
School of Pharmacy & Technology Management, SVKM's NMIMS, Mumbai, Maharashtra-400057, India.

Rima Shah
School of Pharmacy & Technology Management, SVKM's NMIMS, Shirpur Campus, Shirpur, Maharashtra-425405, Ind ia.

J. L. Soto
Hospital Civil de Guadalajara, Salvador de Quevedo y Zubieta No. 750 Esq. Sierra Nevada, Independencia, CP-44340, Guadalajara, Jal., México.

M. M. Srivastava
Department of Chemistry, Faculty of Science, Dayalbagh Educational Institute, Agra, India-282110.

Suren Stolik
Instituto Politécnico Nacional, Unidad Profesional "Adolfo López Mateos", SEPI-ESIME ZAC., Lindavista, CP-07738, D.F., México.

L. Valgimigli
R&D Department, University of Bologna, B&C s.r.l, Via C. Monteverdi-49, 47100 Forli Italy

Bukhtoyarov Oleg Viktorovich
Center for Medical and Social Rehabilitation UFSIN Russia of Kaliningrad region
30A-7, ul. S. Razina-236022, Kaliningrad, Russian Federation.

List of Abbreviations

5-ASA	5-Amino salicylic acid
5-ALA	5-Aminolaevullinic acid
ACA	Acrocentric association
ATP	Adenosine triphosphate
AE	Adverse Events
AMD	Age-related macular degradation
ATCC	American type culture collection
AMPs	Antimicrobial peptides
AFM	Atomic force microscopy
AISRF	Australia-India Strategic Research Fund
CNTs	Carbon nanotubes
CPP	Cell-penetrating peptides
CR	Centric rings
COS	Chito oligosaccharides
CS	Chitosan
CB	Chromatid breaks
CLL	Chronic lymphoid leukemia
CPS	Chronic psycho-emotional stress
CRC	Colorectal cancer
CCS	Comfort chemotherapy scale
CPCSEA	Control and supervision of experiments on animals
CA1	Cornus ammon's field 1
CD	Current subdominants
CF	Cystic fibrosis
DPHP	1-Diphenyl-2-picrylhydrazyl
DSMB	Data safety and monitoring board
DSs	Dermaseptins
DC	Dicentric
DMF	Dimethyl formamide
DMSO	Dimethylsulphoxide
DNSurR9	Dominant negative survivin R9
DESSTINI	Dose escalation safety study in normal individuals
dsRNA	Double-stranded ribo nucleic acid
EPR	Electron paramagnetic resonance
ESR	Electron spin resonance

EPCs	Endothelial progenitor cells
EPR	Enhanced permeability retention
EtOAc	Ethyl acetate
ESF	European Science Foundation
ECM	Extracellular matrix
FGFs	Fibroblast growth factors
FSCP	Fish scale collagen peptides
5-FU	Five-fluorouracil
FAD	Flavin adenine dinucleotide
FRET	Fluorescence resonance energy transfer
FAE	Follicle associated epithelium
FT	Fourier transforms
FTIR	Fourier transform infra red
FR	Fragment
GBM	Glioblastoma Multiforme
GSH	Glutathione
GPx	Glutathione peroxidase
GRx	Glutathione reductase
H-E	Hematoxyline-Eosine
HTAB	Hexadecyl trimethyl ammonium bromide
HIF-1	Hypoxia inducible factor 1
IgG	Immunoglobulin G
IFN-γ	Induce interferon-γ
IAP	Inhibitor of apoptosis protein
ITRI	Institute for Technology Research and Innovation
ICD	Intracalary deletion
IP	Intraperitoneally
ICDH	Isocitrate dehydrogenase
α-KGDH	α-Ketoglutarate dehydrogenase
LPD	Life purpose dominant
LS	Life span
LNCaP	Lymph node carcinoma of the prostate
MRI	Magnetic resonance imaging
MDH	Malate dehydrogenase
MDA	Malondialdehyde
MB	Methylene Blue
miRNAs	Micro ribonucleic acids
MNCEs	Micronucleated normochromatic erythrocytes
MPCEs	Micronucleated polychromatic erythrocytes

MBCs	Minimal bactericidal concentrations
MICs	Minimal inhibitory concentrations
mtDNA	Mitochondrial DNA
MW	Molecular weight
MWCNTs	Multiwalled carbon nanotubes
NALT	Nasal associated lymphoid tissues
NCI	National Cancer Institute's
NDR	Negative differential resistance
NADH	Nicotinamide adenine dinucleotide
NADPH	Nicotinamide adenine dinucleotide phosphate
NOAEL	No adverse observed effect level
NC-AFM	Non-contact atomic force microscopy
nDNA	Nuclear DNA
PILs	PEGylated immunoliposomes
PEM	Photo-elastic modulator
PCF	Photonic-crystal fibers
PVA	Poly(vinyl alcohol)
PGA	Poly glycolic acid
PLA	Poly lactic acid
PLGA	Poly lactic-co-glycolic acid
PQA	Poly quaternary ammonium
PEG	Polyethylene glycol
POMs	Polyoxometalates
PUFAH	Polyunsaturated fatty acid
Pox	Protein oxidation
PDTC	Pyrrolidine dithiocarbamate
QCh	Quaternised chitosan
RNOS	Reactive nitrogen oxygen species
ROS	Reactive oxygen species
rHBsAg	Recombinant hepatitis B surface antigen
RSV	Respiratory syncytial virus
RES	Reticulo endothelial system
RNAi	Ribo nucleic acid interference
SD	Safety dominant
SO	Seed oil
SELEX	Selective Evaluation of Ligands by Exponential Enrichment
shRNAs	Short hairpin ribo nucleic acid
SNPs	Single nucleotide polymorphisms
SWNTs	Single-walled nanotubes

siRNAs	Small interfering ribo nucleic acid
STPP	Sodium tri poly phosphate
SDH	Succinate dehydrogenase
SPION	Superparamagnetic iron oxide nanocrystals
SAWs	Surface acoustic waves
SELEX	Systematic evolution of ligands by exponential enrichment
TMX	Tamoxifen
TS	Taxonomic structure
TGA	Thermogravity analysis
TLC	Thin layer chromatography
TBARS	Thiobarbituric acid reacting substance
TEER	Transepithelial electrical resistance
TGF β)	Transforming growth factor β
TM	Transitional meningioma
TEM	Transmission electron microscopy
TPP	Tri poly phosphate
TNF	Tumor necrosis factor
VEGF	Vascular endothelial growth factor
VHL	Von hippel-lindau
WT	Wavelet transform
WHO	World Health Organization
ZO-1	Zonula occludens-1

Preface

Cancer is a well-known deadly disease that is caused due to the inability of some uncontrollably growing cells to die. More than 100 types of cancer have been identified till date, classified on the basis of the type of the initially affected cell. Cancer usually forms tumors of cells that interfere with the nervous, digestive and circulatory systems of the body and sometimes alter the functions by releasing unwanted hormones. They are usually benign and are limited to a region. The more dangerous is the other kind of tumor, i.e. the malignant ones. It occurs when a cancerous cell manages to travel throughout the body through the circulatory system and destroy healthy tissues in its path. Cancer usually develops due to mutation in the genes of the cell making it to forget to die. The cell goes on multiplying and does not die as it had to. Finally, it starts forming a mass. These mutations are caused by many different stimuli like X-rays, radiations, different chemicals etc. The main factor that affects the successful treatment of cancer is based on the timing of detection. An early detection of the deadly disease greatly improves the odds of successful treatment. Cancer is treated using a number of techniques that include surgery, chemotherapy, radiation, immunotherapy, gene therapy, hormone therapy, holistic medicine etc., that come in the category of oncology. This book discusses how nanomedicine, holistic medicine and other cancer therapies contribute in the treatment of cancer.

Nanotechnology has the power to radically change the way cancer is diagnosed, imaged and treated. Currently, there is a lot of research going on to design novel nanodevices capable of detecting cancer at its earliest stages, pinpointing its location within the body and delivering anticancer drugs specifically to malignant cells. Nanoscale devices smaller than 50 nanometers can easily enter most cells, while those smaller than 20 nanometers can transit out of blood vessels. As a result, nanoscale devices can readily interact with biomolecules on both the cell surface and within the cell. Nanoscale devices are already proving that they can deliver therapeutic agents to target cells, or even within specific organelles. Yet, despite its small size, a nanoscale device is capable of holding tens of thousands of small molecules, such as a contrast agent or drug. The major areas in which nanomedicine is being developed in cancer include: (a) Prevention and control (b) Early detection and proteomics (c) Imaging diagnostics and (d) Multifunctional Therapeutics. Earlier detection of cancer means a better chance of effective treatment.

The holistic approach to cancer involves non-invasive procedures focused upon restoring the health of the human energy fields, based upon a human energy field understanding of disease. Holistic care includes the field of study called energy medicine. An element of energy medicine is present in acupuncture, acupressure, homeopathy, herbal medicine, fresh fruits and vegetables, food supplements, aromatherapy, music therapy, dance therapy, some massotherapy and chiropractic, physical exercise, the martial arts, tai chi, qigong, yoga, meditation, compassionate love, emotional release therapy, touch healing, prayer, and most of the other approaches offered on this web site. Each approach acts to restore the human energy fields to health that then signals the body's biological cells to become healthy. According to researchers in this field, when someone is diseased, the person's human energy field is also diseased, distorted in specific ways that can cause and maintain the disease. Human energy field researchers have long referred to cancer as an energy disease. As the cancer cells grow in number, they begin developing their own energy field system that competes with the human energy field system for control of body functions. In late stage cancer, the cancer energy field system has overwhelmed the normal human energy fields, blocking therapeutic outcomes of both medical and holistic treatment.

Discover the "REAL" truth about cancer and learn about all of the most potent cancer healing therapies in this book. The book enlightens how nanomedicne, holistic medicine and other cancer therapies play their role in treating cancer.

— **Mathew Sebastian, MD**

Chapter 1

Nanotechnological Based Systems for Cancer

Jagat R. Kanwar, Ganesh Mahidhara, and Rupinder K. Kanwar

INTRODUCTION

Carcinogenesis is a multistep process, caused by combination of environmental and genetic factors, leading to a series of genetic and epigenetic changes occurring at various stages in the development and progression of the disease (Aznavoorian et al., 1993). Cancer cells arise from a single transformed cell, which has undergone genetic and epigenetic changes. Thus cancerous state is a result of several sequential events triggered by various factors including genetic predispositions, transformation by viruses, radiation and/or by certain chemicals. Many genetic and cytoplasmic events including de activation of tumor suppressor genes such as P53 or Rb, triggers various events leading to cancer (Harris and Levine, 2005).

Tumor invasion and metastasis is the one of the major causes of treatment failure in cancer patients. Also, tumors have a capacity to generate new blood vessels by using preexisting endothelium and/or endothelial precursor cells, by a process known as angiogenesis (Cavallaro and Christofori, 2000; Folkman, 1995) which in turn involves implication of complex and diverse actions such as extra cellular matrix degradation, proliferation and migration of endothelial cells and morphological differentiation of endothelial cells to form tubes. A range of factors including various growth factors, cytokines, lipid metabolites and cryptic fragments of homeostatic proteins, are involved in angiogenesis (Haas et al., 2000).

There are many anticancer, anti-angiogenic drugs approved and in Phase II clinical trials (http://www.cancer.gov/CLINICALTRIALS). But most of them are chemical and/or fungal derivatives, mainly steroid containing compounds and these have many side effects, when metabolized that is after producing their secondary metabolites. So, natural biodegradable compounds are the best alternative for decreasing patient compliance. In this regard, micro ribonucleic acids (miRNAs) are the ideal candidates to consider. These non-coding RNAs, reported to have many implications in temporal and spatial regulation of genes in different organisms. It has been reported that they have tumor suppressing as well as oncogenic properties. Certain classes of micro RNAs, for instance Let 7 family of miRNAs have been proved to have antitumor properties by inhibiting RAS, a factor involved in cell proliferation. So, it is tempting to use these tiny wonders for antitumor therapies. This chapter discusses about development, progression and metastatic stages in the highly interactive process of tumor development, angiogenic switch and molecular regulators involved in this process with specific emphasis on micro RNA, aptamer biology, von Hippel-Lindau (VHL) tumor suppressor, combinatorial therapy towards eradication of cancer and the possible drug development for future (Aznavoorian et al., 1993; Cavallaro and Christofori, 2000;

Folkman, 1995; Haas et al., 2000; Harris and Levine, 2005; Kerr et al., 1972; Knudson, 1971; O'Rourke and Ellem, 2000; Thompson, 1995; Zapata et al., 2001).

APOPTOSIS

The process of cell death was first recognized in the 19th century, when Carl Vogt first described the process of cell death in the notochord and adjacent cartilage of metamorphic tads. Later on Fleming in 1885 described the same process of cell death as "chromalolysis", in which nuclei of mammalian ovarian follicle broke up and were cleared off spontaneously (Hockenbery et al., 1990; Krammer, 2000). The term apoptosis was first derived from the Greek word describing the process of leaves falling from trees. Many different types of apoptotic pathways contain a multitude of different biochemical components, many of them not yet understood (Wajant, 2002). Any modification/removal of at least one member in a sequential pathway like apoptosis causes disastrous effects, often in the form of a disorder.

Mammalian cells undergo apoptosis by two mechanisms; (1) Extrinsic pathway – mediated by Fas ligand and/or APO1/CD95 and several other proteins such as Fas associated death domain (Krammer, 2000) and caspases 8–10 (Wajant, 2002) and (2) Intrinsic pathway- mediated by Bcl-2 family proteins (Hockenbery et al., 1990; Zapata et al., 2001). These pathways are modulated by definite set of genes, which means apoptosis is a genetically intervened process. Bcl-2 family members regulate apoptosis in response to various death inducing stimuli. Till now, more than 15 members of this large Bcl-2 protein family have been identified. Death antagonists/anti-apoptotic proteins including Bcl-2, Bcl-XL, Mcl1, Bcl-W, and A1 which provide protection, whereas death agonist members including Bax, Bad, Bcl-Xs, Bid, Bim, Bik, and Hrk increase sensitivity to death inducing signals. The ratio of death agonist to antagonist signal determines the susceptibility to death stimuli (Scaffidi et al., 1998). In addition, it is found that members of inhibitor of apoptosis protein (*IAP*) gene family proteins including c-IAP1, c-IAP2, XIAP, NAIP, survivin, apollon, MLIAP/livin, and ILP-2 function as endogenous inhibitors of caspases. Among all the IAP members, survivin and livin are highly expressed in cancer cells and transformed cells but show little or no expression in normal differentiated tissues (Li, 2003; Li and Ling, 2006). Co-localization of survivin antibodies and livin antibodies has been reported in sera of breast cancer patients (Yagihashi et al., 2005). In this regard, we have demonstrated earlier that, combinational therapy using antisense survivin and B7-1 immunogene therapy eradicated EL4 thymic lymphoma tumors (Kanwar et al., 2001a). There are a few reports in using human and/or murine survivin antagonists as anticancer vaccines (Jiang et al., 2006; Paduano et al., 2006).

ANGIOGENESIS AND ITS MECHANISM

Angiogenesis is the formation of new blood vessels from pre-existing blood vessels and/or from EPCs. It has implications in many physiological conditions such as embryo development, ovulation, wound healing, and in some pathological conditions such as arthritis, diabetic retinopathy and of course in metastasis (Figure 1) (Folkman, 1990). It has been observed that some human tumor lines do not form visible tumors when inoculated into immune suppressed mice. Interestingly, when transfected these cells with some pro-angiogenic factors such as vascular endothelial growth factor (VEGF), dormancy was found to be overcome by these microscopic tumors. It has been estimated that more than one third of women between the age 40 and 50 years found to carry *in situ* tumors in their breast tissue by observing autopsy data but only 1% of them diagnosed with breast cancer in later days. Same is the case with prostate cancer in men and with thyroid cancer in certain individuals and patients with Down's syndrome (Folkman and Kalluri, 2004). These examples clearly support the phenomenon of "angiogenic switch". The switch clearly involves more than simple up-regulation of angiogenic activity and thought to be balance of positive and negative regulators. The balance between *in situ* tumor's total output and an individual's total angiogenic balance is what the key factor that determines a tumor to be dormant or not. Also, this is the main reason why all individuals do not develop tumor metastasis.

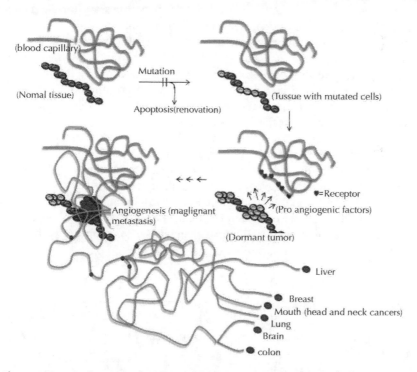

Figure 1. Figure showing various stages in the development of malignant metastatic cancer. A metastatic tumor development is as difficult as development of therapeutic treatments for cancer cure. Healthy cells, if they escape the process of apoptosis by mutations in one or the other among various molecular events related to the programmed cell death, will form a group of cells, normally regarded as a dormant tumor. This tumor then produce various angiogenic factors, balance between pro and anti-angiogenic factors decide the fate of tumor angiogenesis. Once the blood vessel formation occurs, the tumor will now be regarded as malignant tumor, which grows independent of the other tissues, by absorbing nutrients and oxygen required for its growth. Mutated cancer cells from this tissue can travel to various other healthy tissues via the established angiogenic network, before establishing themselves as solid tumors.

Angiogenesis, depending on different physiological processes in which it is involved, can be classified into three major types.

1. *De novo* angiogenesis occurring in embryonic development and in female reproduction.
2. Degenerative angiogenesis in tissue repair and,
3. Pathological angiogenesis occurring in certain disorders such as cancer and diabetic retinopathies.

ANGIOGENESIS AND TUMOR PROGRESSION

Metastasis continues to be a major hurdle to successful and complete treatment of malignant tumors, as portrayed in a number of basic research studies. "angiogenic switch" is the term used to denote the close relationship between angiogenesis and tumor progression (Folkman, 1996). It has been shown that hypoxia induces angiogenesis; high proliferation of tumor cells creates hypoxic areas necessary for the induction of VEGF expression. Also, the identification of transcription factor HIF1 as the up regulator of VEGF under low oxygen conditions proved further insights into the mechanisms of tumor angiogenesis (Maxwell et al., 1997). Hypoxia also has shown to stimulate other angiogenesis supporting growth factors such as PGDF and FGF (Kuwabara et al., 1995). It has been reported that succession of micro metastasis to macro metastasis happens by activation of angiogenic switch. Embryogenic progenitor cells from bone marrow rather than preexisting endothelium were found to be the critical regulators of this angiogenic switch. Immobilization of endothelial progenitor cells (EPCs) by blocking the expression of transcription factor id1 leads to the inhibition of angiogenesis and further reduction in tumor progression (Naumov et al., 2006). The EPCs, interaction between angiogenic factors, their receptors and the interaction between vasculogenesis and lymphangiogenesis are all on and off buttons to the switch. As a result of this, tumor vessels tend to break conventional rules of micro circulation by spreading without organization and changing vessel diameter, with some missing differentiation in arterioles, capillaries and venules.

MODULATORS OF ANGIOGENESIS

Many factors have been found to have implications in the process of angiogenesis termed as positive or negative regulators depending on their respective roles in stimulating or inhibiting action respectively. Some factors related to modulation of angiogenesis are as follows.

Angiogenic Factors

Integrins

Integrins are heterodimeric combination consisting one α and one β -sub units each from 18 different α and β -trans membrane proteins. In one study, blocking integrins α v $\beta3$ and $\alpha1$ $\beta1$ by using specific antibodies showed that antagonists against integrin α v $\beta3$ inhibit pro-angiogenic effects of VEGF and probol esters while antagonists against that of $\alpha1$ $\beta1$ abolish FGF2 and tumor necrosis factor (TNF) α stimulated sprouting of new vessels (Smyth and Patterson, 2002). Angiogenic endothelial cells were shown to undergo apoptosis compared to their resting counterparts, after the α v β3 antibody administration (Brooks, 1996). Defective vascular network as a consequence of injecting α v β3 antibodies in quail embryos shows the role of α v β3 integrins in endothelial cell proliferation (Clark et al., 1996) and in angiogenesis.

Vascular endothelial growth factor

This is the most important factor among angiogenic factors, which was discovered in 1989 by Ferrara and coworkers (Ferrara et al., 2003). It was found that, by disrupting a single VEGF allele in mice ~50% reduction in VEGF and ultimately embryonic death was observed. Six known members of the VEGF family have been discovered viz. VEGF-A, -B, -C, -D, and -E and the placental growth factor, found to be generated by alternative splicing of the *VEGF* gene (Ferrara et al., 2003). The VEGF binds to VEGF R1, R2, and R3 expressed on endothelial cells/lymphatics. After binding to their ligand, VEGF receptors undergo dimerization resulting in mitotic, chemotactic and pro survival signals. Several growth factors such as EGF, TGF α, β FGF, and PDGF; hormones such as estrogen induce VEGF expression.

Angiopoietins

The angiopoetins (Ang-1–Ang-4) have been implicated in the development of vasculature in a wide variety of tumor types (Plank et al., 2004). Among the four known angiopoetins, Ang-1 and Ang-2 are the best characterized cytokines, both exerting their biologic function through binding to the Tie-2 receptor (Maisonpierre et al., 1997). The Ang-1 promotes endothelial cell survival and sprouting and stabilizes vascular networks by recruiting pericytes to immature vessel segments. In contrast, Ang-2, expressed at sites of vascular remodeling, causes the loss of pericytes and exposes endothelial cells to angiogenic factors.

Fibroblast Growth Factors (FGFs)

The FGFs are a family of heparin binding proteins. The FGF-1 (acidic) and FGF-2 (basic) are described as inductors of angiogenesis (Szebenyi and Fallon, 1999). All FGFs bind to heparin sulfate proteoglycans (HLGAGs) of the extracellular matrix (ECM). The FGFs can bind to four transmembrane specific receptor tyrosine kinases inducing receptor dimerization and activation. The FGF-1 and FGF-2 induce endothelial cell proliferation and differentiation of epiblast cells into endothelial cells. Furthermore, FGF-2 stimulates the release of urinary plasminogen activator and collagenases in endothelial cells and acts as a chemoattractant for these cells.

Transforming growth factor β (TGF β)

It has been proposed that TGF β has auto and/or paracrine activity on endothelial cells as well as pericytes (Antonelli-Orlidge et al., 1989). Two isoforms TGF β1 and TGF β2 have been identified, the former acts as pro-angiogenic and the later act as pro-angiogenic at low concentrations and oppositely at high concentrations. Dickson and coworkers found that knockout mice lacking TGF are unable to produce stable vessel walls as well as inadequate tube formation.

CXC-Chemokines

The CC chemokines, that primarily modulate infiltration of monosite/macrophages to the sites of inflammation, have been found to associate with modulation of angiogenesis (Salcedo et al., 2000). Although, underlying mechanism of their involvement in angiogenesis has not been fully validated, an indirect involvement by stimulating monocytes and macrophages, which intern directly produce angiogenic factors has been suggested (Isik et al., 1996). However, recent evidence of endothelial cells expressing of CCL2 receptor CCR2 shows a direct angiogenic modulation by CXC chemokines (Stamatovic et al., 2006; Weber et al., 1999).

Angiostatic factors

Angiostatin

Angiostatin is a 38-kDa plasminogen fragment and systemic injection of angiostatin has been shown to inhibit tumor neovascularization and metastatic growth by inhibition of ECM. Our previous reports have shown that combinatorial therapy of plasmids containing *angiostatin* gene with B7.1 immunogene therapy have reduced solid EL4 lymphomas in syngenic C57BL/6 mice, supports the use of angiostatin in combinatorial therapy (Sun et al., 2001).

Thrombospondin-1

Thrombospondins belong to a family of ECM proteins. The CD36 (also known as GP88, GP IV, GPIIIb) is an important cellular receptor for TSP-1 on microvascular endothelium and is necessary for its anti-angiogenic activity (Tonini et al., 2003). The anti-angiogenic activity of TSP-1 is contained in a structural domain known as the TSP type I repeat which plays a role in endothelial cell apoptosis (Sargiannidou et al., 2001). In addition to CD36-mediated anti-angiogenic effects, TSP-1 can potentially inhibit angiogenesis through an interaction with pro-MMP2/9, MMP-2/9 or induction of cell cycle arrest.

Endostatin

It inhibits endothelial cell migration and induces endothelial cell apoptosis and cell cycle arrest and is encoded by *COL18A1* gene at 21q22.3. In one interesting study, the levels of endostatin was observed in the serum in patients with Down's syndrome along with normal controls and the results were interesting to see that elevated endostatin levels persist in patients with Down's syndrome (Down's syndrome is most commonly caused by trisomy of 21st chromosome) (Shichiri and Hirata, 2001). It has been shown that endostatin directly and specifically acts on endothelial cells in culture to produce intracellular signals such as influx of extracellular calcium, inside the cells (Sargiannidou et al., 2001; Shichiri and Hirata, 2001). Endostatin's application down regulates genes' expression during endothelial cell growth, and exhibited a potent ant migratory effect on endothelial cells *in vitro*, mediated through *c-myc* down regulation (Shichiri and Hirata, 2001). Inhibitory action by endostatin has been proposed to involve binding to the receptor α5β1 (Sudhakar et al., 2003). The cDNA and antibody microarray technology uncovered the full set changes in gene expression following endostatin administration. Endostatin up regulated anti-angiogeneic thrombospondin, kininogen, ATIII, and chromogranin A; while down regulating downstream regulators of anti-apoptotic genes (e.g., *Bcl2, COX2, cMyc*, and *iNOS*) such as *HIF1α, NFkB, Ets-1, id1*, and *STATs*, leading to cell cycle arrest (Abdollahi et al., 2004). Therefore, taking together these evidences, one can articulate that endostatin acts upon one or more receptors, present on endothelial cells, resulting in intracellular signaling which decreases their migratory capacity and/or proliferative ability preventing the vascularization.

As discussed earlier in this review, targeting angiogenesis is the best way to fight with cancer. So, drugs or molecules which can target angiogenic switch are recommended for effective treatment of cancer. Biologically synthesized molecules degraded biologically by host's body; a chemically synthesized molecule, considered foreign to a particular organism, and may cause acute side effects and/or allergic reactions when it gets converted to a metabolite. Therefore, chemicals and/or modified fungal derivatives can be avoided and replaced with the molecules which have fewer side effects. As targeting the specific proteins expressed excessively in tumors and/or angiogenic blood vessels is the key point in developing an antitumor drug, molecules used for this purpose should have certain characteristics as listed below:

(1) Capacity to discriminate between oncogenic, non-oncogenic and/or angiogenic and anti-angiogenic forms of the proteins involved in signaling pathways.

(2) Capacity to quantify the level of expression of the oncogenic forms.

(3) Ideally, be usable both for *in vitro* and *in vivo* purposes

(4) For therapeutic applications, the capacity to block the activity of the oncogene product.

Anti-angiogenic/anticancer peptides, DNA vaccines; oligomers, such as miRNA and siRNA, which control the synthesis of gene product post transcriptionally and small oligomeric aptamers are promising agents in this regard. We consider here micro RNA, aptamers, and certain targeting agents which attracted attention in the recent past.

MICRO RNAs IN CANCER

It has been speculated over a few decades that only 2% of the animal genome encode functional protein coding genes and the remaining is junk. However, recent advances have brought non-protein coding RNAs into spot light. The miRNAs are such kind of non-coding RNAs found to have implications in cell growth, regulation, differentiation, and apoptosis. Nearly, 400 miRNAs have been identified in humans and the number is increasing. By using bioinformatics tools, it has been observed that one miRNA can recognize more than 200 messenger RNAs. Initially miRNAs are transcribed by RNA-polymerase II, as large precursors (Lee et al., 2002), which are further processed by Drosha (an Rnase III enzyme and by a double stranded binding protein DGCR8/Pasha (Gregory and Shiekhattar, 2005; Lee et al., 2003), this processing step produces stem loop structures of nearly 70 nucleotide length. These precursors then are processed by another Rnase III enzyme, Dicer is processed into 22 nucleotide double strand RNA duplex after they got exported from nucleus to cytoplasm by exportin 5 in a Ran guanosine phosphate dependent manner (Yi et al., 2003). This duplex intern is incorporated into the miRISC complex. The RISC-miRNA complex then binds to the corresponding mRNA and represses its translation by blocking translation initiation or by inducing endonucleolytic cleavage of mRNA.

Cloning of first miRNA, lin4, was achieved by doing genetic analysis of the timing of development in *C. alegans* (Ambros, 2001, 2004; Lee et al., 1993) and Reinhart et al. in 1993 identified its prey, lin14 mRNA while doing heterochronic analysis (Reinhart et al., 2000). Recently it has been found that carcinogenesis is strongly associated with inappropriate expression of miRNAs regulating gene expression in translational level. Based on these observations alone, lin4 and let7 miRNAs are thought to be potential tumor suppressors and it has become more interesting after finding that these molecules are conserved in mammals (Kanwar et al., 2010; Pasquinelli et al., 2000). Subsequent reports make it clear that let7 miRNA and miRNAs belong to the family which act as tumor suppressors by targeting 3′ UTR of RAS mRNA, there by effecting RAS protein (Johnson et al., 2005). On the contrary, miRNAs were shown to enhance translation as suggested recently in two different studies (Thai et al., 2007; Tili et al., 2007). It has been observed that miR-155′s over expression resulted in enhanced translation of Tumor Necrosis Factor α alpha (TNF-α), most probably by enhancing the stability of its transcript, and mice over expressing miR-155 in B cell lineage (Eμ-miR-155) which produce more TNF-α alpha when challenged with LPS (Thai et al., 2007). Further research in a realistic approach is needed to confirm the role of miRNAs in enhancing gene expression and translation of proteins. The first evidence for the link between miRNA and cancer came from the work, as reported by Clain and coworkers; deletion in the region coding for miR 15a and miR 16-1 as it is highly likely because of over expression of anti-apoptotic protein Bcl-2 in many chronic lymphoid leukemia (CLL) patients, showing the tumor suppressor functions of miRNA (Calin et al., 2002). There are reports that important group of miRNAs, the Let-7 family were found to regulate RAS and/or MYC oncogene expression at the translational level to be often down regulated in human lung tumors, owing to its growth repression functions (Akao et al., 2006). Recent evidence suggests that miR-143 and miR-145 are frequently down regulated in colorectal tumors (Michael et al., 2003). Down regulation of these miRNAs have also been noted as a common occurrence in breast carcinomas and breast tumor cell lines (Volinia et al., 2006). On the flip side, miRNAs acting as oncogenes have also been identified in the recent past, owing to speculations about their role in tumerogenesis (Tam et al., 2002; Ota et al., 2004). The miR-21 was demonstrated to be up regulated in glioblastoma (Chan et al., 2005). The MiR-372 and miR-373 were found to block RAS induced cellular senescence and potentiate RAS mediated cellular transformation (Voorhoeve et al., 2006).

Various studies earlier reported that micro RNAs have implications in the development and/or regulation of angiogenesis. The miRNA profiles of endothelial cells revealed that let7b, miR-16, miR-23a, miR-100, miR-221, and miR-222 are predominant (Kuehbacher et al., 2007; Poliseno et al., 2006; Suárez et al., 2007), however there was a little work regarding the abundance of these miRNAs in environments that imitate tumor microvasculature conditions. Down regulation of anti-angiogenic genes by miR-130a expressed in HUVECs, in response to addition of serum (FBS) has been reported recently (Chen and Gorski, 2008). Certain classes of micro RNAs, for instance miR17-92 have been proved to have pro-angiogenic properties by inhibiting transcription factors involved in anti-angiogenesis (Dews et al., 2006). Hypoxia is a condition observed in cancer malformation and it has been observed that hypoxia has implications in the formation of blood vessels. It has been shown that hypoxia up-regulates VEGF (Plate et al., 1992; Shweiki et al., 1992), owing both to increased transcription mediated by hypoxia inducing factor-1(HIF-1) and an increase in VEGF mRNA stability dependent on 3′ region of mRNA (Semenza, 1996). Interestingly, a recent study (Kulshreshtha et al., 2007) has shown that a specific spectrum of micro RNAs (including miR-23, -24, -26, -27, -104, -107, -181, -210, and miR-213) is induced in response to low oxygen concentration. A similar study shows miR-120 (induced in hypoxia), over expression enhanced the formation of capillary like structures and migration of endothelial cells (Fasanaro et al., 2008). Promotion of cell survival, tumor growth, and angiogenesis by miRNA-378 was predicted by assaying for the luciferase activity in constructs synthesized containing 3′UTR of it is possible downstream effecter molecules, SuFu and Fus-1 (Lee et al., 2007). In another study, miRNA generation was impaired by silencing the molecules involved in their biogenesis, Dicer and Drosha by siRNA and found a reduced angiogenesis in parallel with decreased spectrum of miRNAs in endothelial cells (Kuehbacher et al., 2007). Similarly, dicer inactivation resulted in altered expression of molecules related to angiogenesis and endothelial biology, including up regulation of Tie-2, Tie-1 receptors and eNOS transcription factor (Suárez et al., 2007). However, one cannot generalize these experiments saying silencing dicer impairs angiogenesis, as it is not about silencing a particular miRNA and observing for a phenotype and the obtained phenotype is an overall result of silencing all miRNAs in an endothelial cell. Also, it has already been demonstrated that dicer itself is required for regulation of angiogenesis (Yang et al., 2005). The miR-126 was found to regulate many aspects of endothelial cell biology (Wang et al., 2008). The mir-126 is found to regulate endothelial cells derived from mouse embryonic stem cells, by promoting VEGF signaling (Fish et al., 2008). It is interesting to see whether these miRNAs have any effect on regulating HIF dependent VEGF and/or other pro-angiogenic factor gene up regulation and further implications in development of metastasis by supporting angiogenesis. In contrast to this, some of the miRNAs are proposed to have anti-angiogenic properties (Poliseno et al., 2006). In summary, identification of miRNAs with dual antitumor and anti-angiogenic effect may lead to discovery of potential anticancer drugs. Also, inhibiting the miRNAs which have implications in enhancing angiogenesis will be other option. One can use molecules such as 2'O-methyl anti-sense oligoribonucleotides directed against a particular pro-angiogenic miRNA. In relation with developing a novel and effective drug towards prevention of cancer progression and metastasis, we are here with providing some biomolecules that can be used to in addition to the above given molecules for increased efficiency, effective targeting and/or for easy penetration of the drug into the systemic circulation.

APTAMERS

Aptamers (Latin; aptus, to fit+ meros, part or region) are composed of oligonucleic acid or peptide molecules which can bind to target molecules that are usually expressed on the surfaces of the membranes. Aptamers are usually created by selecting them from a large random sequence pool, by using specific techniques such as Selective Evaluation of Ligands by Exponential Enrichment (SELEX), developed in the laboratory of Larry Gold in the University of Colorado (Kanwar et al., 2010; Tuerk and Gold, 1990). Natural aptamers also exist in riboswitches. Aptamers are DNA/RNA aptamers and protein aptamers depending on their chemical nature and can bind to a range of molecular targets including nucleic acids, proteins, and small molecules and even to cells. These can be used for both basic research and clinical purposes as macromolecular drugs. Pegaptanib, a nuclease-resistant aptamer used for curing age-related macular degradation (AMD) is one such example. To be able to make these molecules cleaved in the presence of their target, aptamers can be coupled with catalytic RNA (ribozymes). This makes these compound molecules have additional research, industrial and clinical applications, including diagnostics, therapeutics, biosensors and tools for probing fundamental cellular processes (Griffin et al., 1993). Aptamers are more advantageous than antibodies in the sense that they are easy to synthesize in bulk, rather than using cell based expression system. During the phosphoramadite chemical synthesis of aptamers in the lab, fluorescent dyes or chemical modification with functional groups can be achieved. These modifications can further help in *in vivo* applications of the molecules baring the aptamer or for better conjugation of the aptamer on to the other moiety. Aptamers can also be used to probe cellular processes by binding to specific functional groups of proteins (Blind et al., 1999) in contrast to other oligonucleotide agents such as siRNA, RNAi, or ribozymes; aptamers can act on extra cellular targets, that is same as the other entities that have affinity for proteins. But just like other oligo peptides, their biggest limitation is bioavailability—upon oral administration. But the biggest advantage over the peptide and/or antibodies is their low immunogenicity. When comes to therapeutic application, still the progress is in its infancy, however one aptameric drug has been approved by FDA. Pegaptanib, as listed above is a RNA aptamer directed against VEGF, has been implicated for the treatment of all types of neovascular age related ocular vascular diseases. In one study, adeno viral system was used to deliver RNA aptamer (AP50), against $NF_\kappa B$, to overcome non-small cell lung cancer tumor resistance to Doxorubicin, in A539 cells (Mi et al., 2008). However, viral system for drug delivery has its own side effects. More recently, PEGylated, angiopoietin-2 inhibiting RNA aptamers were shown to inhibit tumor angiogenesis and growth, by inhibiting Tie-2 phosphorylation (Sarraf-Yazdi et al., 2008).

VHL

The VHL disease is a familial cancer syndrome caused by autosomal dominant trait, due to mutations in tumor suppressor gene, VHL. It has been observed that, highly vascular tumors especially, glioma, renal cell carcinoma and pheochromocytomas are the most common implications of this disease (Kondo and Kaelin, 2001). It has been shown based on this disease that, application of VHL causes reduced tumor malignancies.

We have previously reported the regression of solid tumors by using a combination therapy of VHL and antisense HIFα It has been observed that VHL inhibits HIF by binding to 1α as well as 2α subunits (Sun et al., 2003a). So it is very promising to use VHL as an antitumor agent in combination therapy.

LACTOFERRIN

Lactoferrin is a natural defense protein, present mainly in milk and bodily secretions. Besides its main function that is iron absorption in the intestine, lactoferrin also plays a role in protection against infections, myelopoisis and against autoimmunity. Previous reports in our lab have shown that 100% iron saturated bovine lactoferrin has augmented the antitumor cytotoxicity of certain chemotherapeutics, in wide range of tumors (Kanwar et al., 2003; Kanwar et al., 2008), by increasing cytokines produced by Th1 family, which includes IL18, IFNγ and TNFα, which in turn helps in infiltration of CTL, CD_4^+, CD_8^+, NK, and NKT cells to the tumor tissue. So using lactoferrin, along with a drug formulation uptake can be increased into systemic circulation and inhibits angiogenesis.

In summary, aptamers that can bind to specific markers on tumor vasculature can be used along with certain tumor, HIF and/or angiogenic inhibitors as discussed above, so as to deliver them to the specified target. However, aptamers are not used that much in the treatment of tumor angiogenesis, although it has same implications as that of retinal angiogenesis; pertaining mainly because of their low bioavailability. One can think of a wonder drug if antitumor peptides and inhibitors of pro-angiogenic factors delivered orally, along with ligands such as aptamers, VHL and Lactoferrin with some protecting aids, to protect them from mucosal and gastric environment. Taken together, combinational therapy is a better approach to target tumor (Baratchi et al., 2009)

DELIVERING ANTI-ANGIOGENIC/ANTICANCER MOLECULES WITH NANOPARTICLES

There are many delivery routes devised for drug administration in different diseases (Baratchi et al., 2009). There are many parenteral and non-parenteral administration routes of drug delivery that have been developed and devised in the past for therapy (Kanwar et al., 2009). However, complications such as thrombophlebitis or tissue necrosis and poor patient compliance have stimulated the investigation of non-parenteral routes (Xin Hua, 1994). Among non-parenteral routes, oral administration is usually preferred because it is noninvasive, most acceptable and convenient for the patient and required no skilled worker for injecting drugs. But oral bioavailability of these prodrugs or enzymes and peptides as well as protein drugs is generally very low, owing to the acidic conditions of the stomach, proteolytic activity of the gastrointestinal enzymes present in the intestinal tract, and poor permeability across intestinal mucosa (Zhou and Li, 1991). Various approaches have been proposed to overcome the biopharmaceutical limitations associated with these drugs, such as inhibition of the enzymatic degradation (Morimoto et al., 1991), chemical modifications (Conradi et al., 1992), *in situ* gel system (Shah and Paradkar, 2005), and the formulation of polymer or microsphere-based carrier systems (Torchilin et al., 1977). Application of nanocarriers for drug delivery, especially RNA, pDNA, prodrugs and bioactive drugs, is an expanding area of research that provided the design of biomaterials with controlled rates of drug release (Prokop et al., 2002). Recent advancements in chemotherapy are using nanomaterials of broad range of chemistry, including PEGylated, hydrophobicated, glycol chitosan moieties and other poly esters. These nano wonders are reported to protect the drug from the extremities of the pH and enzymatic degradations. Drug delivery is one of the promising biomedical applications of nanotechnology. Several nano based cancer drugs for example, Doxil and Abraxane are in clinical trials, to be able to use in cancer chemotherapy. Ideally speaking, a good nanocarrier will have minimal side effects and greater hangover time in blood. Nanocarriers made up of two or more different polymers can spontaneously assume various shapes in specific solvents and bring several advantages to the nanocore like size, stability, drug loading, and release efficiencies. Blood vessels in tumor vasculature are found to be leaky and have pores in the range of 10-100s of nanometers (Kanwar et al., 2009). This fact can be exploited for drug delivery to the tumor site, which was being named as enhanced permeability retention (EPR) effect (Matsumura and Maeda, 1986).

USES OF NANO PARTICLES IN CANCER TREATMENT

A nanocarrier ideally shall have a diameter from 1–100 nm and can carry multiple drugs. As they will have high surface to volume ratio, one can think of a better drug, tagging more ligands on their surfaces. Also, nanocarriers can better exploit EPR effect posed by the tumor vasculature, for improved drug delivery (Peer et al., 2007). Of late, natural and synthetic polymers are used as drug delivery vectors. Various nanocarriers used along with polymer conjugates include polymeric nanoparticles, lipid based carriers such as liposomes and micelles, dendrimers, carbon nanotubes and inorganic nanoparticles. There has been increased attention towards the development of biodegradable, polymeric nanoparticles for the diagnosis and treatment of cancer, in the scientific field. As mentioned above, anticancer biomolecules targeted along with nanocarriers especially polymeric nanocarriers and dendrimers is being done at pace. In recent past, some formulations have been tested by using chemotherapeutic drugs, along with polymeric nanoparticles. A formulation with two distinct layers of biodegradable polymers with inner nucleus containing antitumor agent, Doxorubicin and the PEGylated outer envelope with anti-angiogenic agent, has been successfully tested (Sengupta et al., 2005). In another development, nanoparticles that co-deliver Paciltaxil and Ceramide to overcome multi drug resistance in tumors, using the same formulation, developed PEO-PCL nanoparticles with tamoxifen and paciltaxil encapsulated with poly ethelene oxide modified poly-ε-caprolactone, to overcome MDR in breast cancer cell lines (Devalapally et al., 2008). Anticancer drug nutlin-3a has been actively targeted using EpCAM antibodies, loaded on to poly(lactide-*co*-glycolide), has been successfully tested (Das and Sahoo, 2010). Lodamin was the mPEG-PLA modification of TNP-470, using methylated poly ethelene glycol (PEG) and poly lactic acid (PLA), which have fewer side effects compared to its counterpart, TNP and was tested successfully in melanoma and LLC cell lines (Benny et al., 2008) and was reported to be a promising oral administrative, for anti-angiogenic therapy. In addition, there were some polymer conjugates which are under clinical use such as Zinostatin, stimalmer, oncaspar, and Neulasta for cancer treatment (Duncan, 2006).

To develop an oral administrative, careful design of the core and exterior coat is required. Recent developments in bone marrow tissue engineering, dentistry, orthopedics, and plastic surgery are making use of these kinds of composites in the macro scale; utilizing the same principle in nanoscale ensuring more promising drug development (Kanwar et al., 2009). Ceramic nanocores are being designed in order to assist protein adsorption on them and various layers of biodegradable polymers are then coated on their surface, as discussed below, in order to protect them, from lytic or gastrointestinal enzymes and for obtaining sustained release kinetics of the loaded drug. Ceramics can be defined as solid compounds that are formed by chemical reaction between a metal and a nonmetallic elemental solid or between a nonmetal and nonmetallic elemental solids (Benny et al., 2008; Cevc, 2004; Duncan, 2006; Foley et al., 2002; Martin and Kohli, 2003; Rawat et al., 2006, 2008; Mahidhara et al., 2011). Some of the ceramic composites are discussed below.

Calcium phosphate ceramics
Various forms of calcium phosphate ceramics are being used for last 3 decades, which include hydroxyapatite, beta tri calcium phosphate, biphasic calcium phosphate amorphous calcium phosphate, carbonated appetite, and calcium deficient hydroxyapatite (Mahidhara et al., 2011).

Calcium phosphate cements
They consist of powder phase of calcium and/or phosphate salts together with an aqueous phase, react at room or body temperature and form a calcium phosphate crystal that sets by entanglement of crystals.

Bioactive glass
It is produced like a conventional glass, in which basic components are SiO_2, Na_2O, CaO, and P_2O_5. It is commercially available as Bioglass®.

Characteristics of these include high mechanical strength, good body response, and strong binding ability with proteins, which helps in a sustained release. However, they are less biodegradable, which may be a draw back and this can be overcome by adding biopolymers such as chitosan, which not only improve their biodegradability but also increases tolerance towards variations in pH and protects towards enzyme action in the gut. Polymers widely used are listed here.

1. Poly lactic acid/poly glycolic acid polymers such as poly lactic acid (PLA, PLLA, PDLLA), poly glycolic acid (PGA), poly (lactic-*co*-glycolic acid) (PLGA) and poly-caprolactones.
2. Natural proteins such as collagen, gelatin, fibrin, and casein.
3. Carbohydrates and their derivatives such as chitin, chitosan, alginate, cellulose, starch, hyaluronan, and amylopectins.

Recently Saraf et al. (Rawat et al., 2006, 2008) have developed nanoparticles, which can be used for oral delivery of peptides. However, to the best of our knowledge no one has used these ACNC carriers for pDNA or RNAi delivery for gene targeting in any disease *in vitro* or *in vivo* in human or animal systems. It is tempting to expand the utility of nanocarriers for delivery of therapeutic enzymes, because particles larger than 20 μm are prone to be washed out, being inefficient for mucosal delivery (Lameiro et al., 2006) and to maintain the native structures (Cleland, 1997). In this regard, innovative techniques have led to the use of ceramics in high-tech applications like delivering chemicals and biologicals effectively *in vitro* and *in vivo* (Cherian et al., 2000). We recently for the first time used the covalently cross-linked CPP (R9 and Tat peptides) complexed with siRNA to survivin, an inhibitor of apoptosis which over expressed in tumors and inflammation (unpublished observations). We designed covalently cross-linked CPP (R9-siRNA to survivin and Tat peptides-siRNA to survivin peptides) complexed with siRNA to survivin on to design ACNC for effective loading and protection of active acid-labile and alkaline-labile large nanocarriers for oral administration. We tested these nanocarriers loaded targeted nanoparticles in human colon cancer cells (Caco-2 and HT-29) in transwell assays. As an attempt towards increasing the bioavailability and conformational stability, we have loaded covalently complexed CPP with survivin siRNA into ACNC with no effective protection, mucoadhesiveness, and sustained release (Mahidhara et al., 2011). The prolonged activity was obtained due to slow release of the protein or RNA from the ACNC and the intact structure without denaturation or dehydration during delivery and storage. The encouraging results obtained in this study could propose ACNC for future *in vivo* studies, especially in the delivery of RNA, DNA, protein, peptide and drugs. These novel nanocarriers were found to be promising for protection of the spatial qualities for exhibiting better therapeutic effect. But further studies in terms of pharmacokinetics, toxicology, and animal studies are required for clinical utility of the formulation. More recently, we were able to load cell permeable dominant negative survivin R9 (DNSurR9) (Bawa 2009; Baratchi et al., 2010; Cheung et al., 2006) and survivin and HSP-90 antagonists, "shepherdin" on alginate gel-encapsulated, chitosan ceramic nanocarriers (ACNC-NPs) and were able to induce apoptosis and disintegrate the mitochondria of colon and breast cancer cell lines (but not normal control cells) more efficiently in *in vitro* cell based assays. In this study, we loaded non-covalently cross-linked CPP (R9-siRNA to survivin and Tat-peptides-siRNA to survivin peptides) complexed with siRNA to survivin and oncogenic antisense microRNA-27a (as-miR-27a) on ACNC-NPs and transferred to human breast cancer MDA-MB-231 and MCF-7 cell lines by endocytosis, as outlined. Our results show that both R9 and Tat CPP peptides covalently complexed with as-miR-27a loaded ACNC-NPs exhibits oncogenic activity. Suppression of miR-27a inhibits breast cancer cell growth and invasion. Simultaneous covalently complexed CPP (R9 and Tat-peptide) with siRNA to survivin and oncogenic as-miR-27a loaded ACNC-NPs results in down expression of genes that are important for cell survival and angiogenesis faster and more efficiently than the monotherapy. In addition, these responses were accompanied by decreased expression of survivin and angiogenic genes, including survivin isoforms, VEGF, and VEGF receptor 1(VEGFR1). We also demonstrated the down regulation of survivin expression in Western blot in the covalently complexed CPP (R9 and Tat-peptide) with siRNA to survivin and oncogenic as-miR-27a loaded ACNC-NPs treated cells. The TUNEL assay, caspase activity assay and changes in mitochondrial membrane potential reveal that cell death was mainly through intrinsic apoptosis pathway. Oral delivery of siRNA to survivin and oncogenic as-miR-27a loaded ACNC-NPs induced apoptosis, necrosis, and cytotoxicity in the xenograft breast cancer model. Oral administration of covalently complexed CPP (R9 and Tat-peptide) with siRNA to survivin and oncogenic as-miR-27a ACNC-NPs in combination regress tumor growth faster and inhibits angiogenesis in the xenograft breast cancer mouse model as compared to monotherapy (Bawa, 2009). We also compared our results with the doxorubicin and taxol loaded ACNC-NPs (Figure 2). Taken together, our results are highly encouraging for the development of combination nanotherapeutic strategies that combine gene silencing and drug delivery to provide more potent and targeted therapeutic, especially in late and metastatic breast cancer.

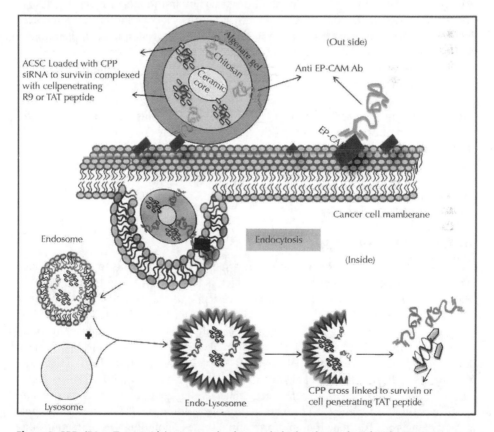

Figure 2. CPPs (R9 or Tat peptide) were covalently cross linked and complexed with siRNA to survivin and oncogenic antisense microRNA-27a then loaded on nanoparticles alginate gel-encapsulated, chitosan ceramic nanocores (ACNCs). These ACNCs were protected from various gastric enzymes *in vitro* and *in vivo* studies. ACNCs were transcytosise in to gut cells and present in circulation and make available of siRNA to the tumor sites for knockdown of survivin gene. siRNA loaded ACNC nanoparticles coated with alginate can be endocytosed easily and can be used for oral therapy, as they can sustain intestinal pH. These nanoparticles can enter blood circulation by transcytosis in intestinal villi before encountering a cancer tissue via the blood stream.

GENE DELIVERY TO TARGET CELLS

The RNAi-mediated gene-silencing effect is limited in the cells reached by RNAi effectors, which makes the delivery of RNAi effectors to target cells important in achieving RNAi-based therapeutic treatment. Lots of *in vivo* delivery methods of RNAi effectors have been developed, including those developed and optimized for the delivery of plasmid DNA (pDNA) for gene therapy for inhibiting angiogenesis and/or immunomodulation by co-stimulatory pDNA immunogene therapy (Luo et al., 2006; Sun et al., 2005, 2003b; Kanwar et al., 1999, 2001b; Cheung et al., 2006). Early studies on *in vivo* RNAi often used the expression of reporter genes that were expressed from vectors co-administered with RNAi effectors (Bartlett and Davis, 2006; Kobayashi et al., 2004; Wooddell et al., 2005). Similarly, suppression of tumor cell growth by efficient RNAi induction in tumor tissue by intratumoral injection has also been studied (Zhang et al., 2008). In contrasts to this, a few studies have reported successful induction of gene silencing in target cells after systemic administration of shRNA-expressing pDNA. The shRNA-expressing plasmids, which are encapsulated in the interior of 85 nm PEGylated immunoliposomes (PILs), can suppress the gene expression in tumor cells intracranialy inoculated into the brain (Maliyekkel et al., 2006; Zhang et al., 2003). Among the non-viral carriers are cell-penetrating peptides (CPP), which have the ability to enter cells by crossing the plasma membrane directly or through uptake by the endocytotic pathway (Meade and Dowdy, 2008). We (Krissansen et al., 2006) and many other research groups have demonstrated the effective use of CPP (Meade and Dowdy, 2008; Schaffert and Wagner, 2008; Zhang et al., 2007; Zuhorn et al., 2007). Here we summarize CPP-based RNA delivery strategies, and focus on recent improvements that enhance the release of siRNAs trapped in endosomes into the cytosol.

RNAI FOR CANCER THERAPY

Double-stranded RNA (dsRNA) containing a sequence homologous to a specific gene causes sequence-specific gene silencing, which is termed RNA interference (RNAi). The RNAi was first discovered in *Caenorhabditis elegans*, an organism in which gene expression is down regulated by long dsRNA (Fire et al., 1998). Remarkably, the basic molecular mechanism of RNAi is conserved in mammalian cells, and the applicability to mammalian systems was recently discovered using short dsRNAs (19–23 base-pairs), termed small interfering RNAs (siRNAs) and short hairpin RNAs (shRNAs) (Caplen et al., 2001; Elbashir et al., 2001; Paddison et al., 2002). The RNAi-mediated gene-silencing is now an essential strategy in analyzing gene functions due to its high specificity, high efficiency, and great facility. In addition, it offers one of the most attractive methods for gene therapy for many diseases, including viral infectious diseases and cancers (de Fougerolles et al., 2007; Devi 2006). Many types of diseases have been demonstrated to be potential targets for RNAi-based therapy in laboratory experiments.

Appropriate systems that enable safe and efficient RNA delivery to target cells or organs are required to further expand the use of RNAi to therapeutic applications. Several kinds of RNA delivery systems have been developed and improved upon, including viral vectors and non-viral carriers, such as cationic lipids, polymers and dendrimers. These have been reviewed earlier (Schaffert and Wagner, 2008; Zhang et al., 2007; Zuhorn et al., 2007). Among the non-viral carriers are CPP, which have the ability to enter cells by crossing the plasma membrane directly or through uptake by the endocytotic pathway (Meade and Dowdy, 2008). We (Krissansen et al., 2006) and many other research groups have demonstrated the effective use of CPP and observed the efficient down regulation of gene expression by CPP-based siRNA delivery, although the numbers of reports regarding CPP-based delivery are much less than those of viral or lipid-based delivery (Schaffert and Wagner, 2008; Zhang et al., 2007; Zuhorn et al., 2007). However due to inherent problems of viral vectors and liposome's here in this review, we summarize CPP-based RNA delivery strategies, and focus on recent improvements that enhance the release of siRNAs trapped in endosomes into the cytosol. The CPPs are already utilized in many biological and biotechnological studies to deliver various kinds of biologically active molecules into cells. The CPPs were first used for the delivery of proteins that were genetically fused to CPPs. Subsequently, CPPs have been used for the delivery of many types of cargo molecules, ranging in size from small inorganic or organic molecules (Josephson et al., 1999; Lewin et al., 2000; Liang and Yang, 2005; Rothbard et al., 2000) to large liposomes (diameter = 200 μm) (Khalil et al., 2006; Torchilin et al., 2001), by conjugating the cargo to the CPP.

CONCLUSION

The ability to precisely and differentially target functionally bio-relevant molecular signals in patient's cancers will establish a new paradigm in cancer management; one which focuses on defining the uniqueness of each patient's tumor and tumor-host processes and interactions following rational target prioritization using computational systems biology algorithms. This, then, would allow for exploitation of the "attack vulnerability" of the rewired cancer network by deconstructing essential hubs and linkages, multiply targeting and eliminating them. Both siRNA and shRNA effectors are attractive opportunities. The capability of potentiating activity using a bifunctional design may further enhance safety and efficacy. Though shRNA seems ideal for cancer related therapeutic development, new technology such as bifunctional RNA interference may provide an even greater opportunity for enhancement in potency as well as heightening safety thereby increasing the opportunities for multiple target therapy. This, of course, is contingent on optimization of delivery and minimization of off-target effect which will need to be established through early clinical testing. The RNAi has rapidly been established as an experimental tool and is expected to be used as a therapeutic treatment for various diseases beside cancer. Besides siRNA, shRNA-expressing pDNA is also a promising candidate for RNAi-based therapeutic treatment. As shRNA-expressing pDNA and siRNA possess advantages and disadvantages, they should be chosen on a case-by-case basis. There are still difficulties in the successful therapeutic application of RNAi. However, considering the pace of new findings and developments in the application of RNAi, we believe that these problems will be solved and that RNAi will become a major therapeutic treatment in the near future. The RNA delivery for RNAi-mediated gene silencing is a comparatively new area of CPP-mediated molecular delivery. Endosomal entrapment of RNAs delivered by CPPs is a problem that must be overcome for practical CPP-based cellular RNA delivery. A few groups have addressed this problem by using endosomolytic peptides and reagents, as well as photoinduced endosomal escape strategies. In addition, strategies targeting the CPP-cargo complex to a specific organ, to cancer, or to virus-infected cells, will be necessary for therapeutic applications. Recently, there has been a great advance toward therapeutic applications, in particular through the use of non-covalent strategies to form cargo-CPP complexes. The photoinduced RNAi strategy may also be useful as a targeting strategy for therapeutic applications. As RNAi is one of the most promising strategies for gene therapy, further advances in CPP-based RNA delivery with nanocarriers are expected in the near future.

KEYWORDS

- **Angiogenesis**
- **Angiostatin**
- **Apoptosis**
- **Bioactive glass**
- **Integrins**
- **Micro ribo nucleic acids**

ACKNOWLEDGMENT

This work was supported by Department of Innovation Industry Science, Research, and Commonwealth of Australia (BF030016). We are also gratefully acknowledging the financial support from Centre for Biotechnology and Interdisciplinary Sciences (BioDeakin), Institute for Technology Research and Innovation (ITRI), Deakin University.

Chapter 2

In vivo Spectroscopy for Detection and Treatment of GBM with NPt Implantation

José de la Rosa, Diego Adrián Fabila, Luis Felipe Hernández,
Edgard Moreno, Suren Stolik, Gabriela de la Rosa, Mayra Álvarez,
Alfonso Arellano, Tessy Lypez, R. Mercado, J. L. Soto, L. Arredondo,
J. Bustos, A. Mosqueda, and I. Rivero

INTRODUCTION

Nowadays, cancer is one of the main human causes of death worldwide. In 2007, 7.9 million deaths were due to this disease. The World Health Organization (WHO) estimates that 84 million people will die in the 10 year period from 2005 to 2015 due to cancer (IARC, 2008). In Mexico, from 1922 to 2001, the increase in the cancer-related grew from 0.6 to 13.1% of all the deaths occurring in the overall population (Kuri et al., 2010). Cancer types vary from one country to another, and specialists estimate that if current tendencies are maintained, the rate of incidence will rise all over the world. Since the incidence of most cancers increases with age, these Figures are going to rise if life expectancy continues to increase.

BRAIN TUMORS

Brain tumors are graded on the basis of their histological characteristics from I to IV; this Figure which provides an approximate prognostic guide. Grade I grows slowly. It is circumscribed or encapsulated. Histologically, the tumor cells are well-differentiated, resembling the origin or native cell. For this category, mitosis is absent or very rare and blood vessels are scanty and normal. In a remarkable contrast, a Grade IV tumor grows fast, is highly invasive, destroys the local tissue, and is found surrounded by edema. In this category, the tumor cells are anaplastic (undifferentiated), and pleomorphic (varied in shape, size, and pattern), and mitosis is common and often atypical. In addition, the blood supply is rich with abnormal vessels, and hemorrhage and necrosis are common.

Astrocytic constitute the largest group of intracranial tumors. Based on their histological features, the WHO distinguishes four grades of astrocytic tumors. Glioblastoma multiformes (GBM) is the most malignant and fastest-growing glioma, and constitutes 50–60% of astrocytic tumors. It most commonly occurs in mid- and late-midlife, with an average clinical course from 12 to 18 months. This tumor is commonly situated in the hemispheres, preferentially in the lobes (frontal and temporal) and appears circumscribed, though borders are ill-defined.

For GBM-affected tissues, cut surfaces have a multicolored appearance; they contain pinkish-gray viable tissue, yellow necrosis, cystic degenerations, and rusty and reddish areas associated with old and fresh hemorrhages, respectively. Since GBM is a fast-growing tumor, extensive edema and mass effects are prominent.

Histologically, GBM is characterized by high cellularity, with a great degree of anaplasia and pleomorphism. Some cells are small, round to ova or elongated, slender and spindle-shaped. Others are large, with one or multiple hyperchromatic nuclei, while giant cells are not uncommon. This tumor exhibits high mitotic activity and, a rich vascular supply; the blood vessels display endothelial and adventitial proliferations and thrombotic occlusions. A glomeruloid appearance of the proliferated capillaries is also typical. The GBM presents extensive necrotic regions. Smaller occurrences are surrounded by tumor cells in a pseudopalisading pattern. When GBM reaches the subarachnoid space or the ventricles, it may disseminate along the CSF pathways, forming small nodules or diffuse infiltrates. It seldom metastasizes outside the nervous system to the lymph nodes, lung, liver, and bone marrow (Haberland, 2007).

The GBM is a tumor that has a consistently heterogeneous pattern spreading over the neighboring cerebral tissue. The solid component is an easily distinguishable mass but the boundaries between tumor and cerebral tissue are difficult to differentiate because of the tumoral cells' infiltration. This non-evident infiltration pattern is also of great interest in low-grade gliomas because these other tumors have significant proportion of this infiltrative component. Although metastatic or multicentric recurrences could happen, in up to 90% of the cases tumors typically recur within 2 cm of the tumor resection bed (Hochberg and Pruitt, 1980; Wallner et al., 1989).

While therapies for high-grade gliomas are helpful, existing treatments cannot cure these tumors. The two major reasons for this are that tumor cells infiltrate into surrounding brain tissues and thus cannot be completely removed by the surgeon, and that most glioma cells are at least partially resistant to radiation and chemotherapy. The conventional regimen of treatment consists of surgery, followed by chemotherapy or radiotherapy. The main difficulty is the distinguishing of tumoral tissue and healthy tissue under normal surgical conditions. During surgical removal of the tumor, functional areas of the brain must be conserved, in order to protect vital functions of the patient. Nevertheless, in many cases surgical removal is virtually impossible due to the location of the tumor. No significant increase in survival has been observed in patients that have received surgery plus chemotherapy/radiotherapy regimens intended to treat GBM (Burger and Green, 1987).

Many attempts have been made in order to prolong life in patients with GBM. In the cases where surgery has not been an option, combined coadjuvant chemo/radiotherapy regimens have been tested in clinical trials with differing results in the treatment of adults (Frappaz et al., 2003). Temozolomide and radiotherapy is perhaps the most commonly used because Temozolomide is the most effective and well-tolerated drug for GBM. A random, controlled prospective study showed that the benefit of this regimen is very poor, with an increase of just 2.5 months of survival, compared with a radiation only treatment (Stupp et al., 2005). Another trial proposed repeated surgery and Temozolamide administration; in this study the median survival reached

15.1 months, higher than the 9 months that had initially been estimated (Terasaki et al., 2007).

Chemotherapeutic agents have several adverse side effects due to the impossibility of being able to differentiate between healthy and tumoral tissue. Among those effects are nephotoxicity, headache, vomiting, edema, and alopecia; all of them causing the patient to lose quality of life. Research regarding this pathology has been focused on the development of more effective and less toxic chemotherapeutic agents, as well as on the design of new diagnostic techniques and surgical instruments intended to allow neurosurgeons a higher degree of accuracy during neurosurgical procedures.

Nanotechnology has become a good alternative for the treatment of this GBM tumor. López et al. (2008, 2010) have reported on the preparation of novel nanostructured biocatalysts with antitumor activity. Catalytic nanomedicine has shown that it is possible to use a nanosized inorganic biocompatible catalyst inside tumors to reach significant shrinkage (López et al., 2008, 2010). The main advantage of these novel biocatalysts is the lack of adverse side effects, because nanoparticles are selective and also because they are locally infiltrated.

Optical biopsy refers to the detection of a cancerous state in a tissue using, optical methods. This is a new area, offering the potential to use noninvasive or minimally invasive *in vivo* optical spectroscopic methods to identify a cancer at its various early stages and to monitor its progression. The basic principle utilized for the method of optical biopsy is that absorbance, reflectance, and fluorescence emission are strongly influenced by the composition and cellular structure of tissues. The change in tissue from normal state to cancerous state has been shown to alter those properties.

Both auto fluorescence spectroscopy at UVA-Blue excitation (320, 337.1, 360, 366, 370, 405, 410, 440, 470, and 490 nm) and visible emission (400–700 nm) have been studied for the purpose of demarcating brain tumors (Butte et al., 2005; Chung et al., 1997; Croce et al., 2003; Lin et al., 2001; Marcu et al., 2004; Saraswathy et al., 2009). After the emission and absorption spectra of biological material in the brain, (see Figure 1 in (Wagnieres et al., 2003)), NAD(P)H (located principally in the mitochondria and throughout the cytosol), FAD (located in the mitochondria), and porphyrin (located in the blood) could be considered the main fluorophores responsible for healthy brain tissue autofluorescence emission at 365 nm excitation (Policard, 1924). In Table 1, the absorptivity and quantum yield of these components are summarized.

Table 1. Molar absorptivity (ε) and fluorescence quantum yield (Q) of principal fluorophores in brain tissue at 365 nm.

	ε $Lmol^{-1}cm^{-1}$	Q
NAD(P)H	6.3×10^3 (DaCosta et al., 2003)	0.019 (Scott et al., 1970)
FAD	9.6×10^3 (Ball, 1998)	0.03 (DaCosta et al., 2003)
Porphyrin	1.71×10^4 (Rimington, 1960)	0.1 (Ricchelli, 1995)

Fluorescence measurements excited at 366 nm in GBM have shown that the main responsible fluorophore for brain autofluorescence emission is the NAD(P)H (Croce et al., 2003). The measurement of *in vivo* continuous and time-resolved fluorescence, requires high intensity levels of light and high-sensitivity detectors due to the poor fluorescence characteristics of the NAD(P)H and FAD. The reported experiments used high pressure Hg lamps and spectrographs with OMA systems (Croce et al., 2003), and N_2 lasers with PMT's (Butte et al., 2005). In the case of time-resolved spectroscopy high speed electronics are necessary (Butte et al., 2005). Fluorescence in the red spectral region (>600 nm), which was noted in tumors as early as 1924 (Katz and Alfano, 1996), was originally attributed to bacteria, but is now thought to be secondary to endogenous porphyrins. Lin et al. (2001) reported that measurements of UV fluorescence spectroscopy and optical diffuse reflectance from 400 to 800 nm, in a pilot clinical trial consisting of 26 brain tumor patients, gave a sensitivity and specificity of 100 and 76%, respectively.

Usually, in fluorescence measurements with a fiber optic, the reflected excitation light is filtered out in order to have a better sensitivity in the fluorescence interval. In this work, we have reported the spectroscopic reflected scattering and fluorescence from GBM tumors, captured in the same signal. A portable fluorescence system, based on a recently-introduced high-power commercial UV-LED, a mini-spectrometer, and a bifurcated fiber optic was used. The measurements were obtained under continuous wave excitation at 365 nm. In agreement with previous studies (Lin et al., 2001), it was observed that the fluorescence intensity is lower in the cancerous tissue than in the cortex and white matter. Likewise, it was observed that the reflectance is higher in healthy tissue than at tumor borders, and that it almost disappears in the kern of the tumor. In order to complement these observations, biopsies were taken for further histopathological analysis.

EXPERIMENTAL

Nanoparticles

Nanostructured biocatalysts used in the tumors were prepared as previously reported (López et al., 2008, 2010). The powders were lightly pressed onto a sterile amalgam setter in such a way that, once inside the tumor bed, the cylindrical device made of nanoparticles crumbles when it comes into contact with the brain mass and CSF.

Histology

In order to compare the observed fluorescent behavior with pathologic diagnostics, biopsies of different tumor regions were taken after the *in situ* fluorescence measurements. The samples were fixed in paraffin wax and sections were stained by conventional Hematoxyline-Eosine (H-E) and Masson methods for microscopic study. The H-E is the most commonly used microscopical light stain in histology and histopathology. The staining method involves application of a basic dye hematoxylin dye, which colors basophilic structures with a bluish-purple hue, and alcohol-based acidic eosin, which colors eosinophilic structures a bright pink. The basophilic structures are usually the ones containing nucleic acids, such as ribosomes and chromatin-rich cell nuclei, and the cytoplasmic regions rich in RNA. Masson is a trichromic stain. The trichromic staining allows selective visualization of muscular fibers, collagen fibers, fibrin, and erythrocytes by employing three different coloring solutions. The selection of the employed colorants, which are differentiated by their molecular size, produces a distinguishable coloration of the different tissue compounds. In this study, H-E and Masson techniques were used to visualize any morphological change in both normal and tumor tissue, in order to observe the nanoparticle effect.

Spectrofluorometer

Figure 2 shows the experimental arrangement used to measure the steady-state fluorescence spectra from the brain. The system consists of an excitation light source with variable radiation power from 2 to 200 mW, a bifurcated optical fiber probe for delivery (six 200 μm channels) and collection (one 200 μm central channel) of light, a mini spectrometer, and a laptop computer. The excitation light is directly coupled to the bifurcated fiber-optic probe (R200-UV/VIS manufactured by Ocean Optics) with an efficiency of 18 (± 0.2)%. After sample excitation, part of the emitted fluorescence light is captured by the central channel of the bifurcated fiber-optic probe and guided into the entrance slit of a HR4000CG-UV-NIR or USB4000 spectrometer manufactured by Ocean Optics.

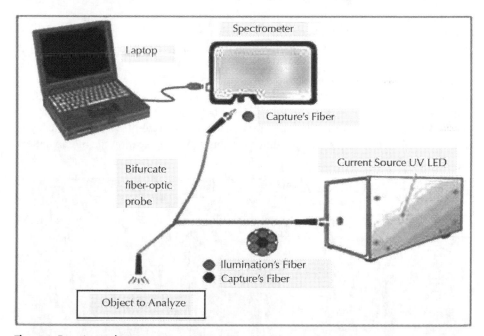

Figure 1. Experimental setup.

The electrical output from the spectrometer is sent, *via* a USB port to laptop for its analysis. For this study, we used a 200 mW light emitting diode (NCSU033A LED manufactured by Nichia Co.), which shows a peak emission in the UV-A at 365 nm, a band width of 9 nm, and a radiation angle of 100°. The LED is powered by a DC current supply regulated from 10 to 500 mA in order to produce a variable radiation power from 2 to 200 mW. The radiation power emitted by the LED is displayed on an LCD (2X16). The emitted power was calibrated with a UV light meter YK-34UV from Digital Instruments. A 12 V regulated DC power supply was used, which could be replaced by a battery to have a completely portable spectrofluorometer. The system is controlled from the laptop by a program written in the graphical language "G" from LabVIEW, which generates and processes the spectra in real time.

DISCUSSION AND RESULTS

As it was mentioned above, the first therapeutic option for brain tumors is surgery; craniotomy being considered one of the most common surgeries for treating these tumors. This procedure consists of the surgical removal of a section of bone (bone flap) from the skull, allowing neurosurgeons access to the brain for tumor removal and surgical repair. Preoperative MRI, CT, or arteriogram imaging studies is required to identify the most appropriate site for the procedure (see Figure 2). The head is clamped in place to avoid any movement during surgery, and the neurosurgeon shaves and marks the scalp where flap will be cut to expose the skull bone. Several small, interconnected burr holes are drilled into the skull. A craniotome is used to cut from one hole to the next to create a removable bone section. The section is then removed, forming a window that allows access to the tumor. Through that window, neurosurgeons can directly access and remove the tumor using microsurgical techniques. The bone section is replaced after surgery, and the scalp muscle and skin are stitched over the replaced bone. Although a craniotomy is considered a common procedure, it has some risks like such as infection, bleeding, seizures and added neurological deficits caused by the tumor removal. During tumor excision many vessels are cut: thus it is important for the surgeon to avoid hemorrhages. To prevent them, vessels are cauterized (by radiofrequency or laser) with an electrocautery as the tumor is being removed, sealing the blood vessels.

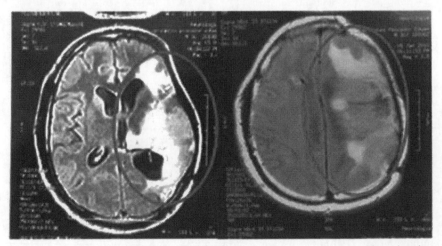

Figure 2. The RMI of two different patients before surgery. By this technique infiltrated malignant cells are not visible.

Optical spectra emissions of non-neoplastic and neoplastic tissue were taken during surgery on patients with GBM that were under clinical trial with NPt (46/09 INNN). The tested regions were the GBM solid portion; the cerebral border infiltrated by the tumor and apparently healthy brain tissue. Biopsies from pathological tissue were taken for the purpose of microscopy correlation after each spectral reading. Following Croce et al. (2003), before each measurement, the probe tip was washed with a saline solution and the investigated site was also rinsed with this solution to remove blood accumulation at the tissue surface. During measurements, the fiber probe tip was kept perpendicularly in contact with the tissue surface, without any pressure being exerted, by the neurosurgeon (see Figure 3). The room lights were temporarily turned off during spectral acquisition. The irradiation power was varied between 6 and 15 mW.

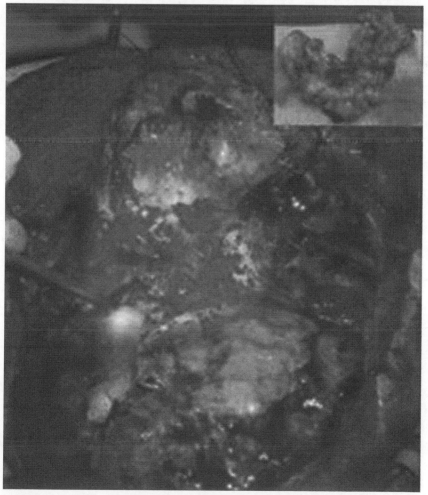

Figure 3. Results of the *in vivo* fluorescence measurements. The inset shows a portion of extracted tumor. Note the morphological difference between healthy brain tissue and tumor.

In a patient with a widespread GBM, infiltrating almost half of the brain (see Figure 4), the neurosurgeon selected three different regions to place the probe: the cerebral cortex, white matter that was considered healthy tissue, and the tumor region. The results of the fluorescence and reflection measurements are shown in Figure 5.

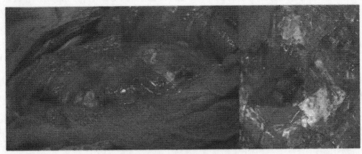

Figure 4. Wide-spreading high grade GBM. The cavity size is approximately 7 cm (right image).

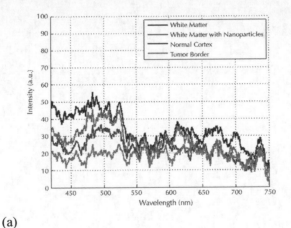

(a)

(b)

Figure 5. (a) Brain tissue fluorescence and (b) Diffuse reflectance. In this case, the GBM tumor was infiltrating a large part of the brain.

Figure 5(a) shows that a fluorescence spectrum in the range of 400–550 nm with a maximum emission around 490 nm is produced by the cerebral cortex and white matter. This result can be attributed to the effect of NAD(P)H and FAD. White matter also shows fluorescence in the range of 600–750 nm; this is principally due to the presence of porphyrins. Additionally a weaker fluorescence signal was detected in the tumor region. In Figure 5(b), the excitation light reflection in both the cerebral cortex and in the white matter was stronger than in the tumor region.

In a well located GBM that reaches the most external part of the brain (see Figure 6) the excitation light reflection in normal cortex tissue is also stronger than in the tumor region (see Figure 7). As the measurement region approach the GBM kern, the excitation light decreases reflection until it almost disappears in solid the portion of the tumor.

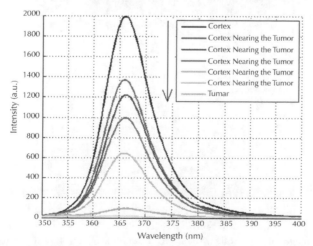

Figure 6. Typical example of a well located GBM.

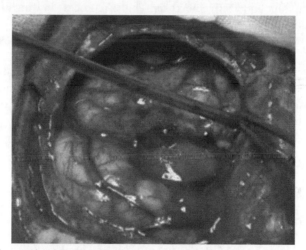

Figure 7. Diffuse reflectance spectra in a patient with a well located tumor reaching the most external part of the brain.

HISTOPATHOLOGY

In Figure 8(a) (40x), a control region of the tumor that corresponds to the surface temporal region is shown. Here coagulative necrosis was observed, with a "ghostly" appearance of the cells. In Figure 8(b), we can see the presence of nanoparticle aggregates (in the middle of the picture). These particles divided the tumor into two delimited zones; in the left zone viable tumors cells can be clearly observed, whereas on the right side some differences can be noticed. At higher amplification (Figure 8(c)), supporting tissue damage is evident and the necrotic process observed in herein liquefactive. This is a type of necrosis which is characteristic of focal bacterial or fungal infections, in which the affected cell is completely digested by hydrolytic enzymes. However, in the case of the brain, a hypoxic death of cells within the central nervous system also results in liquefactive necrosis. This is a process in which lysosomes turn tissues into a soup, as a result of the lysosomal release of digestive enzymes in the bacterial-onslaught phase. Loss of tissue architecture means that the tissue is essentially liquefied. Figure 8(d) is a close-up of the right side of Figure 8(c) revealing the presence of macrophages as well as neutrophiles (basophils). Masson stain (see Figure 8(e) and Figure 8(f)) was used in order to complement the obtained information from H-E. With this technique, we confirm the damage in supporting tissue as the soft-pink colored zones indicate.

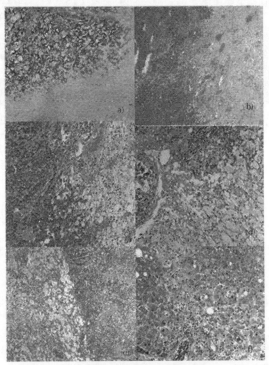

Figure 8. The H-E images of (a) necrotic tissue from the temporal region (40x), (b) the temporal region where nanoparticles were administrated (40x), (c) 100x, (d) right side of c (100x); (d), and (e) Masson stained sections at 40x and 100x, respectively.

The graded anaplasia of the glioma group reaches its extreme in GBM. Most authors consider this lesion to be a neoplasm of astrocytes because (1) the glioblastoma merges as a clinical entity with the two better-differentiated astrocytomas and anaplastic astrocytomas, (2) pathologically, the gioblastoma sometimes evolves out of a better differentiated astrocytic tumor, and (3) it often contains neoplastic astrocytes.

One of the main features observed, after NPt treatment, is related to the type of necrosis. As a result of the tumor growth, commonly the growth is so fast that in some cases cells die and some necrosis can be observed. However, this common necrosis is coagulative. In the region where nanoparticle aggregate can be clearly detected, a liquefactive necrosis area appears which can be associated with the action of the NPt. It is important to note that in this case neither inflammatory cells nor an abscess appears. These features are common to this type of process. Moreover, the damage caused to the malignant tissue (as the slimming of the support tissue shows), provides evidence that the NPt which were previously put inside the tumor, are acting against malignant cells inducing cell death.

With regard to fluorescence measurements, it was observed that even healthy white matter has a high absorption coefficient in the range from 300 to 600 nm; as a result that can be attributed to the porphyrin content in the blood (Roggan et al., 1995). The high vascularization in GBM tumors could be the reason for low reflection measurements related to the higher absorption in this tissue. So, reflection measurements can be used to demarcate the GBM border tumors. As the reflection measurements are more sensitive than those of the fluorescence, they can be used as a better criterion for finding tumors and cancer infiltrated tissue in the brain. The observed reflectances for the different brain areas could be an excellent tool for the *in situ* infiltration of nanoparticles, improving the odds of the survival after the surgical resectioning of malignant and infiltrative tumors like GBM.

CONCLUSION

In the present study, *in vivo* measurements of the reflectance and fluorescence of very-well- demarcated Glioblastoma tumors at 365 nm UV-light have been presented. As the measurement region approaches a non-neoplastic zone to the plain tumor, the reflectance decreases until it completely vanishes in the tumor. The measurements of the reflectance at 365 nm could be used to demarcate the resection or nanoparticle-infiltration zone during a surgical procedure.

The use of nanotechnology for the treatment of malignant tumors is an emerging research field that may offer more effective treatments that will increase patients' life expectancy beyond today's records. Moreover, the use of tools for *in situ* demarcation of highly invasive tumors could open new possibilities of more precise surgical procedures for tumor excision, and, at the same time, allow the precise administration of local antitumor agents like NPt. The simultaneous use of both detection and treatment tools will enhance the performance and results of surgical procedures, reducing collateral side effects.

KEYWORDS

- **Brain tumors**
- **Fiber-optic probe**
- **Glioblastoma multiformes**
- **Masson**
- **World health organization**

ACKNOWLEDGMENT

We acknowledge the FONCICyT-CONACyT 96095 project for their financial support. Also, the authors are grateful to UAM, H. C. Guadalajara, and INNN for the use of their facilities.

Chapter 3

Nanobiotechnology for Antibacterial Therapy and Diagnosis

Jagat R. Kanwar, Kislay Roy, and Rupinder K. Kanwar

INTRODUCTION

The development of structures and devices on a nanometer scale and their application in several fields is referred to as nanotechnology. One of these fields is medicine, better known as nanomedicine. Nanomedicines have many descriptions ranging from, "the use of materials", of which at least one of their dimensions that affects their function is in the scale range 1–100 nm, for a specific diagnostic or therapeutic purpose (Kostarelos, 2006) through to "the science and technology of diagnosing, treating and preventing disease and traumatic injury, of relieving pain, and of preserving and improving human health, using molecular tools and molecular knowledge of the human body" (Hermerén et al., 2007) as described by the European Science Foundation (ESF).

Due to a constant exposure to any pathogen there is need for an efficient antibacterial therapy. Most of the prevalent methods have proven to be ordinary by the increasing population of multi-drug resistant bacteria (Zampa et al., 2009). Study done by Matthews et al. (2010) explains the inefficiency of current bacterial diagnostics and discovery of new and innovative therapeutics and diagnostics. This study highlighted implementation of nanomaterials and nanotechnology for antibacterial medical therapeutics and diagnostics. Introduction of nanomedicine in field of antibacterial therapeutics has brought a revelation and the unmet medical need for new treatments has motivated the drug industry to search for new antimicrobial agents. Single stranded DNA or RNA known as aptamers have found their way into specifically targeting microbes (Kanwar et al., 2010). Aptamers have been selected using systematic evolution of ligands by exponential enrichment (SELEX) specifically for microbes such as *Bacillus anthracis* (Sterne strain) to diagnose and target them (Bruno and Kiel, 1999). This method is much specific when compared to any other technology. The review discusses some of these pioneering studies in which nanomedicines have been or are undergoing evaluation as potential therapeutic and diagnostic applications (Yacoby and Benhar, 2008). This review chapter will be arranged into two main categories; *antibacterial therapeutics* and *antibacterial therapeutics with diagnostic potential,* of these two main categories there will be sub-categories containing each application reviewed.

ANTIBACTERIAL THERAPEUTICS

Carbon Nanotubes and Fullerenes

Carbon nanotubes (CNTs) and fullerenes are the most commonly approached methods in nanotechnology. Yacoby and Benhar (2008) describe an investigation done by Kang et al. (2007) consisting the interaction of well-characterized, low metal content, narrowly distributed, pristine single-walled nanotubes (SWNTs) with a model bacterium (Kang et al., 2007). This study claimed to provide the first direct evidence that highly purified SWNTs can exhibit strong antimicrobial activity. Another carbon-based nanomoiety evaluated was the fullerene C60. Yacoby and Benhar (2008) explained how Lyon et al. (2005) investigated the interactions between nano-C60 and two common laboratory bacteria; *Escherichia coli*, gram-negative bacterium and, *Bacillus subtilis*, a gram-positive bacterium. The results of the tests performed showed both gram-negative and gram-positive bacteria were affected by nano-C60, with the minimal inhibitory concentrations (MICs) and minimal bactericidal concentrations (MBCs) (Lyon et al., 2005). The authors proposed three possible hypotheses for the mechanism of toxicity: the first was that nano-C60 disrupts electron transport, second was that nano-C60 punctures bacterial membranes and the third being nano-C60 produces radical-oxygen species that are toxic (Yacoby and Benhar, 2008). Emerging technology has brought a revelation in the modern trends in nanomedicines. Multiwalled carbon nanotubes (MWCNTs) functionalized with covalently bonded lysozyme were prepared and characterized by thermogravimetery, Raman spectroscopy, transmission electron microscopy (TEM) and cyclic voltametry (Table 1). It was estimated that per 4000 C atoms there is binding of 1 lysozyme residue. The MWCNT-lysozyme nanocomposite showed higher antibacterial activity in the gram positive *S. aureus* when compared to the free lysozyme (Merli et al., 2011) (Figure 1). Although this technology has been refined well and has many applications more research is required to determine its future safety and applications.

Table 1. Various antibacterial therapeutics and their mechanism of action.

Antibacterial therapeutics	Examples	Developed Against	Mechanism of action	Reference
carbon nanotubes	single walled nano-tubes (SWNT)	bacterial model	Punctures cell membrane, produce toxic free radicals, disruption of electron transport chain.	(Kang 2007)
fullerenes	fullerene C60	*E. coli,* *B. subtilis*		(Lyon et al. 2005)
	Multi-walled carbon nanotubes (MWCNT)-lysozyme	*S.aureus*	hydrolytic action	(Merli et al 2011)
Bioactive glasses	SiO_2-Na_2O-CaO-P_2O_5	*E. coli,* *P. aeruginosa,* *S. aureus*	created high PH in surrounding	(Yacoby and Benhar 2008)

Table 1. (Continued)

Antibacterial therapeutics	Examples	Developed Against	Mechanism of action	Reference
Biopolymers	quaternised chitosan (QCh)	wide range	chelating transition metals and inhibiting enzymes	(Ignatova et al. 2006a, 2006b)
	poly vinyl alcohol (PVA)	wide range	-	(Ignatova et al. 2006a, 2006b)
	Fish scale collagen peptides (FSCP)/ chito oligosaccharides (COS)	*S. aureus, E. coli*	disrupts cell membrane	(Wang et al. 2011)
Bacteriophages as drug carriers	chloramphenicol-phage-target specific peptides-IgG	broad range antibiotic	protein synthesis inhibitor	(Yacoby et al. 2007)
	aminoglycoside antibodies-phage-solubility enhancing peptides	broad range	cell membrane disruption	(Yacoby 2006)
Nanoemulsions	NB-401(oil in water)	*Burkholderia cepacia*	-	(LiPuma et al. 2009)
Aptamers	DNA aptamer	*Bacillus anthracis* (sterne strain)	targets bacterial spores	(Kanwar et al. 2010)

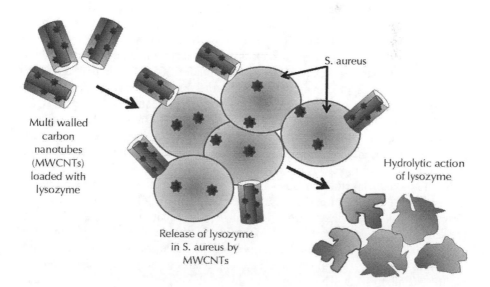

Figure 1. The Figure 1 shows antibacterial activity of lysozyme loaded Multiwalled carbon nanotubes (MWCNT). The nanotubes localize inside the bacteria *S.aureus* and release the lysozyme which due to its hydrolytic action destroys the bacteria (Merli et al. 2011).

Bioactive Glasses

The antimicrobial activity of bioactive glasses (SiO_2-Na_2O-CaO-P_2O_5 systems) has been established. Once suspended in aqueous solutions they release their ionic compounds over time which is the cause of the antimicrobial activity. Bioactive glasses show some promise as dentin disinfectants; however, the antibacterial effectiveness of calcium hydroxide in human teeth is much superior to that of the bioactive glasses. Yacoby and Benhar (2008) describe previous attempts to spike bioactive glass with silver to increase its antimicrobial efficacy using *E. coli*, *Pseudomonas aeruginosa* and *Staphylococcus aureus* as test microorganisms. Tests showed that concentrations of silver oxide (Ag_2O) bioactive glass (in the range of 0.05 to 0.20 mg/ml) of cultured medium inhibited the growth of these bacteria. The release of Na^+ and Ca^{2+} ions from, and the incorporation of H_3O^+ protons into the corroding bioactive glasses results in a high pH environment in closed systems (Sepulveda et al., 2002), which is not well tolerated by micro biota (Allan et al., 2001). The author explained that the introduction of nanometer scale particles led to more than a 10-fold increase in specific surface area and, consequently a stronger antimicrobial effect than the currently applied micron-sized material (Waltimo et al., 2007; Yacoby and Benhar, 2008).

Biopolymers

Nanoparticles of biological origin also exhibit antibacterial activity either in their natural state or once they are modified. The first example involves an additional application of electrospun nanofiber mats spun from polysaccharide chitosan. Polymers with intrinsic bacteriostatic and bactericidal activity and in particular, polysaccharides that are considered as promising for wound-healing and wound-dressing applications were reported. The natural polysaccharide chitosan was reported to possess several biological properties, such as hemostatic activity, non-toxicity, biodegradability, intrinsic antibacterial properties and the ability to affect macrophage function which contributes to a faster wound healing process (Balakrishnan et al., 2005; Muzzarelli et al., 2005). Yacoby and Benhar (2008) covers a study performed by Ignatova et al. (2006a) on the antibacterial properties of NPs that were fabricated from quaternised chitosan (QCh) and poly (vinyl alcohol) (PVA). The QCh derivatives illustrated a higher activity against bacteria, broader spectrum of activity and higher killing rate when compared with those of chitosan. The preparation of QCh-containing nanofibers was carried out by electrospinning of mixed QCh/PVA aqueous solutions and the antibacterial properties of photo-cross-linked electrospun QCh/PVA mats were studied. It was found that the antibacterial activity of photo cross-linked electrospun QCh/PVA mats was found to have a "reduction of bacterial growth by 98% (after 120 min of exposure)" (Yacoby and Benhar, 2008). In a recent study, nanofibrous membranes of 50–100 nm were formed using 2:1 ratio of low molecular weight fish scale collagen peptides (FSCP)/ chito oligosaccharides (COS) which had antibacterial activity and were designed to be used for wound dressing. These nanofibres showed good antibacterial activity against gram positive S. aureus and gram negative *E. coli*. Sensitivity for *S. aureus* was found to be much higher when compared to *E. coli*. The antibacterial activity of the nanofiber was due to its ability to disrupt the cell membranes of the bacterias. However when tested on human cells, the fibers proved biocompatible and supported the proliferation of human skin fibroblast cells. Such studies mark the further advance of biopolymers in the medicinal field (Wang et al., 2011).

Bacteriophage Drug-carrying Platforms

Filamentous bacteriophages (phages) were applied as targeted drug-carrying platforms aiming to eradicate the pathogenic bacteria and other cells which carry any infection or disease (Yacoby and Benhar, 2008). Authors describe phage NPs as nanoneedles with a diameter of ~8 nm, capable of delivering a large dose of a cytotoxic drug to the target cells. In order to make the procedure successful against pathogenic bacteria a drug was linked to the genetically modified phage by means of chemical conjugation through an esterase-cleavable linker subject designed to control release by serum esterases. The specificity of the drug-carrying phages to target cells was enhanced by genetic expression of a targeting moiety on the phage coat. This approach may re-enable the use of drugs that are not in use, owing to their toxicity or low specificity, and have been excluded from clinical use (Yacoby and Benhar, 2008). The capability of this approach was demonstrated using chloramphenicol (as it is rarely used to treat patients systematically due to its toxicity) (Yacoby and Benhar, 2008; Yacoby et al., 2007). The nanoparticle targeting was accomplished by using two different targeting moieties: target-specific peptides and antibodies linked to the phage via an immunoglobulin G (IgG) Fc-binding ZZ domain. The process had drawbacks such as restricted ability to inhibit bacterial growth due to the limited loading capacity of less than 3,000 drug molecules per phage (Yacoby et al., 2007). To overcome these limitations, a modified system was developed based on the application of hydrophilic aminoglycoside antibiotics as branched, solubility-enhancing linkers using unique drug conjugation chemistry (Yacoby, 2006); replacing the loading methodology and modifying the antibody-phage conjugation method, which improved the system for targeting a broad range of pathogenic bacteria. The new drug-conjugation approach led to an arming rate of over 40,000 chloramphenicol molecules/phage (Yacoby and Benhar, 2008). The results obtained were from within an artificial closed system and did not reflect an in vivo application (Yacoby et al., 2007), although this did offer great possibilities for the future of in vivo treatments. It was concluded that the drug-carrying phages represent a therapeutic NPs with wide range of applications that, may become an important general targeting drug-delivering platform "owing to the chosen coating, by the simplicity of which it can be equipped with a targeting moiety, and massive drug-carrying capacity", (Yacoby and Benhar, 2008).

ANTIBACTERIAL NANOEMULSION

Researchers at the University of Michigan (USA), have developed a nanoemulsion with an immaculate antibacterial activity against ~99% of the resistant bacteria that commonly cause respiratory tract infections in patients suffering with cystic fibrosis (CF). The primary cause of death in persons with cystic fibrosis is respiratory tract infection involving opportunistic bacteria having broad-spectrum antibiotic resistance (LiPuma et al., 2009) and treating these patients is made more complicated by the thick sputum present within the lungs which is caused by this disease. These infections are caused by bacterial strains highly resistant to common antibacterial agents like the *Burkholderia cepacia* complex. A topically administered surfactant-stabilized (oil-in-water) nano-emulsion, named NB-401 was developed. When this nanoemulsion was tested on 150 bacterial strains, all but two showed sufficient bactericidal activity; irrespective of their resistance, the growth of all strains was inhibited by NB-401. No decrease in the level of activity was observed against multi-drug or panresistant strains as well and NB-401 also proved to be effective against planktonic strains growing in human sputum or against strains that grew in biofilm. The nanoemulsion also overcame difficulties in the administration of systemic antibiotics. This topical or inhaled (nebulizer) therapy can achieve high level concentrations of the drug that could never be achieved with an oral systemic drug because of the systemic toxicity (LiPuma et al., 2009).

Antibacterial Therapeutics with Diagnostic Potential-pluronic Block Copolymers as Micellar Nanocarriers

This study investigated the specific arrangement of polymeric molecules at the na-noscale. They enhance the chances for safe and efficient delivery of various drugs, several biomolecules and genes and can be used for imaging and biosensing as well. The diameter of Pluronic micelles normally ranges from 10–100 nm (Kabanov et al., 1995). The core of the micelles consists of hydrophobic poly (propylene oxide) blocks that are separated from the aqueous exterior by the shell hydrated of hydrophilic poly (ethylene oxide) chains. The core represents the carrier ship for the incorporation of various therapeutics and diagnostic reagents (Batrakova and Kabanov, 2008). Pluronic block polymers with respects to various antibacterial and antifungal drugs showed enhanced bioactivity against many microorganisms (Croy and Kwan 2004, 2005; Saski and Shah, 1965a, 1965b). Much work in this field is still under clinical evaluation and several fascinating developments in this area are expected in the coming years (Batra-kova and Kabanov, 2008).

Multifunctional Nanoplatforms

It is very difficult to diagnose and treat a biofilm infection as most of the infections are resistant to the prevalent treatments and the infectious pathogens stay dormant for quite some time and infect sporadically producing the symptoms of infections (Costerton et al., 1999). Multifunctional nanoplatforms such as protein cage architectures can utilize the infection-specific magnetic resonance imaging (MRI) markers that can be used to identify and characterize the centers of biofilm infections. It has been established that both therapeutics (Flenniken et al., 2005) and imaging agents (Allen et al., 2005; Flenniken et al., 2006) have been delivered efficiently by protein cages. It is however important that the size of such nanostructures be in such a range that it can efficiently pass through the biofilm barriers and yet deliver a sufficient amount of the desired drug (Suci et al., 2007). More research has to be done to determine the immune system response and the mechanism of action of these nanostructures before they can be put to use clinically (Zhang and Falla, 2006).

Dermaseptin 01 Antimicrobial Peptides

A new family of antibiotics namely antimicrobial peptides (AMPs) was investigated by Zampa et al. for clinical applications (Zampa et al., 2009). Dermaseptins (DSs) is a member of AMP family isolated from the secretion of frog skin (*Phyllomedusa* genus) (Brand et al., 2006; Leite et al., 2008). It consists of cationic molecules 24–34 amino acids long that can fold into amphiphilic helices when in contact with hydrophobic media. The DS polypeptide chains are "gene encoded as part of larger precursor molecule compromising a signal peptide of 22 residues, followed by an acidic pro-peptide, a typical pro-hormones processing signal, and a DS progenitor sequence". Zampa et al. (2009) from previous research works explained that DSs has cytolytic action against numerous microorganisms and are considered as promising agents to fight viral diseases, drug-resistant bacteria, protozoa, yeast, and filamentous fungi. Adding to its benefits these peptides do not cause significant cytolysis against mammalian blood cells. The DS 01, collected from the skin of *P. oreades* and *P. hypochondrialis* frogs, has demonstrated high antibacterial activity against gram-positive and gram-negative bacteria (Brand et al., 2006). Due to their lack of stability in serum and plasma as a big drawback the DS peptides are easily degraded by the proteolytic enzymes *in vivo* but their efficiency is high in *in vtiro*. It is however observed that the Multimeric forms of the DS peptides are much stable *in vivo* when compared to the monomeric peptides (Pini et al., 2005; Tam et al., 2002). Immobilization of DS 01 within a nanostructured (nickel tetrasulfonated phthalocyanine nanostructure, film-forming electroactive molecule) thin film was used to serve as a biosensor. The results showed that DS 01 appeared to be the most promising irreversible anti-parasitic peptides. The growth inhibition in accordance with death of *Leishmania chagasi*, clearly shows the Leishmanicidal activity of DS 01. Enhanced detection was demonstrated using cyclic voltammetry suing the AMP-containing films as electrodes. It was observed that inclusion of slight modifications in the assay time and the signal to noise ration may enhance the sensitivity and efficiency of this method. Both high sensitivity and specificity are reflected by enhanced pathogen detection (Zampa et al., 2009). Nanoparticles are commonly used as delivery systems for various drugs. Most nanoparticles have sustained drug delivery due to enhanced permeability retention (EPR) effect and thus the drug can be released over a long period of time reducing the options of multiple dosages. Various nanoparticle systems have been established as antibacterial drug carriers such as silver nanoparticles (Sondi and Salopek-sondi, 2004), metal oxide nanoparticles including magnesium oxide (Huang et al., 2005), zinc oxide (Jones et al., 2008), silicon dioxide (Jia et al., 2008), chitosan nanofiber (Ignatova et al., 2006b), poly-l-lactide nanoparticles (Salmaso et al., 2004), gold nanoparticles (Faulk and Taylor, 1971), quantum dots (Edgar et al., 2006), magnetic nanoparticles (Faulk and Taylor, 1971) and many more. Magnetic nanoparticles consisting of Fe_3O_4 core and coated with antibacterial compound poly (quaternary ammonium) (PQA) have been prepared and well characterized by various methods including Fourier transform infrared (FTIR), thermogravity analysis (TGA), TEM. These nanoparticles showed 100% biocidal efficiency against *E. coli* (10^5 to 10^6 *E.coli*/mg nanoparticle) and after use the nanoparticles could be collected again under influence of external magnetic field (Dong et al., 2011) (Figure 2). Thus a wide range of work has been done in the field of nanoparticles based delivery.

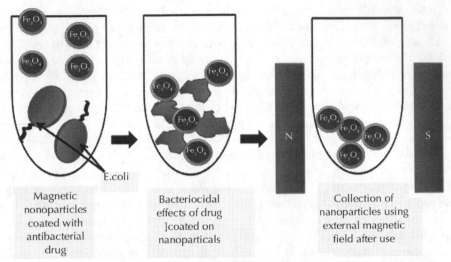

Figure 2. The magnetic nanoparticles (Fe_3O_4) loaded with antibacterial compound PQA are shown in the Figure. These nanoparticles target the bacteria *E.coli* and kill them due to the antibacterial activity of PQA. After the use the nanoparticles can be recollected under the influence of external magnetic field. Thus these nanoparticles are referred to as the recyclable nanoparticles (Dong et al. 2011).

CONCLUSION

With new strains of multi-drug resistant bacteria and viruses always presenting themselves, the need for antimicrobial defenses is required on a daily basis. These studies reviewed were aimed at informing the reader of new and modified antibacterial, therapeutic and diagnostic methods that are being developed. With a lot of these potential antibacterial nanomedicines still being researched, the possibilities are ever increasing. The applications, such as bacteriophage drug-carrying platforms will soon shift diagnosis to a pre-symptomatic stage and allow pre-emptive therapeutic measures, or the treatment of high-resistant pathogens using multifunctional nanoplatforms as a less invasive method. Pluronic block polymers as micellar nanocarriers and DS 01 antimicrobial peptides would improve diagnostic methods for bacterial infection, as well as treating them. Introduction of aptamers as nanomedicines has changed the scenario of drug development and effective targeting. But for these future technologies to succeed and be of use, they will need to be cost-effective with higher performance in terms of resolution, sensitivity, specificity, reliability, reproducibility, and integration.

KEYWORDS

- **Biopolymers**
- **Carbon nanotubes**
- **Cystic fibrosis**
- **Dermaseptins**
- **Diagnostic**
- **Nanomedicines**
- **Nanotechnology**
- **Quaternised chitosan**

ACKNOWLEDGMENT

The work was supported by the grants from Institute of Biotechnology, Institute for Technology & Research Innovation and the Australia-India Strategic Research Fund (AISRF) Department of Innovation Industry Science, Research, and Commonwealth of Australia (BF030016), and BioDeakin, ITRI, Deakin University.

Chapter 4

Chitosan Nanoparticles

Divyen Shah, Vaishali Londhe, and Rima Shah

INTRODUCTION

Natural polymers are having advantages like biodegradability and biocompatibility, which make them favorable for most of the drug delivery system (Schmidt, 2009). Nanoparticle drug delivery system is used because of its high bioavailability, reduced dosage and toxicity, targeted delivery, and so on. Chitosan (CS) is one of the commonly used naturally obtained polymers with various therapeutic uses. Chitosan ((1→4)-2-amino-2-deoxy-β-D-glucan), a linear polyamine with a high ratio of glucosamine to acetyl-glucosamine units, is a natural mucoadhesive cationic polymer, which is obtained by partial deacetylation of chitin (Banerjee et al., 2002). Chitosan (pKa = 6.5) is solubilized in acidic medium (Chen, 2003). The primary amino groups lead to special properties that render chitosan very interesting for pharmaceutical applications like development of controlled release drug delivery systems like chitosan gels, tablets, capsules, microspheres, microcapsules, and nanoparticles for parenteral, nasal, ophthalmic, transdermal, and implantable delivery of drugs, proteins, peptides, and gene materials (Chen et al., 2007). The free amino functional group in chitosan makes it possible to form nanoparticles by cross-linking, emulsion cross-linking, spray drying, desolvation with cationic salts, ionic complexation/coacervation or ionic gelation method by interacting with various other reactive groups such as alginates, dextran sulphate, sodium tri poly phosphate (STPP), polyethylene glycol (PEG), different ligands, antibodies, DNA and pH sensitive moieties, and so on. (Kumar, 2000) Chitosan can enhance the transmucosal absorption by increasing the paracellular permeability of intestinal epithelia. Chitosan nanoparticles are having good potential for the ocular drug delivery system because of its mucoadhesive nature (Campos, 2001). It has been extensively used in nasal drug and vaccine delivery (Csaba, 2008). Main advantage of chitosan nanoparticle is it can be used for hydrophilic drug entrapment. The hydrophilic nanoparticle remains in circulation for long time without PEGlyation, by avoiding reticulo endothelial system (RES). The other advantage of using chitosan nanoparticles is that they do not require any organic solvent or any other extreme conditions mainly in ionotropic gelation or complex coacervation technique which results in more stabilization of proteins and peptides.

Ionic gelation and complex coacervation are almost same except that, ionic gelation uses electrolyte such as tri poly phosphate (TPP), whereas in complex coacervation oppositely charged ionic polymer such as alginate are used. Ionic gelation method using TPP is more common for entrapment of hydrophilic drugs, proteins and plasmids. By ionotropic gelation method, we can obtain size from 100 to 1000 nm and zeta potential between +20 to +60 mv by varying the ratio of chitosan/STPP (Soppimath et al., 2001). The structure of chitosan and STPP is given in Figure 1.

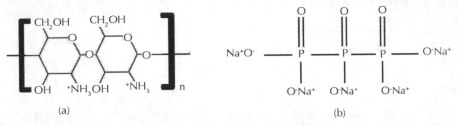

(a)   (b)

Figure 1. Structure of (a) Chitosan and (b) Sodium tri poly phosphate.

Size, surface charge, release characteristics and percentage drug entrapment efficiency of these chitosan/STPP nanoparticles can be modulated by (i) using different molecular weight chitosan, (ii) by incorporating additional polymers such as poloxamer, hyaluronic acid, cyclodextrin and so on. or (iii) by using chemically modified chitosan derivatives, such as N-trimethyl chitosan (Csaba, 2008).

Figure 2 explains chitosan's application as biomedical material along with percentage contribution in various fields (Issa, 2005).

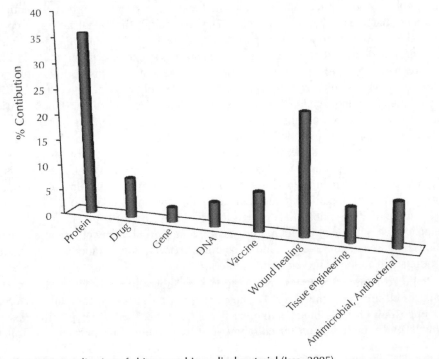

Figure 2. Main application of chitosan as biomedical material (Issa, 2005).

METHODS OF CHITOSAN NANOPARTICLE PREPARATION

Chitosan-based nanoparticles can be prepared by following methods.

1. Ionic gelation
2. Covalent cross-links
3. Complex coacervation
4. Desolvation method
5. Emulsion-droplet coalescence method
6. Reverse micellar method

We will mainly discuss ionotropic gelation method in detail. Other methods are discussed in brief.

Ionic Cross Linking (Ionic Gelation)

This method is the most common technique to prepare chitosan nanoparticles. In this method, only aqueous phases are used and no organic solvent is used, and thus the chances of degradation of peptides are decreased. Chitosan is dissolved in one phase, and in other phase negative charge generating ployanion like STPP is dissolved. Both the phases are mixed under magnetic stirring at room temperature which generates gel like nanoparticles. The nanoparticles are formed due to intra and inter molecular linkage between chitosan and STPP. The schematic representation of preparation is given in Figure 3. The pH of both the phases can play important role on particle size and percentage entrapment efficiency. Generally the method does not require any stabilizer or surfactants and the nanoparticles generated are stable in nature (Yang et al., 2009a).

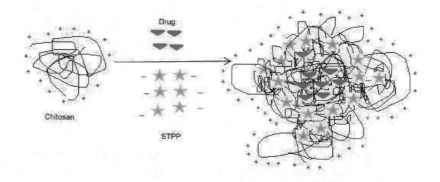

Figure 3. Schematic representation of chitosan/STPP nanoparticle.

To obtain high yield of chitosan-TPP nanoparticles, the chitosan: TPP weight ratio should be between 3:1 and 6:1. The nanoparticles can also be made by introduction of other hydrophilic polymer. Even it may increase versatility for association and delivery of proteins. In nanoparticles of chitosan and diblock copolymer of ethylene oxide and propylene oxide, PEO-PPO is attached to surface of particle which was confirmed by transmission electron microscopy (TEM). In general, protein loading can be obtained as high as 50%. Highest loading efficiency can be obtained when pH of solution is above isoelectric point of protein, so that it has negative charge. In addition to ionica crosslinking with TPP, other mechanisms may also work for association of macromolecules, because insulin nanoparticles prepared at pH where insulin is positively charged, showed 30% entrapment efficiency. These mechanisms could be hydrogen bonding, hydrophobic interaction and other physicochemical forces. Even the drug release profile of insulin varies with pH medium. Cross-linking induced by incorporation of TPP will make the nanoparticles compact and resistant to freeze drying (Janes et al., 2001).

The cross-linking density, crystallinity, and hydrophilicity of cross-linked chitosan can allow modulation of drug release. Even the swelling behavior of cross-linked chitosan depends on pH of TPP. Cross-linked chitosan shows higher swelling ability (Bhumkar, 2006).

There were some studies in which the effects of cationic surfactant like cetyltrimethylammonium bromide were studied. The addition of cationic surfactant might reduce the size, while increasing the zeta potential. The decreased size may improve permeability through extracellular membrane. The increased surface charge density may facilitate absorption efficiency and may prevent nanoparticles from enzymatic degradation (Bao, 2008).

Covalent Cross-links

The process involves the precipitation of the polymer followed by chemical cross-linking by oppositely charged polymer. Precipitation can be done by sodium sulfate followed by chemical cross-linking using formaldehyde, glutaraldehyde or even using a natural crosslinking agent such as genepin. Later on the solvent is removed by rotary evaporator and dry nanoparticles are obtained. In this method, the drug is immobilized on nanoparticles instead of encapsulation (Hamidi, 2008).

Complex Coacervation

The process is spontaneous phase separation which occurs upon mixing of oppositely charged polyelectrolyte in aqueous medium. This method is almost similar to ionic gelation method, but here opposite charge generating polymers like alginate or dextran sulfate are used. The mechanical strength is comparatively higher than that of ionic gelation method (Chen et al., 2007).

Desolvation Method

In this method, a more water soluble polymer or water miscible nonsolvent for chitosan is added drop wise under stirring and then liquid particles are hardened by chemical cross-linking with glutaraldehyde. These nanoparticles can be prepared by either o/w or w/o/w emulsion (Chakravarthi, 2007).

Emulsion-droplet Coalescence Method

As chitosan is having solubility in acidic medium (below its pKa= 6.5), it will precipitate when it will come in contact with other alkali medium. In this method, two emulsions are prepared. In one emulsion, only chitosan is dissolved along with the drug while in other emulsion, the chitosan is dissolved along with little quantity of sodium hydroxide. Finally, both the emulsions are mixed at high speed resulting in formation of small solid chitosan nanoparticles due to collision between the two emulsions (Agnihotri, 2004).

Reverse Micellar Method

In this method, chitosan and drug solutions are added to organic solvent having surfactant. The transparency of the solution should be maintained by adding water additionally if required. Cross-linking agent is added to above system and is stirred continuously to evaporate the organic solvent to obtain transparent dry mass. Then, the obtained transparent material is dispersed in water and then suitable salt is added to precipitate out the surfactant which was separated by centrifugation. The obtained supernatant is having drug loaded nanoparticles. By dialyzing the solution, free drug is removed and the remaining solution is lyophilized (Patel, 2009).

APPLICATIONS OF CHITOSAN NANOPARTICLES

Chitosan nanoparticles are having tremendous application in various fields which are as follows:

Molecular Imaging

Chitosan-based system such as microbubble, micelles and liposomal nanoparticles are used in molecular imaging. The incorporation of hard and brittle calcium phosphate or hydroxyapatite with chitosan yields a bioresorbable composite with favorable mechanical property for bone and cartilage tissue engineering. Particles with ferric oxide can be used in MRI for hepatocyte targeting imaging. The chitosan coated superparamagnetic iron oxide nanocrystals (SPION) are used as MRI contrast agent, which can have high labeling efficiency and high uptake efficiency by stem cells. Water soluble chitosan-linoleic acid conjugate can be used as contrast agents to target hepatocytes. Gadolinium-loaded chitosan nanoparticles displayed prolonged retention in tumor tissue after *in vivo* intratumoral injection (Agrawal, 2010).

Protein Delivery

It can be done *via* oral route and *via* nasal route.

Via Oral Route

a. As vaccination

The n-trimethyl chitosan-TPP nanoparticles prepared by ionic gelation method for protein delivery system by oral route have shown promising results. They have reduced the transepithelial electrical resistance (TEER) or have increased the paracellular transport to the cells. They have shown good systemic immune response when immunized with urease loaded nanoparticles (Chen et al., 2008).

The adsorption of protein on chitosan nanoparticles is giving high loading capacity. Hydrophilic nanoparticle with negative surface charge (excess sodium alginate) can be uptaken by Rat Peyer's patches, which can be used as carrier of mucosal vaccination (Borges et al., 2006).

Using Bovine serum albumin, the loading efficiency can be obtained as high as 68%. As the deacetylation degree increases, the loading efficiency also increases but the drug release rate decreases. As the molecular weight of chitosan was increased, the loading efficiency was increased but the drug release rate was decreased. The PEG addition can accelerate the drug release (Chun, 2007).

The M cell represents a potential portal for oral delivery of peptides and for mucosal vaccination because of their transcytotic capacity. Alginate modified trimethyl chitosan nanoparticles were used for loading of urease. Nanoparticles may influence their ability to enhance drug permeation through paracellular pathway. The systemic and mucosal immune responses were also good (Prego et al., 2010).

Recombinant hepatitis B surface antigen (rHBsAg) as a model was used to prepare hepatitis B vaccine, in which chitosan nanoparticles were prepared by chitosan-TPP ionic gelation method. Normal vaccines prepared by using alum as adjuvant, were unstable when there was slight temperature change, and thus stable vaccine was needed. Chitosan-based nanoparticles were stable, and protected the associated antigen during storage, either as an aqueous suspension under different temperature conditions (+ 4°C and − 20°C), or as a dried form after freeze-drying the nanoparticles. Even the IgG level was 9-fold higher than conventional alum adsorbed vaccines (Prego et al., 2010).

b. For Hyperglycemia

Insulin loaded chitosan-TPP nanoparticles were prepared at controlled pH by ionotropic gelation method for oral route delivery with 63% entrapment efficiency (Ma, 2002).

Insulin was entrapped by alginate and calcium chloride, and then chitosan formed polyelectrolyte complex with alginate. They protected insulin from aggressive environment of GIT, when administered orally. Insulin was released in pH dependent manner. The glucose level was decreased by more than 40% for 18 hr with 50 IU/kg. Confocal microscopy study confirms that nanoparticles adhere to intestinal epithelium (Sarmento et al., 2007).

Via Nasal Route

a. As Vaccination

Chitosan-DNA nanoparticle complexes were prepared for vaccination purpose of flu, in which hemagglutinin and Influenza A virus were used as plasmids. Even measles and respiratory syncytial virus (RSV) by nasal route were also prepared (Illum et al., 2001).

Even they are effective for targeting to nasal associated lymphoid tissues (NALT) in nasal vaccine delivery (Nagamoto et al., 2004).

Trimethyl chitosan nanoparticles can increase the M cell dependent uptake and enhance the association of the antigen with dendritic cells (Slutter et al., 2009).

Nanoparticles transport through M cell co-culture model is 5-fold higher than intestinal epithelial monolayer, with atleast 80% chitosan-DNA nanoparticles uptake in 30 min (Kadiyala et al., 2010).

Chitosan nanoparticles and chitosan-ethylene oxide- propylene oxide polymer blocks were used for association and control release of bovine serum albumin, tetanus and diphtheria toxoid. Protein was released at constant rate which matches with the intensity of protein loading. Tetanus vaccine was released for atleast 15 days (Calvo et al., 1997).

b. For Hyperglycemia

As chitosan is having mucoadhesive nature, it will intensify the contact between insulin and nasal mucosa, leading to increased concentration at absorption site. The nanoparticles were prepared by ionic gelation method, which were having average size of 300–400 nm and 55% insulin loading efficiency. The molecular weight of chitosan had no impact on drug release profile or on the level of blood glucose level, but the nanoparticles were able to reduce blood glucose level in rabbit due to increased nasal absorption (Urrusuno et al., 1999).

The chitosan concentrations, osmolarity, medium and absorption enhancers in chitosan nanoparticles have significant effect on the insulin nasal delivery. As the concentration increases, the insulin transport increases. The permeability will also increase in hypo or hyper osmotic medium compared to iso-osmatic medium (Yu et al., 2004).

For Anti-fungal Delivery

The amphotericin B is the ideal candidate for many fungal infections. But it is very less soluble and its bioavailability is poor by oral route. Thus it needs to be given by parenteral route, which is causing nephrotoxicity. The nanoparticles were prepared by chitosan-dextran sulfate coacervation method using zinc sulfate as stabilizing agent. Loading efficiency of 65% was obtained by this method. More importantly, the nephrotoxicity was reduced when checked by *in vivo* renal toxicity study (Tiyaboonchai, 2007).

For Gene Delivery System

The chitosan and DNA interaction is electrostatic, which is strong enough that they do not dissociate until they have entered in to cell. Even the mucoadhesive and cationic nature of chitosan play important role in adhesion to cell and lysosomal escape of DNA. They are divided in two categories depending on mechanism of formation. The complex can be protected from DNAse to improve bioavailability of plasmid DNA.

a. Chitosan-DNA Complexes

Gentle mixing followed by incubation of chitosan and DNA solution can generate chitosan-DNA complexes with size from 100 to 600 nm depending on the molecular weight of chitosan, in which proportion of chitosan is in excess. The stability depends on positive amino group of chitosan to the negative phosphate group of DNA, and is also having direct effect on surface charge and particle size. Higher charge ratio can give better stability along with good transfection efficiency (Janes, 2001).

b. Chitosan-DNA nanosphere

In this method, chitosan and DNA solutions are mixed with controlled speed of mixing and temperature with addition of dilute salt in to DNA solution which works as a desolvating agent for polymer. They are having size of 200–500 nm with loose rod-like and toroidal structure. These nanoparticles may be entering to cell via endocytic pathway (Janes, 2001).

The size of chitosan-DNA complex decreases as the molecular weight (MW) of chitosan decreases. High MW chitosan are superior to those of low MW chitosan in enhancing the stability of complex, giving protection to DNA in cellular endosomal/lysosomal compartments, but on other side, it restricts release of DNA. Higher deacetylation of chitosan will result in increase positive charge enabling a greater DNA binding capacity and cellular uptake. Chitosan in salt form have higher transfection efficiency than chitosan-base alone. The pH below pKa value of chitosan favors DNA association and dissociation (Mao, 2010).

Der p 2- a house dust mite's dermatophagoides pteronyssinus is responsible for asthma, perennial rhinitis and atopic dermatitis. Thus allergic diseases can be characterized by sensitization of allergen specific Th2 cells and IgE production. The chitosan pDer p 2 nanoparticles have shown 100% encapsulation efficiency with sufficient protection of plasmid. They are able to induce interferon-γ (IFN-γ) in serum, and thus prevent allergic response caused by Th2 sensitization (Li et al., 2009).

Generally chitosan-DNA vaccines are applied through traditional high pressure gene guns which elicit high titres of protective immunity, but will cause inevitable pain. To overcome this, a low pressure gene guns were used. The vaccine for Japanese encephalitis virus was prepared, which have produced specific antibodies, and have maintained high survival rate (Huang et al., 2009).

Chitosan lactate and chitosan acetate have also been used as carrier of pSV β-galactosidase plasmid, have shown cell viability of more than 90% (Weecharangsan et al., 2006).

For Hepatitis Treatment

Glycyrrhetic acid is an aglycone and an active metabolite of glycyrrhizin which is having anti-inflammatory, anti-hepatotoxic, anti-tumorigenic activity, and is used in chronic hepatitis. It is having side effect of aldosteronism. Glycerrhetic acid is metabolite of glycyrrhizin and is active in nature. But bioavailability of glycerrhetic is very less when given as such. Thus the nanoparticles of ammonium glycyrrhizinate were prepared by PEGlated chitosan-TPP ionic gelation method, which was having 82% entrapment efficiency (Wu et al., 2005).

For Anti-microbial Agents

Chitosan-alginate nanoparticles were prepared for Polymixin B, a potent peptidic antibiotic having effect on gram negative bacteria. They also showed uptake by M cells.

Polymixin B was earlier given by parenteral route because it was absorbed very less by oral route (Coppi et al., 2006).

Amoxicillin- a broad spectrum antibacterial is having very short half-life suggesting frequent dosing. To overcome this, a controlled drug delivery system of chitosan-TPP nanoparticle was developed (Singh, 2010).

Chitosan nanoparticles and copper loaded nanoparticles have shown antibacterial activity against *E. coli, S. choleraesuis, S. typhimurium,* and *S. aureus* and the results state that minimum inhibitory concentration is 0.25 µg/ml, and minimum bactericidal concentration is 1 µg/ml. Exposure of *S. choleraesuis* to nanoparticles disrupt the cell membrane and causes leakage of cytoplasm, which was later on confirmed by atomic force microscopy (Qi et al., 2004).

For Tumor Targeting
Doxorubicin is one of the potent anti-cancer agents having cardio toxicity. The nanoparticles prepared by chitosan-dextran have shown reduction in side effects and improved efficacy in treatment of solid tumor. The size of 100 ± 10 nm was obtained which favors the enhanced permeability and retention effect observed in solid tumors (Arhewoh, 2005).

The doxorubicin was not released in cell culture, and it had entered to cell while remaining associated with nanoparticles, which was later confirmed by confocal microscopy. The positive charge carrier of nanoparticle will be useful in the treatment of solid tumor. Even the biodistribution and organ accumulation pattern will be changed when given by intravenous route (Janes et al., 2001).

The 5-amino salicylic acid (5-ASA), an anti-inflammatory agent used in ulcerative colitis, Crohn's disease which may provide protection against development of colorectal cancer in patient suffering from inflammatory bowel disease. It is metabolized in intestine and eliminated from there. If given orally, adverse effects like hepatitis, blood dyscrasias, pancreatitis, pleuropericarditis, and intestinal nephritis can be seen. Chitosan-Ca-alginate matrix in which 5-ASA is dispersed can be used for targeting colon because chitosan is insoluble in pH above 6.5 and is mucoadhesive in nature. In colon, chitosan is degraded by microflora and free drug is available (Mladenovska et al., 2007).

Gadolinium neutron capture therapy utilizes photon and electrons emitted *in vivo* as a result of nuclear neutron capture reaction with administered gadolinium-157 and non-radioelement. It is having highest thermal neutron capture cross section, and release of gamma rays and electron by neutron-capture reaction. Gaopentetic acid loaded chitosan nanoparticles were prepared for gadolinium neutron capture therapy and MRI diagnosis by emulsion droplet coalescence technique. The nanoparticles have not released gadolinium in phosphate buffer and retained gadolinium in tumor for long time *in vivo* after intratumor injection (Tokumitsu, 1999).

Epirubicin is an effective anti-cancer agent. Chitosan was carboxymethylated and bound covalently on Fe_3O_4 nanoparticles *via* carbodiimide activation. Thus, chitosan-magnetic nanoparticles were prepared for diagnosis and targeted therapy; it could be used in biomedicine (Chang et al., 2005).

The 5-flourouracil (5-FU) is mainly used in colon cancer. The 5-FU loaded n-succinyl chitosan nanoparticles were prepared by emulsification solvent diffusion method. It was having 19% loading capacity with 61% release in 24 hr. They have shown good anti-tumor activity against sarcoma 180 solid tumor with reduced toxicity (Yan et al., 2006).

Heparin, a known anticoagulant, is known to interact with diverse groups of proteins having heparin binding domain which regulates cell proliferation, differentiation and inflammation. It exhibits anti-cancer activity in process of tumor progression and metastatis. It binds with vascular endothelial growth factor (VEGF) and inhibits angiogenesis required for tumor growth. Free heparin molecules within cells interacts with transcription factors which plays important role in cell survival and growth, ultimately leading to apoptotic cell death *via* caspase dependent pathway. Chitsan-PEG-heparin polyelectrolyte complexes were prepared which were having higher toxicity against B16F10 cells. The cancer cells show higher internalization of complex, so higher cellular uptake of heparin resulting in dramatic cell death (Bae et al., 2009).

Colorectal cancer is having very short survival time because early detection is not excellent. The 5-aminolaevullinic acid (5-ALA) loaded chitosan-TPP nanoparticles were prepared to detect colorectal cancer at early stage. The 5-ALA is zwitterionic drug, so the entrapment efficiency by this method was greatly affected by pH of solution. The 5-ALA is degraded to protoporphyrin IX. The protoporphyrin IX is having different decomposition rate in cancer cell and normal cells, and is a photosensitive flourophore, and thus it can be used for detection of colorectal cancer. Even nanoparticles were able to escape from bacterial uptake in GIT. Fluorescence microscope showed that nanoparticles are engulfed by caco-2 colon cancer cells (Yang et al., 2009b).

Arginine rich hexapeptide are blocking the growth and metastasis of VEGF, which secretes human carcinoma cells. It shows significant inhibition of angiogenesis induced by VEGF in chorioallantoic membrane and rabbit cornea neovascularization. Thus it is useful in human tumor and angiogenesis dependent diseases which are related to action of VEGF. The peptide was encapsulated by chitosan-dextran sulfate nanoparticles by coacervation process, with 75% entrapment efficiency with sustained release characteristics (Chen, 2003).

Tamoxifen (TMX) is used in breast cancer, is having side effect for vaginal symptoms, thrombotic events, stroke, endometrial cancer and drug resistance. The TMX chitosan nanoparticles prepared shows uptake by Peyer's patch. The nanoparticles are transported to breast cells *via* lymphatic system reducing the toxicity (Coppi, 2009).

Catechin like polyphenolic compound is having anti-oxidant property, by which heavy metals can be chelated and lipid peroxidation can be prevented, which can reduce many side effects in cancer treatment. They undergo high first pass metabolism. The catechin loaded nanoparticles were prepared by ionic gelation method, which showed entrapment efficiency of 90% along with 32% drug release in 24 hr (Dudhani, 2008).

For Buccal and Sublingual Delivery System

Chitosan and trimethyl chitosan were even able to increase macromolecule permeation across buccal epithelium, which was later on confirmed by confocal laser microscopy, histopathology analysis, and immunohistochemistry reaction. The increase in permeability was quantified by Franz diffusion cell using isolated buccal epithelium (Sandri et al., 2006).

For Articular Joint Therapy

Macrophages are responsible for increased tissue permeability at inflammation site, including rheumatoid arthritis. Thus, their selective elimination from such inflammatory site may be beneficial. Photodynamic therapy is used in such cases which involves nontoxic photoactivable dye known as photosensitizer along with harmless visible light of defined wavelength. When photosensitizers are activated, they form reactive oxygen species resulting into destruction of macrophages along with cellular death. The phototoxicity of photosensitizers entrapped in Hyaluronate chitosan nanogels was decreased considerably. The nanogel encapsulated photosensitizers were retained in inflamed joint for long time compared to rapid clearance from joints of free photosensitizers. The treatment showed better result than the standard corticosteroid therapy for inflammation (Schmitt et al., 2010).

For Ocular Delivery System

Topical application to eye is limited due to protective physiological mechanism which exists at precorneal area resulting into drug loss, which ultimately results in to less effective concentration at site of action. The chitosan nanoparticles were stable against lysozyme and did not affect the mucin viscosity. They also prolonged the retention time on eye surface. Confocal microscopy study has confirmed that nanoparticles penetrate corneal and conjuctival epithelia with 100% cell survival (Campos et al., 2004).

Pilocarpine is choice of agent in open angle glaucoma. The drop causes frequent dosing schedule, while gels because blurred vision. Picocarpine loaded chitosan carbopol nanoparticles were prepared which improve interaction with negatively charged biological membrane along with sustained release property (Kao et al., 2006).

Indomethacin reduces post-operative inflammation and decreases intraocular irritation, cataract extraction and cystoid macular edema with side effects such as burning sensation, irritation and epithelial keratitis. Using chitosan-TPP nanoparticles, the residence time of indomethacin was increased on cornea and thus the bioavailability was also increased. With loading efficiency of 85%, minimum 76% drug release was observed in 24 hr. The nanoparticles were able to treat chemical ulcer in rabbit eyes (Badawi et al., 2008).

Cyclosoprin A is effective in extraocular disorders like caratoconjuctivitis sicca or dry eye disease, with very slow partition rate at corneal epithelium. Nanoparticles were prepared by ionotropic method having 79% association efficiency. In vivo study on rabbit cornea suggested that therapeutic concentrations were achieved for 48 hr, while negligible level was observed in inner ocular structure, blood and plasma (Campos, 2001).

Gatifloxin is fourth-generation fluoroquinolone antibiotic which inhibits bacterial enzyme DNA gyrase and topoisomerase IV. A chitosan-sodium alginate nanoparticulate reservoir for ocular delivery was developed, which has average size of 205–572 nm and zeta potential from +17.6 mV to 47.8 mV. Nanoparticles have shown sustained release by non- Fickian diffusion process for ocular delivery. The TEM and Atomic force microscopy (AFM) confirms that nanoparticles are spherical and dense in nature (Motwani et al., 2008).

For Brain Delivery

Alzheimer's disease, a neurodegenerative disease, is becoming public health issue. Tacrine- acetylcholinestarase inhibitor, affects by reversible inhibition of cholinesterase, which increases level of acetylcholine in CNS. It is having high first pass metabolism, which result in poor oral bioavailability of 17 ± 3% only. Tacrine loaded chitosan nanoparticles were prepared by spontaneous emulsification method, with good drug loading capacity. They have shown continuous slow release of drug. They have provided good result in Alzhemier disease (Wilson et al., 2010).

MECHANISM OF NANOPARTICLE TRANSPORT

With development of nanoparticles system, *in vitro* model has been performed for the transport studies which lack the clinical studies. There are mainly two pathway by which nanoparticle can be transported (Rieux et al., 2006) (Figure 4)

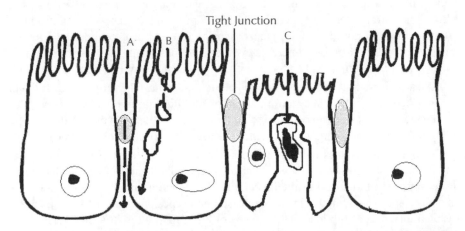

Figure 4. Particle Transport Mechanism (a) Paracellular transport, (b) Enterocytes and (c) M cells.

1. Paracellular pathway
2. Transcellular pathway

Paracellular Transport

The paracellular transport can be enhanced by interaction with negative charge of cell membrane or by complexing calcium ion involved in structure tight junction. Chitosan is having effect on depolymerization of cellular F-actin and tight junction protein Zonula occludens-1 (ZO-1). It can act *via* activation of protein kinase C.

Chitosan decrease cellular toxicity or damage because its effect on caco-2 cell line is reversible in nature.

Transcellular Transport

It occurs by transcytosis- particles are taken up by cells, which begins with endocytosis and ends at the time of release at basolateral pole. Absorption occurs by mainly two kinds of cells: enterocytes and M cells, located on Payer's patch. The M cells are able to absorb large range of materials. Some strategies for uptake of nanoparticle is given below

Non-specific Uptake of Nanoparticles:

a. By epithelial cells

Transcellualr transport can start by one of these endocytosis processes: pinocytosis, macropinocytosis and clathrin mediated endocytosis. All the activity is active transport, which requires energy. Phagocytosis and clathrin mediated endocytosis are receptor mediated, while pinocytosis is non-receptor mediated transport process.

Mucoadhesive materials improve transport by increasing residence time in contact with epithelium, thus increasing the concentration at site of absorption.

Chitosan nanoparticles may enhance oral uptake by crossing the epithelium, or that chitosan molecules release the drug at the apical pole of epithelial cells, facilitating somehow their transcytosis. Even it can be due to interaction of chitosan with tight junctions or adsorptive endocytosis which is saturable, energy and temperature dependent in nature. They may cause decrease in TEER value.

b. By M cells

Particle transport by M cells is energy dependent and transcellular which occurs by fluid phase endocytosis, adsorptive endocytosis and phagocytosis. Many factors like nanoparticle size, hydrophobicity, targeting moiety on surface, and so on can play important role for nonspecific transcellular uptake. Particles below 1 μm are taken up by M cells and transported to basal membrane, while particles larger than 5 μm are taken up by M cells but they remain entrapped in peyer's patch.

Specific Uptake of Nanoparticles

a. By epithelial cells

The most popular approach is modification of nanoparticle surface. It can be done by use of lectins, wheat germ agglutinin, Concanavalin A, tomato lactin. The level of targeting and uptake is directly proportional to the amount of targeting agent attached to particles. Targeting is a specific phenomenon, which is greatly reduced in presence of free lectin or specific sugar. Chitosan nanoparticles were prepared using glucomanan, which facilitates interactions of nanoparticles with mannose receptors present in epithelial cells.

b. By M cells

The most popular approach is modification of nanoparticle surface. Most effective ligand is ulex europaeus agglutinin-1 lectin, which is highly specific for α-L-fucose, located on apical membrane of M cells. Lectins derived from *Sambucus nigra* and *Viscum album* were able to selectively label the surface of human follicle associated epithelium (FAE), and therefore could be used as ligands to human drug delivery applications.

Another strategy can be mimicking some pathogen bacteria, such as *Yersinia*, *Salmonella*, and *Shigella* species that are able to hijack the mucosal immune system, by using M cells to invade the intestinal mucosa. These bacteria present microbial adhesions at their surface, which are responsible for their binding and internalization by M cells. Immunoglobulins, particularly IgA, can specifically interact with M cell surface. Gangliosde GM1 could be used for targeting.

CONCLUSION

Chitosan is natural biodegradable, biocompatible, mucoadhesive and water soluble polymer, which can be used in the form of nanoparticles for ocular, nasal, oral delivery for drugs, antigens, DNA with improved bioavailability and improved stability. Chitosan nanoparticles protect material from bacterial uptake and are highly target specific including their use in diagnosis *via* MRI, PET, and so on. Main advantage is that they do not require any stabilizer particularly in ionic gelation method which generates stable nanoparticles. Still further development is required for commercialization of chitosan nanoparticles.

KEYWORDS

- **Chitosan**
- **Doxorubicin**
- **Glycerrhetic acid**
- **Nanoparticles**
- **Natural polymers**
- **Protein**
- **Tamoxifen**

Chapter 5

Synthesis and Biomedical Application of Silver Nanoparticles

M. Saravanan and V. Anil Kumar

INTRODUCTION

Nanoscience nowadays is a fast developing field focusing on wide spectrum of synthesis and application of different nanomaterials. This emerging field (Ahmad et al., 2003) is considered to be a conclusion for solving many stiff-necked problems in multi disciplinary fields such as pharmaceutical sciences, applied physics, material sciences, colloidal sciences, device physics, supramolecular chemistry, mechanical, and electrical engineering, and so on. Nanomaterials have received much attention because of their structure and properties varing from those of atoms, molecules, and bulk materials (Rosei, 2004) and there by having many potential applications (Chen et al., 2009; Papp et al., 2008). The nanoparticles have significant properties and are used in optical detectors, laser, sensor, imaging, display, solar cell, photocatalysis, photo chemistry, biomedicine (Zhang, 2009), pharmaceutical applications (Chan and Nie, 1998), magnetic materials and information storage (Gopidas et al., 2003; Jortner and Rao, 2002; Kamat, 2002; Maxwell et al., 2002; Shon et al., 2003; Walter et al., 2002) and so on. owing to their vast application an immense demand to obtain these nanoparticles in non agglomerated, uniform with a well controlled mean size and narrow distribution has arisen (Brust and Kiely, 2002; Jana et al., 2001; Pileni 2001).

Nanoparticles are referred to those particles with size up to 100 nm (Simi and Abraham, 2007; Willems and van den Wildenberg, 2005). Silver, gold, copper and so on are some of the noble metals which are being used for metal nanoparticles synthesis (Leela et al., 2008a). Among all the nanoparticles, silver nanoparticles have great applications in various fields especially in the fields of biological systems, living organisms, medicine (Parashar et al., 2009) environmental, and biotechnology (Hussain et al., 2003; Virender et al., 2009). These nanoparticles have important properties like catalytic activity, surface enhanced raman scattering effect (Chen et al., 2005; Kearns et al., 2006; Li et al., 2006; Setua et al., 2007; Smith et al., 2006) good conductivity, chemical stability, antibacterial activity (Cao et al., 2002; Rosi and Mirkin, 2005; Tessier et al., 2000), therapeutics (Elechiguerra et al., 2005; Rai et al., 2009), degrading pesticides (Kuber and D'Souza, 2006), filtration (Cao, 2004), biolabeling (Hayat, 1989) and nanocoated medical devices (Furno et al., 2004). So, a keen viewed attention has been drawn in synthesis of silver nanoparticles (AgNps) in several ways. Considering the overall scenario of silver nanoparticles among multidisciplinary fields, the production of them in bulk amount has a great criterion in this field of nanotechnology.

A number of physical, chemical, and biological approaches are available for the synthesis of silver nanoparticles (Goia et al., 1998; Panacek et al., 2009). In a broad view, the physical synthesis procedures involve evaporation, condensation, laser abla-tion, and the chemical procedures involve reduction of metal ions in the solution to form small metal clusters or aggregates (Egorova and Revina, 2000; Khomutov and Gubin, 2002; Oliveira et al., 2005). Based on the reducing agent used, the chemical methods are subdivided into classical chemical method that involves chemicals like hydrazine, sodium borohydrate, hydrogen and so on with (Toshima et al., 1993) or without stabilizing agents (Liz-Marzan and Philipse, 1995) and radiation chemical method, where the reduction process is initiated by solvated electrons generated by the ionizing radiation (Joerger et al., 2000).

On the other hand, silver metal nanoparticles are synthesized using a variety of methods including hard template (Zhou et al., 1999), bioreduction (Canizal et al., 2001) and solvent phase evaporation (Sun et al., 2003; Yu et al., 1997). In one way the techniques for synthesis are categorized into top-down and bottom-up methods (Rocio Balaguera-Gelves, 2006). The top-down approach use silver in bulk form and reduces its size mechanically to nano scale by lithography and laser ablation (Bae et al., 2002). In case of bottom-up approach, in other words self-assembly method, involves the addition of reducing agent into a silver salt solution followed by addition of a stabiliz-ing agent to prevent agglomeration on synthesized nanoparticles. As these processes use solvents and reducing agents they show great impact on the physical and mor-phological characteristics. Other physical and chemical modes of silver nanoparticles synthesis are a dielectric approach where magnetron sputtering, ion exchange sol-gel deposition and convective methods are followed. One of the most commonly used fab-rication methods is the ion implantation (Kishimoto et al., 2004; Stepanov et al., 2000; Townsend et al., 1994) which provides the controled synthesis of metal nanoparticles, reduction of metal salts in the solutions (Krishna and Dan, 2009; Pal et al., 2007; Pillai and Kamat, 2004; Rosemary and Pradeep, 2003; Tripathi et al., 2010b), chemi-cal and photochemical reactions in the reversible micelles (Maillard et al., 2002; Taleb et al., 1997; Xie et al., 2006), thermal decomposition of silver compounds (Kim et al., 2005; Navaladian et al., 2007) as solvothermal synthesis (Starowicz et al., 2006), ra-diation assisted (Henglein, 2001) like ultra sonic radiation (Salkar et al., 1999) laser irradiation (Abid et al., 2002) and radio lysis (Ershov et al., 2007; Soroushian et al., 2005), electrochemical methods (Mazur, 2004; Rodriguez-Sanchez et al 2000; Tang et al., 2001; Zhu Jian et al., 2005), sonochemical approach (Esau et al., 2010; Zhang et al., 2004; Zhu et al., 2000), facile methods (Nidhi et al., 2009) and microwave as-sisted processes (Patel et al., 2005, 2007) are being carried out. Now there is a great need to develop environmentally safe processes for the synthesis of nanoparticles that avoid toxic chemicals in the synthesis protocols (Whitesides, 2003). Luoma (2008) over viewed about silver and the environment including the expected quantities to be released, source of release, expected pathways, and the toxicity. Biosynthetic meth-ods employing microorganisms and plant extracts have emerged as a simple and vi-able alternative to chemical synthetic procedures and physical methods (Revathi and Prabhu, 2009) and hence a green chemistry route for synthesis of nanoparticles has started. It has been known for a long time that in nature a variety of nanomaterials are synthesized by biological processes from microbes such as bacteria (Beveridge and Muuray, 1980; Brierley, 1990; Golab, 1981), yeast (Huang et al., 1990), fungi (Frilis and Myers-Keith, 1986; Niu et al., 1993; Volesky, 1990) and algae (Darnall et al., 1986; Sakaguchi et al., 1979) are able to adsorb and accumulate metals used in recovery of metals from waste, few examples are the magnetotactic bacteria synthesize intracellular magnetite or greigite nanocrystals (Blakemore, 1982) and some other diatoms synthesize siliceous materials (Kroger et al., 1999; Mann, 1993). Even at high concentrations, microorganisms can overcome metal stress and can survive due to their ability of efflux systems, alteration of solubility and toxicity *via* reduction or oxidation, biosorption, bioaccumulation, extracellular complexation or precipitation of metals and lack of specific metal transport systems (Beveridge et al., 1997; Bruins et al., 2000,).

METHODS FOR SILVER NANOPARTICLE SYNTHESIS

The synthesis of metallic nanoparticles is an active area of "application research" in nanotechnology. A variety of chemical and physical procedures could be used for synthesis of metallic nanoparticles. However, these methods are fraught with many problems including use of toxic solvents, generation of hazardous by products, and high energy consumption. Accordingly, there is an essential need to develop environmental friendly procedures for synthesis of metallic bionanoparticles. A promising approach to achieve this objective is to exploit the array of biological resources in nature. In deed, over the past several years, plants, algae, fungi, and bacteria, have been used for production of low-cost, energy-efficient, and nontoxic metallic bionanoparticles.

Microbial Synthesis of AgNPs

Recently many studies were conducted to explore the synthesis of AgNPs using microorganisms as a potential bio source; Basavaraja et al. (2007) used *Fusarium semitectum* for biosynthesis of AgNPs. Sastry et al. (2003) have also reported that when the fungi *Fusarium oxysporium* and *Verticillium* sp. were exposed to Ag$^+$ ions, were formed AgNPs. New enzymatic approaches using bacteria and fungi in the synthesis of nanoparticles by both intra and extra cellularly have been expected to play a key role in many conventional and emerging technologies.

Silver ions and silver based compounds are highly toxic to microorganisms and hence show strong bactericidal effects in many common species of bacteria including *E.coli* (Windt, 2009). The AgNPs were found to accumulate in the bacterial membranes, in some way interacting with certain building elements of the bacterial membrane thus causing structural changes, degradation and finally cell death. It is well known that many organism can provide inorganic materials either intra or extracellularly (Mann, 1996) but it is very important to develop AgNPs in an eco-friendly and easier manner. Silver bionanoparticles can be produced by physical and chemical methods (Burda et al., 2005; Kowshik et al., 2003) whereas they can also be produced in biological methods specifically by bioreduction (Porter et al., 2006). As the physical and chemical methods use toxic chemicals in their synthesis, it raises great concern for environmental reasons. Extracellular synthesis of silver nanoparticles from microorganisms has been proved fruitful because it possesses antimicrobial activity (Ahmad et al., 2003; Anil Kumar et al., 2007; Bhainsa and D'Souza, 2006; Mukherjee et al., 2002). Another reason to use AgNPs over bulk silver metals is because of its high specific surface area and high fraction of surface atoms; hence it has been proved to be a good antimicrobial agent for pathogenic microorganisms (Cho et al., 2005).

Mechanism for microbial synthesis: Extracellular enzyme shows an excellent redox properties and it can act as an electron shuttle in the metal reduction. Many other compounds other than extracellular enzymes like hydroquinones, napthoquinones, and anthroquinones (Baker and Tatum, 1998; Bell et al., 2003; Duran et al., 2002; Medentsev and Alimenko, 1998) act as electron shuttle in metal reduction (Newman and Kolter, 2000). Previous studies have indicated that NADH- and NADH-dependent enzymes are important factors in the biosynthesis of metal nanoparticles and the initiation of metal reduction seemed to be the transfer of electron from NADH by NADH- dependent reductase as electron carrier (Ahmad et al., 2003; Duran et al., 2005; Mukherjee et al., 2002). Shankar et al. (2005) reported that Ag^+ ion is a highly active chemical agent which binds strongly to electron donor groups and these bindings with biomolecules like protein could restrict the size of the particle. Gericke and Pinches (2006) stated that the rate of intracellular particle formation to an extent can be controlled by altering the parameters such as pH, temperature, substrate concentration, and exposure time to substrate. Even at high metal ion concentration microorganisms have tolerance against, metal stress by efflux systems, alteration of solubility and toxicity, biosorption, bio accumulation, extracellular complexation or precipitation of metals and lack of specific metal transport systems (Beveridge et al., 1997; Bruins et al., 2000; Fortin and Beveridge, 2000; Rouch et al., 1995; Summers and Silver, 1978).

Table 1. The different fungal strains used for the biosynthesis AgNPs for the last one decade.

Biological entity (Fungal stains)	Size (nm)	Ref.
Trichoderma reesei	5–50	Vahabi et al. (2011)
Aspergillus clavatus	550–650	Saravanan and Nanda (2010)
Aspergillus flavus	8.92±1.61	Vigneshwaran et al. (2007)
Aspergillus fumigatus	5–25	Bhainsa and D'Souza, (2006)
Cladosporium cladosporioides	10–100	Balaji et al. (2009)
Neurospora crassa	11	Castro-Longoria et al. (2011)
Phoma sp.	71–74	Chen et al. (2003)
Verticillium sp.	25±12	Medentsev and Akimenko (1998) Mukherjee et al. (2001a) Senapati et al. (2004)
Nitrate reductases - Fusarium oxysporium	10–25	Kumar et al. (2007)
Penicillium sp. K_1	10–100	Maliszewska and Sadowski (2009)
Penicillium sp. K_{10}	18–100	Maliszewska and Sadowski (2009)
Trichoderma asperellum	13–18	Mukherjee and Sadowski (2008)
Trichoderma viride	5–40	Amanulla et al. (2010)

Table 1. (Continued)

Biological entity (Fungal stains)	Size (nm)	Ref.
Fusarium oxysporum	5–60	Ahmad et al.(2003)
		Duran et al. (2005)
		Senapati et al. (2005)
		Souza et al. (2004)
		Oksanen et al. (2000)
Fusarium oxysporum PTCC 5115	50	Karbasian et al. (2008)
Fusarium acuminatum	5–40	Ingle et al. (2008a)
Fusarium solani (USM-3799)	5–35	Ingle et al.(2008b)
Cladosporium cladosporioides	10–100	Balaji et al. (2009)
Volvariella volvacea	15	Daizy (2009)
Phoma sp. 3.2883	67.6–74.52	Chen et al. (2003)
Verticillium sp.	12–37	Mukherjee et al. (2001a) Sastry et al. (2003)
Pencillium brevibacterium WA 2315	23–105	Nikhil et al. (2009)
Yeast strain MKY$_3$	2–5	Kowshik et al. (2003)
Morganella sp.		Parikh et al. (2008)

Table 2. The different bacterial strains used for the synthesis AgNPs for the last one decade.

Biological entity (Bacteria)	Size (nm)	Ref.
Pseudomonas stutzeri	200	Joerger et al. (2000)
Staphylococcus aureus	160–180	Nanda and Saravanan (2009)
Klebsiella pneumonia	5–32	Shahverdi et al. (2007)
Escherichia coli	50	Gurunathan et al. (2009)
Plectonema boryanum UTEX 485	200	Lengke et al. (2007)
Brevibacterium casei	10–50	Kalishwaralal et al. (2010)
Bacillus subtilis	5–60	Saifuddin et al. (2009)
Bacillus sp.	5–15	Pugazhenthiran et al. (2009)
Bacillus lichenformis	50	Kalimuthu et al. (2008)
Corynebacterium strain SH09	10–15	Haoran et al. (2005)
Pseudomonas stutzeri AG259	100–200	Klaus et al. (1999)
		Wei and Qian (2008)
Pseudomonas AG4	60–150	Wei and Qian (2008)

Phytosynthesis of Silver Nanoparticles

Green synthesis of AgNPs follows benign protocols and materials, which is cost effective and involves bulk synthesis. As the synthesis procedures involve no high pressure, energy, temperature, and toxic chemicals (David, 2004; Mohanpuria et al., 2008), the green chemistry methods are aided for the synthesis and for many biomedical applications.

Usually synthesis of AgNPs refers to synthesis from vascular plants leaf extracts (Gardea-Torresdey et al., 2002; Parashar et al., 2009). Jain et al. (2009) reported the synthesis from fruit extracts for the first time. Using plant for the synthesis can be advantageous over other biological processes by eliminating the elaborate process of maintaining the cell cultures (Shankar et al., 2004). Phytosynthesis involves preparation of plant extract and then reduction of silver ions into nanoparticles. Extraction procedure is usually by boiling of the air dried leaf pieces followed by decantation or filtration. To this extract, silver nitrate is added and then incubated to produce nanoparticles. Shankar et al. (2004) reported that the terpenoids are believed to be surface active molecules stabilizing the nanoparticles and the reaction of the metal ions is possibly facilitated by reducing sugars in neem leaf broth. Li et al. (2007) reported that proteins which have amine groups played a reducing and controlling role during the synthesis procedure in *Capsicum annum*. Ahmad et al. (2011) reported that *Desmodium* contain chemically different groups, water soluble scavenging super-oxide anion radicals and 1, 1-diphenyl-2-picrylhydrazyl (DPHP) radicals present in the plant extract can be responsible for the reduction of silver and the synthesis of nanoparticles. However, the exact mechanisms about the plant extract and the synthesis of the nanoparticles are not been concluded.

Leela and Vivekanandan (2008b) reported the synthesis of AgNPs from plants belonging to basellaceae, asteraceae and poaceae and their rates of reduction of silver nitrate. Among the plants used, the spectrometric analysis of sunflower reaction mixture exhibited strong absorption between 400–500 nm and the particles are characterized by XRD. Parashar et al. (2009) reported the advantage of reduction of silver ions in nanoparticles by using *Menthapiperita* leaf extract, as it occurs very fast within 15 min and 90% of Ag ions are reduced to nanoparticles (7–50 nm). Linga Rao and Savitramma (2011) reported the phytosynthesis of AgNPs from *Svensonia hyderabadensis* which belongs to Verbenaceae family and is listed under the rare texa. Roy and Barik (2010) reported bioreduction property of three aquatic weed leaf extract such as *Ipomoea aquatic* (convolvulaceae), enhydrafluctuans (asterceae) and *Ludwigia adscendens* (onagraceae) in the synthesis of AgNPs. It was considered to be the advantageous work due to the use of unwanted plants in synthesizing nanoparticles and for many biomedical applications. Govindaraju et al. (2010) reported the stability of synthesized AgNPs from *Solanum torvum* which have unchanged surface Plasmon absorbance even after 6 months. Elumalai et al. (2010) described the synthesis of Ag-NPs using *Euphorbia hirta* L and stated that the leaf extracts act as a reducing as well as capping agent. Singh et al. (2010) reported the synthesis of AgNPs using Argemone *Mexicana* for the first time. Prabhu et al. (2010) reported the phytosynthesis of AgNPs from Ayurvedic herbs *Oscimum sanctu* and *Vitex nigundo*, and their antibacterial effect on *Proteus vulgaris* and *Vibrio cholera*.

Table 3. The choice of Plant Materials used for the Phytosynthesis of AgNPs.

Biological entity (Plant)	Size(nm)	Ref.
Azadirachta indica	50–100	Shankar et al. (2004)
Aloe vera	15–20	Chandran et al. (2006)

Table 3. (Continued)

Biological entity (Plant)	Size(nm)	Ref.
Emblica officinalis	10–20	Ankamwar et al. (2005a)
Cinnamomum camphora	55–80	Huang et al. (2007)
Tamarind(leaf extract)	20–40	Ankamwar et al. (2005b)
Carcica papaya	25–50	Devendra et al. (2009)
Parthenium hysterophorus L	40–50	Vyom et al. (2009)
Diopyros kaki	15–19	Jae and Beom (2009)
Camellia sinensis	30–40	Alfredo et al. (2008)
Eucalyptus hybrid	50–150	Manish et al. (2009)
Aloe vera	15.2±4.2	Chandran et al. (2006)
Emblica officinalis	10–20	Ankamwar et al. (2005a)
Jatropha curcas(seed)	15–20	Harekrishna et al. (2009b)
Jatropha curcas(latex)	10–20	Harekrishna et al. (2009a)
Cinnamomum camphora (dried leaf)	55–60	Huang et al. (2007)
Pine apple (leaf extract)	15–500	Jae and Beom (2009)
Persimmon (leaf extract)	15–500	Jae and Beom (2009)
Ginkgo (leaf extract)	15–500	Jae and Beom (2009)
Magnolia (leaf extract)	15–500	Jae and Beom (2009)
Platanus(leaf extract)	15–500	Jae and Beom (2009)
Azadirachta indica	20	Tripathi et al. (2010a)
Geranium(Pelargonium graveolens) leaf extract	16–40	Shiv Shankar et al. (2003)
Hibiscus sabdariffa	25	Kamala Nalini (2008)
Phoma glomerata	60–80	Birla et al. (2009)
Cinnamomum camphora	5–40	Huang et al. (2008)

Chemical Synthesis of AgNPs

The chemical synthesis of colloidal nanoparticles started with the pioneering work of Farady which paved the way for the synthesis of nanoparticles.Three concepts involved in the "wet" chemical reduction of silver ions. The first one involves the radiation reduction of silver ions with γ-rays (Henglein and Giersig, 1999), UV or visible light (Huang et al., 1996, Yanagihara et al., 2001, Callegari et al., 2003), microwave (Gao et al., 2005), or ultra sound irradiation (Xiong et al., 2002). Second concept refers to the formation of silver colloids with relatively strong reducing agent such as hydrazine (Taleb et al., 1997). Thirdly it involves reduction of silver by prolonged refluxing in the presence of weak reducing agents such as glucose (Raveendran et al., 2003), ascorbic acid (Lee et al., 2004) and polyols (Sun et al., 2002).

A variety of techniques have been developed based on the above mentioned concepts to synthesize metal nanoparticles, they are as follows: chemical reduction (Petit et al., 1993; Tan et al., 2002; Vorobyova et al., 1999; Yu, 2007), aerosol technique (Harfenist et al., 1996), electro chemical or sonochemical deposition (Liu et al., 2001; Zhu et al., 2001,), photochemical reduction (Darroudi et al., 2009), laser irradiation technique (Abid et al., 2002), chemical vapour deposition (Szłyk et al., 2001), heat evaporation (Bae et al., 2002, Smetana et al., 2005), reversible micelles process (Maillard et al., 2002; Xie et al., 2006), salt reduction (Pillai and Kamat, 2004), microwave dielectric heating reduction (Patel et al., 2005), ultrasonic irradiation (Salkar et al., 1999), radiolysis (Ershov et al., 2007; Soroushian et al., 2005,), and solvo thermal synthesis (Starowicz et al., 2006).

Some of the chemical reductants used are $NaBH_4$, N_2H_4, ethanol, ethylene glycol, sodium citrate, *N,N-* dimethyl formamide (DMF) and other polyols (He et al., 2001; Link et al., 1999; Mallin and Murphy, 2002; Pal and Maity, 1986; Petit et al., 1993; Pastoriza-santos and Liz-Marzan, 2002; Sun and Xia, 2002; Sun et al., 2003), while the most reduction is by the amines (Chaki et al., 2002). Some of the surfactants used for chemical synthesis procedure such as sodium dodecyl sulphate (Kuo and Huang, 2005), cetyl trimethyl ammonium borate (Jana et al., 2001a; Sau and Murphy, 2004), sodium bis-(2- ethyl hexyl) sulfonyl succinate (Mandal et al., 2005) and poly-(oxyethylene) iso octeyl-phenyl ether (triton X-100) (Ghosh et al., 2003), but a majority of these surfactants assisted synthesis of nano sized silver use seed-mediated growth strategy (Jana et al., 2001b; Sau and Murphy, 2004). After synthesis of the nanoparticles, they are stabilized by stabilizing agents (quaternary ammonium) proposed by Bonnemann et al. (1998) typical redox synthesis methods however use hazardous chemicals as reducing agents or require significant energy input (Cushing et al., 2004) and hence raises a great concern for environmental reasons (Kowshik et al., 2003).

Biomemetric Synthesis of Silver Nanoparticles
Rajesh et al. (2002) reported an advanced approach for the synthesis of silver nanoparticles which uses a combinatorial way to identify silver binding peptides from a phage display library of random peptides instead of using the conventional molecular biology procedures for isolating silver binding proteins from bacteria. Sequencing was done by using an ABI 310 automated sequencer of over thirty independent clones, but only three peptide sequences AG3 AG4 AG5 were confirmed to be silver binding peptides.

Polyoxometalates Method
Weinstock (1998) and Troupis et al. (2002) reported the potential use of polyoxometalates (POMs) for the synthesis of AgNPs as they act as photocatalysts, reducing agent and as a stabilizer, due to the ability to dissolve in water, undergoing stepwise multi-electron redox reactions without disturbing their structure. Zhang et al. (2007) have mentioned a one step synthesis and stabilizing of silver nanostructures with mixed valence POMs in water at room temperature.

Synthesis of Silver Nanoparticles from Saccharides

Silver nanoparticles that are prepared utilizing water as solvent and polysaccharides as reducing agent, in some cases serve as both reducing and capping agent. Sreeram et al. (2008) reported the usage of starch as a template/reducing agent and effect of synthetic strategy- uncontrolled/controlled heating, microwave synthesis on size and shape of nanoparticles. Darroudi et al. (2011) reported the usage of D-Glucose as reducing agent and gelatin as a stabilizer for the synthesis of nanoparticles. Vigneshwaran et al. (2006a) stated the synthesis of stable silver nanoparticles by autoclaving $AgNO_3$ solution with starch at 15 Psi, 121°C for 5 min. Raveendran et al. (2003) reported starch as a capping agent and β D-glucose as reducing agent for the synthesis of starch silver nanoparticles in a gently heated system, and then the synthesized particles are separated from starch at high temperatures. Panacek et al. (2006), mentioned about the synthesis of silver nanoparticles in controlled sizes with two monosaccharides (Glucose and Galactose) and disaccharides (Maltose and Lactose). Purwar and Pokharkar (2011) stated the use of sulphated polysaccharides for the synthesis of Ag-NPs and confirmed SPR at 404 nm. The reduction mechanism involves a sulphate group attached to the primary hydroxyl group of sulphated polysaccharide, which disappeared after synthesis of silver nanoparticles.

Irradiation Method

Eutis et al. (2005) reported a photosensitizing technique for the synthesis of AgNPs using benzoquinone. Sudeep and Kamat (2005) studied the visible light irradiation for synthesis of AgNPs using thiophene as photosensitizing dye. Zhang et al. (2003) carried out AgNPs production by illumination of Ag $(NH_3)^+$ in ethanol. Microwave radiation and ionizing radiation can also promote reduction of Ag^+ ions in Ag NPs synthesis, and it was reported by Chen et al. (2008) and Long et al. (2007) respectively. Phong et al. (2009) reported a rapid synthesis of silver colloidal solution by using microwave irradiation and nontoxic chemistry substances like silver nitrate, oxalic acid, poly vinyl pyrolidone (PVP; MW = 55000).

Tollen's Method

It is a one step process for the synthesis of AgNPs with a controlled size (Kvitek et al 2005; He et al 2006; Sato et al., 2003; Yin Yadong et al., 2002). Tollens reaction involves the reduction of $Ag(NH_3)_2^+$, a tollens reagent by an aldehyde

$$Ag(NH_3)_2^+(aq) + RCHO(aq) \rightarrow Ag(s) + RCOOH(aq)$$

Sato et al. (2003) and Kvitek et al. (2005) developed a modified method to reduce Ag^+ ions to saccharides in the presence of ammonia, yielding silver nanoparticle films in the order 20–50 nm and silver nanoparticles in different shapes. The AgNPs of different morphologies with less than 10 nm diameter were synthesized by adjusting the concentrations of N-n hexadecyl trimethyl ammonium bromide (HTAB) and tollens reagent ($Ag(NH_3)_2^+$) in water at 120°C (Yu and Yam, 2004; Yu and Yam, 2005).

BIOMEDICAL APPLICATIONS OF AgNPs

The first recorded medical use of silver was reported during 8th century (Moyer, 1965). Silver vessels were used in ancient times to preserve water and wine whereas silver powder for beneficial healing and anti disease properties like ulcer treatment believed by Hippocrates (father of modern medicine). But later the silver compounds have emerged for medical practice. The ever living facts about silver compounds used as disinfectant for wound healing in World war-I. In 1884, Crede German obstetrician introduced 1% silver nitrate as an eye solution for prevention of Gonacoccal opthalmia neonatorum, which is perhaps the first scientifically documented medical use of silver (Russell and Hugo, 1994). The disinfectant property of silver is being exploited for hygienic and medical purposes in treatment of mental illness and infectious diseases like syphilis and gonorrhea (Gulbranson et al., 2000). Other applications include jewels, utensils, currency, dental alloy, photography, clothing (Chen et al., 2009), and explosives and so on. In higher concentrations, silver is toxic to the human beings whereas in low concentration it is non-toxic (Pal et al., 2007).

Historically silver compounds and ions were extensively used for both hygienic and healing purposes (Chen and Sehlueseiner, 2008). Li et al. (2008) reported that wide ranges of applications were developed in consumer products ranging from disinfecting medical devices and home appliances to water treatment. Melaiye et al. (2005) anticipated that the nano silver particles are found to be a possible antimicrobial agent. Roy et al. (2008) stated that antimicrobial activity of silver nanoparticles is comparable or better than the broad spectrum of most prominent antibiotics used world wide, and is dependent on the size of nanoparticle. Silver sulfadiazide is listed by the World Health Organization as an essential anti-infective topical medicine. Silver has varied *in vivo* and *in vitro* applications (Haes and Van Duyne, 2002; Mc Farland and Richard P. Van Duyne, 2003) as it has the highest bactericidal activity and bio compatibility among all the known antibacterial nanoparticles and it also is more advantageous since it does not require any photocatalytic agent for bactericidal action as required by TiO_2, ZnO, CdSe, ZnS, and so on. (Kloepfer et al., 2005; Qourzal et al., 2006). Dunn and Edwards Jones (2004) stated that some nano silver applications have received approval from the US food and Drug administration. The mechanism of the antimicrobial action of the silver ions is closely related to their interaction with thiol groups. Furr et al. (1994) mentioned that interaction of silver ions with thiol groups in enzymes and proteins also plays an essential role in its antimicrobial action although other cellular components like hydrogen bonding may also be involved.

Silver is known to have effective bactericidal properties for centuries and now silver nanoparticles are found to have inhibitory and bactericidal effects extending its application as an antibacterial agent (Atiyeh et al., 2007; Chu et al., 1988; Deitch et al., 1987; Law et al., 2008; Silver, 2003). The biologically synthesized silver nanoparticles could be of immense use in medical textiles for their efficient antimicrobial function (Vigneshwaran et al., 2006b). The sterile cloth and materials play an important role in hospitals, where often wounds are contaminated with microorganisms; in particular fungi and bacteria, like *S. aureus* frequently occur (Lee et al., 2003). Thus, to reduce or prevent infections, various antibacterial disinfection techniques were developed for all types of textiles. Silver ions and silver nanoparticles have inhibitory and lethal effect on bacterial species such as *E.coli*, *S.aureus* and even yeast (Gogoi et al., 2006, Kim et al., 2007). Morones et al. (2005) defined the antibacterial activity of AgNPs against four types of Gram negative bacteria *E. coli*, *V.cholera*, *P. aeruginosa* and *S. typhus*.

Antimicrobial resistance is becoming a major factor in virtually all hospitals, since the acquired infection became untreatable which led to a serious public health problem (Gad et al., 2004). These concerns have headed to major research effort to discover alternative strategies for the treatment of bacterial infection (Salata, 2004). Nanobiotechnology is an upcoming and fast developing field with potential application for human welfare. An important area of nano-biotechnology is to develop a reliable and eco-friendly process for synthesis of nanoscale particles through biological systems (Deendayal et al., 2006). Many organisms including unicellular and multi cellular microorganisms have been explored as potential bio factory for synthesis of metallic nanoparticles (gold, silver, Cadmium sulfide) either intracellularly or extracellularly (Ahmad et al., 2003; Klaus et al., 2004; Kowshik et al., 2003; Mukherjee et al., 2001b; Nair and Pradeep, 2002; and Vigneshwaran et al., 2006a). Recently few studies have been conducted for characterization and antimicrobial effect of silver nanoparticles. Souza et al. (2004) showed that the bulk counterparts of AgNPs are an effective antimicrobial agent against various pathogenic microorganisms. Shrivastava et al. (2007) has reported that the range of 10–15 nm of AgNPs has increased stability and enhanced antimicrobial potency.

Bactericidal effect of AgNPs against multidrug resistant bacteria like *Pseudomonas aeroginosa*, ampicillin resistant *E.coli* and erythromycin resistant *Streptococcus pyogenes* was mentioned by Lara et al. (2010) and Matsumura et al. (2003). Ahmad et al. (2007) confirmed about the combination effect of AgNPs with different antibiotics and proved that the antibacterial activities of penicillin G, amoxicillin, erythromycin, clindamycin, and vancomycin increases in the presence of AgNPs against *S. aureus* and *E.coli*.

The possible mechanism of antibacterial effect of AgNPs involves the release of K^+ ions from the bacteria and thus the bacteria plasma or cytoplasmic membrane which is associated with many important enzymes and DNA is an important target site of silver ions (Miller and McCallan, 1957; Rayman et al., 1972; Schreurs and Rosenberg, 1982). Kim et al. (2005) reported the possibility of free radical involvement in the antibacterial activity of AgNPs but the underlying mechanism and characteristics remain unclear. Corinne et al. (2000) studied the interaction between relative oxygen species (ROS) and bacterial cell death. The AgNPs when interact with bacterial DNA or mitochondria releases ROS such as superoxide anion (O_2^-), hydroxyl radical (OH) and singlet oxygen ($^1O_2$) with subsequent oxidative damage. In many studies, direct electron microscopic view determined the structural change of bacterial cell, confirming the cell damage. Lara et al. (2010) suggested that the mode of action of silver nanoparticles is similar to that of silver ions, which complex with electron donor groups containing sulfur, oxygen or nitrogen atoms normally present as thiols or phosphates on amino acids and nucleic acids. In addition to their effect on bacterial enzymes, silver ions cause marked inhibition of bacterial growth and they get deposited in the vacuole and cell wall as granules (Brown and Smith, 1976).

Candida species is one of the most common fungal pathogens causing hospital acquired sepsis with a mortality rate of about 40% (Patterson, 2007). Prophylaxis with antifungal may lead to the raise of many drug resistant strains. Just a few studies on antifungal efficacy of AgNPs were published (Falletta et al., 2008; Roe et al., 2008; Zeng et al., 2007), but the fungicidal effect and mode of action of silver ions remained obscure (Kim et al., 2008). By 1980, four classes of antifungal agents—polyenes, azoles, morpholines and allylamines were identified, but till now only one oral drug Ketoconazole was introduced for the treatment of systemic fungal infections (Kauffman and Carver, 1997). Panacek et al. (2009) studies revealed the antifungal activity of AgNPs against *Candida* sp. which has no cytotoxicity effect on human fibroblast at a concentration of 1 mg/l of Ag. It was reported that SDS stabilized nanoparticles penetrated into the cell wall and cytoplasmic membrane to inhibit the activity of various enzymes such as ATPase activity of P-glycoprotein or lecitin/cholesterol acyltransferase. Kim et al., 2008 made a study on antimicrobial effect of nano silver on clinical fungal isolates and ATCC strains of *Trichophyton mentagrophytes* and *Candida* species and stated that mycelial forms of fungi is responsible for pathogenicity due to the dimorphic transitions from yeast to mycelia form which is found primarily during the invasion of host tissue and he also finally concluded that the potential activity of nano Ag inhibit the dimorphic transition. Young et al. (2009) discussed about the biocidal effect of AgNPs on phyto pathogenic fungi *B. sorokiniana* and *M. grisea* in fields and other soil borne sterile fungi that rarely produce spores.

CONCLUSION

Nanotechnology is an emerging field in the 21st century which is the root cause for the next industrial revolution. Synthesis, characterization, manipulation and application of nanomaterials are being rapidly used in development of nanotechnology. Nanoparticles are the building blocks of nanotechnology as they play vital role in their applications. The application of nanoscale materials and structures may provide solutions to technological and environmental challenges in the areas of solar energy conversion, catalysis, and medicine. With the increased efficiency of pathogenic microorganisms resistant to multiple antimicrobial agents in this urbanized environment, demands have increased for better disinfection methods. The use of nanoparticles nowadays have proved to be a better alternative for antimicrobial properties and although more experiments have to be done on this, the properties of Ag^+ ions were known since ancient times and are used widely as bactericide in catheters and wounds. The concept to eclipse the multidrug resistant pathogens is a great deal in the field of nanomedicine. The development of multidrug resistant clinical pathogens like MRSA and MRSE have become a major factor in all hospital acquired infections which are untreatable and inturn causing severe public health problem. These concerns have led to major research effort to discover alternative strategies (using Nanobiotechnology tools) for the treatment of multi drug resistant bacterial infections (Nanda and Saravanan, 2009). The regular monitoring of antimicrobial susceptibility pattern of pathogens and formulation of a definite antimicrobial policy may be helpful for reducing the incidence of these infections. The biomedical application of AgNPs on selected synthetic process was reported in this chapter. In future, nanobiotechnologists will go into the deeper level of understanding on the biochemical and molecular mechanisms of nanoparticles formation and achieve better control over size and polydispersity of the nanoparticles.

KEYWORDS

- **Antimicrobial**
- **Dimethyl formamide**
- **Nanomaterials**
- **Nanoparticles**
- **Nanoscience nowadays**
- **Nanotechnology**
- **Polyoxometalates**
- **Silver ions**

Chapter 6

Recent Advances in Cancer Therapy Using Phytochemicals

Hullathy Subban Ganapathy, Rajakani Senthil Nagarajan, and Hirotaka Ihara

INTRODUCTION

Cancer is the most devastating disease with more than 10 million new cases every year around the world. It is well known that environmental factors and chemical carcinogens play a predominant role in the induction of DNA lesions and other genomic abnormalities which causes the cancer. Currently, several chemotherapeutic agents are being used in the treatment of cancer, including alkylating agents, antimetabolites antagonists, anticancer antibiotics, and plant-derived anticancer agents. However, chemotherapy, being a major treatment method used for the control of advanced stages of malignancies and metastasis, is known to exhibits severe toxicity (Markowitz and Bertagnolli, 2009). Because of high death rate associated with cancer and because of the serious side effects of chemotherapy and radiation therapy, many cancer patients seek alternative and/or complementary methods of treatment. Phytochemicals are one of fast growing anticancer agents for such alternative therapies. Basically, phytochemicals are large variety of plant-derived chemical compounds, which are present in fruits and vegetables that may reduce the risk of cancer, possibly due to dietary fibers, polyphenol antioxidants, and anti-inflammatory effects. There are many plant-derived phytochemicals which have been used as anticancer drugs and it has been shown to inhibit cancer cell growth efficiently. Moreover, they are known to maintain the health and vitality of individuals, and also cure different diseases, without causing toxicity (Chung et al., 1995; Tyagi et al., 2010). More than 50% of all modern drugs in clinical use are of natural products, many of which have the ability to control cancer cells (Chao et al., 2005). A recent survey showed that more than 60% of cancer patients use vitamins or herbs as therapy. Interestingly, an important and well known cancer drug, Taxol (paclitaxel), is a phytochemical, initially extracted and purified from the Pacific yew tree (*Taxus brevifolia*) (Tyagi et al., 2010). Pharmacologically safe phytochemicals that have been identified from plants or their variant forms can modulate these molecular targets. These phytochemicals include *genistein, resveratrol, dially sulfide, S-ally cysteine, allicin, lycopene, capsaicin, curcumin, 6-gingerol, ellagic acid, ursolic acid, betulinic acid, flavopiridol, silymarin, anethol, catechins and eugenol* (Aggarwal et al., 2004). Because of their pharmacological safety, these agents can be used alone to prevent cancer and in combination with chemotherapy to treat cancer. These herbal medicines have been increasingly accepted universally, and they have an impact on both world health and international trade (Park et al., 1998). The plant-based traditional medicines are widely used in India and China. Very recently, for alternative therapy, National Centre for Complementary and Alternative Medicine has been established in USA. The herbal products have been classified under "dietary supplements" and are included with vitamins, minerals, amino acids, and "other products intended to supplement the diet". The National Cancer Institute collected about 35,000 plant samples from 20 countries and has screened around 114,000 extracts for anticancer activity. Of the 92 anticancer drugs commercially available prior to 1983 in the US and among worldwide approved anticancer drugs between 1983 and 1994, 60% are of natural origin. In this instance, natural origin is defined as natural products, derivatives of natural products, or synthetic pharmaceuticals based on natural product models (Cragg and Newman, 1997). Other important phytochemicals such as *Allium sativum, Actinidia chinensis, Aloe vera, Ananas comosus, Angelica sinensis, Annona species, Arctium lappa, Astragalus membranaceus, Betula utilis, Catharanthus roseus, Chlorella pyrenoidosa, Colchicum luteum, Combretum caffrum, Curcuma longa, Echinacea angustifolia, Fagopyrum esculentum, Glycine max, Glycyrrhiza glabra, Gyrophora esculenta, Lentinus edodes, Panax ginseng, Linum usitatissimum, Picrorrhiza kurroa, Mentha species, Podophyllum, and Withania somnifer* are known to control the growth of cancer cells (Sakarkar and Deshmukh, 2011). In this article, we aim to provide an overview the recent advances in the research based on phytochemicals for cancer therapy.

MEDICINAL PLANTS AS CANCER DRUGS

In the recent past, numerous cancer research studies have been conducted using traditional medicinal plants in an effort to discover new therapeutic agents that lack the toxic side effects associated with current chemotherapeutic agents. Table 1 shows list of important phytochemicals studied for different cancers (cell lines and type of cancer) and the potential bioactive compounds present in these plants. These plant-derived compounds play an important role in the development of clinically useful anticancer agents and more than 3,000 plant species have been tested against the cancer *in vitro* and *in vivo* models (Cragg and Newman, 2004). One of the more versatile plants used as a source of flavonoids is the root of the traditional Chinese medicinal herb baikal skullcap (*Scutellaria baicalensis*), a member of the mint family (Chung et al., 1995). Traditionally, the dried roots of *S. baicalensis* were extracted and used in a Chinese herbal medicine "Huang Qin" to treat a variety of ailments (Maloney, 1998) and *S. baicalensis* has remained an important herb in both Chinese and Japanese traditional prescriptions, such as "Xiao-Chai-Hu-Tang" which is used in the treatment of viral hepatitis and a variety of tumors (Fei et al., 2002). Various flavonoids isolated from this traditional Chinese medicinal plant were shown to have antiandrogenic and growth inhibitory activity against prostate cancer cells *in vitro* and *in vivo* (Bonham et al., 2005; Sandava and Winesburg, 2005). In addition, extracts and isolated flavonoids from this herb have been shown to relieve oxidative stress and immune dysfunction associated with the onset and progress of cancer. Studies have also demonstrated that flavonoids from *S. baicalensis* have the ability to arrest the cell cycle of tumor cell lines that are resistant to multiple chemotherapeutic drugs (Choi et al., 1999) and act as inhibitors of key steps necessary for the progression of tumor angiogenesis

(Liu et al., 2003). Methanolic extracts from seven *Plantago* sp. used in traditional medicine for the treatment of cancer were evaluated for cytotoxic activity against three human cancer cell lines recommended by the National Cancer Institute (NCI, USA). The results showed that *Plantago* sp. exhibited cytotoxic activity, showing a certain degree of selectivity against the tested cells in culture. Since the flavonoids are able to strongly inhibit the proliferation of human cancer cell lines, it was identified that the compound, luteolin-7-*O*-β-glucoside as major flavonoid present in most of the *Plantago* sp. These results could justify the traditional use of the *Plantago* sp. and topoisomerase-mediated DNA damage might be a possible mechanism by which flavonoids of *Plantago* exert their cytotoxicity potential (Gálvez et al., 2003). *D. nobile* is an orchid plant, which has compound gigantel that have antimutagenic activity and the flower extract of *D. nobile* release the diversified antioxidants, which destroy the cancer cells. The cytotoxic effect of plant-derived components was tested with DLA cell lines (Uma Devi et al., 2009).

Botanical name	Name of the bioactive compound	Cancer Type		Ref.
		Type	Cell lines	
Scutellaria baicalensis	Flavanoids	Breast	MCF7	(Fei et al., 2002)
		Prostate	PC3	
Plantago	Flavanoids	Breast	MCF7	(Gálvez et al., 2003)
		Renal	TK-10	
		Melanoma	UACC-62	
Azadirachta indica (Neem)	Tannin, β-sitosterol, nimbin, quercetin and carotne	Breast	MCF-7/ADR.	(Tepsuwan et al., 2002, Nanduri et al., 2003, Arivazhagan et al., 2004, Subapriya et al., 2005)
		Colon	SW620	
	Alkaloid and inositol	Lung	H522	
	Tannin and phenolic compounds	Melanoma	M14	
		Ovarian	SKOV3	
		Prostate	DU145	
		Renal	A498	
Andrographis paniculata	Flavonoid, Andrographin and andrographolide	Breast	NCI/ADR-RES	(Singh et al., 2001 Kumar et al., 2004, Pfisterer et al., 2010)
		Colon	HT29,SW620	
		Lung	H522	
		Melanoma	M14	
		Ovarian	SKOV3	
		Prostate	DU145	
		Renal	A498	
		CNS	U251	
Abrus precatorius	Methyl ester on N, N-dimethyl tryptophan metho-cation and picatorine	Antitumor activity against Yoshida ascites sarcoma	-	(Kathiresan et al., 2005)
Cajanus cajan	Benzophenone and β-Sitosterol	Breast	MCF-7	(Ashidi et al., 2010)
		Lung	COR-L23	
		amelanotic melanoma	C32	

Botanical name	Name of the bioactive compound	Cancer Type		Ref.
		Type	Cell lines	
Calophyllum inophyllum	Polyphenols, Carotene, Epigallo-catechin-3-gallage	gastric	SGC-7901	(Dai et al., 2010)
Camellia sinensis	Ascorbic acid, Xanthine and Inositol and β-sitosterol ,	Ovarian	SKOV 3	Zhang et al., 2002, Hsu et al., 2002, Su and Arab, 2002, Lu et al., 2010)
		Oral cavity	GN56, CAL27, HSG1, HSC-2	
		Colon	RKO	
		Stomach	CNE 2, MGC-803, Hela	
		Prostate	LNCap, DU-145, CWR22Rν1, and PC3	
Cassia absus	Hydrocyanic acid, Cyaniding	Breast	MCF-7	(Bingfen et al., 1994)
		Colon	HCT-15, SW-620, COLO 205	
		Lung	HOP-62	
		Ovarian	OVCAR-5	
		Prostate	PC-3	
		cervix	SiHa	
Careya arborea	Methanol extract	solid tumor	DLA	(Natesan et al., 2007)
Cissus quadrangularis	Flavonoid, flowers, Limooid, Tangeretin	GastricUlcer	-	(Jainu and Shyamala Devi, 2003)
Ceiba pentandra	Tetracyclic triterpenoid and β-sitosterol	liver	-	(Bairwa et al., 2010)
Citrus limon	Resin, Essential oils, Coumarins	Breast	-	(Hirano et al., 1995, Heber, 2004)
		Prostate	-	
		Lung	-	
		Leukemia	HL60	
Eugenia caryophyllata	Dimethlsulfone, caffeic acid	Cervical	Hela	(Kouidhi et al., 2010)
		Colon	HT 29	
		Lung	A549, MRC-5	
Glycerrhiza glabra	C-oxidase, Catalase, Caffeic acid, Oleic, Lauric, and Palmitic acid	Colon	-	(Lee et al., 2007)
Ipomoea batatas	Essential oils, (menthol, menthone, limonene)	Lung, colon	-	(Konczak-Islam et al., 2003, Konczak et al., 2004)
Mallotus philippensis	Vitamins (A,C)	Colon	HT 29	(Sharma, 2011)
Mentha arvensis	Quercetin, β-Sitosterol, saponin and Glucoside	Cervical	HeLa,	(Janin et al., 2011)
		Breast	MCF-7,	
		Leukemia	Jurkat,	
		colon	HT-29	

Botanical name	Name of the bioactive compound	Cancer Type		Ref.
		Type	Cell lines	
Moringa olifera	Essential oil, crystal-line Furocoumarin	Leukemia	HL60,HCT-8, CEM	(Costa-Lotufo et al., 2005)
Piper sps	Ca, Fe and Vitamins (A,B,C)	Breast colon	MCF-7	(Sakpakdeejaroen and Itharat, 2009)
Tetragonia tetragoni-oides	β-Sitosterol , Flucoside	Liver carcinoma	HepG2	(Kyung-A et al., 2011)
Thespesia populnea	Lupeol, and β-Sitosterol	Oral colon	-	(Dhanarasu et al., 2010)
Vaccinium macrocarpon	flavonols, proanthocy-anidin, oligomers, and triterpenoids	Breast	MCF-7	(Seeram et al., 2004, Sun and Hai Liu, 2006, Neto et al., 2007, Dhanamani et al., 2011)
		Colon	HT-29, HCT116, SW480, SW620	
		Prostate	RWPE-1, RWPE-2, 22Rvl	
		Oral	KB, CAL27	
Vernonia cinerea		Colon		(Dhanamani et al., 2011)

Many of the naturally derived anticancer agents originally discovered using such assays, have been shown to exert their cytotoxic action through interaction with cancer cells. Additional phytochemicals with such anticancer capabilities on different cancer cells with the literature citation are listed in the Table 1.

Carcinogenesis is a multistep process consisting of tumor initiation, promotion, and progression. Phytochemicals can act at any of the stages. Initiation is the conversion of a normal cell to a cancer cell after exposure or uptake of a carcinogen and its interaction with the cellular DNA. Cancer-blocking agents prevent carcinogens from reaching the cell, or prevent the carcinogen from interacting with cellular components. Examples of phytochemicals that block initiation include ellagic acid, indole-3-carbinol, sulphoraphane, and flavonoids. Cancer-suppressing agents, on the other hand, block the promotion stage, which is the slow multiplication of cancer cells to pre-neoplastic cells, or to the progression stage, which is the conversion to neoplastic cells that can invade tissues and metastasize (spread). Examples of cancer-suppressing phytochemicals include β-carotene, curcumin, epigallocatechin gallate, genistein, resveratrol, gingerol, and capsaicin (Joon Surh, 2003). Most of these cancer-suppressing phytochemicals act on signaling molecules that have been abnormally activated or silenced. These signaling molecules, which are kinase enzymes, are responsible for the activation of genes that regulate cell growth, differentiation, and apoptosis.

CONCLUSION

The use of alternative medicine and natural approaches and the value of natural healing substances have been largely acknowledged and gained popularity in the recent years. However, though there is increasing evidence from several model systems from cell lines to animal models in demonstrating an anticancer role for herbal drugs, the underlying mechanisms and molecular players in this field still remain largely unknown, and therefore further research is needed to address these questions. Although, the clinical trials showed that herbs were helpful against cancer, these outcomes require further confirmation with rigorously controlled clinical trials. Though many of researchers have demonstrated that herbs are helpful against cancer, especially useful in improving survival and quality of life in patients suffering from advanced cancer, the lack of controls and reporting bias have been severe flaws. In certain cases, excessive dosage or inappropriate administration of certain herbs could result in severe toxicity as well. Hence, it is very important that scientists pay attention to the scientific basis of such studies using herbal drugs in the future, so as to improve the status, because plants could actually be sometimes dangerous to the human body if not used correctly. Furthermore, special emphasis should be given to understanding herb-drug interactions, if being prescribed at the same time (Das, 2002; Romero-Jimenez et al., 2005; Sakarkar and Deshmukh, 2011).

KEYWORDS

- **Cancer**
- **Cancer-suppressing**
- **Carcinogenesis**
- **Flavonoids**
- **Phytochemicals**

ACKNOWLEDGMENT

Funding was supported by a Grant-in-Aid for Scientific Research from the Ministry of Education, Culture, Science and Technology of Japan (KAKENHI: No. 2324501801).

Chapter 7

Mitochondrial Dysfunction and Cancer: Modulation by Palladium α-Lipoic Acid Complex

C. V. Krishnan, M. Garnett, and F. Antonawich

INTRODUCTION

Cancer is the uncontrolled multiplication of subtly modified or mutated normal human cells. While surgery, radiation, and chemotherapy are all commonly used to treat cancer, chemotherapy is the only option if the cancer has metastasized and spread through the body. To minimize side effects, one need cancer-specific cytotoxic drugs, including DNA-binding agents, alkylating agents, and antimetabolites that interfere with DNA replication.

The numerous side effects as well as the cost associated with modern medicine have driven cancer patients to look for other treatments, collectively termed as alternative or holistic medicine. Holistic medicine's ostensible aims include addressing the physical, mental, emotional, and spiritual problems of the body. The medical systems that make up holistic medicine include herbal medicine including ayurveda, homeopathy, acupuncture, yoga, and others. There are different philosophies driving each of these diverging systems, with the tenets of each often conflicting. There is a general reluctance on the part of practitioners of modern medicine to accept the tenets of holistic medicine, partly due to lack of rigorous clinical investigation. But there is a modern trend to accept some of these treatments as a complementary or adjuvant therapy to attain a feeling of maximum wellness, one that goes beyond recovery. In that sense a symbiotic relationship is slowly developing between modern medicine and its less tested brethren.

Our research is based on a holistic approach of a different kind. It addresses the need for modern medicine to include the role played by the mitochondria in optimal cellular function. It is different from traditional holistic medicine in that the results presented in this chapter are based on substantial investigations of mitochondrial effects. Mitochondria are involved in energy metabolism, calcium regulation and apoptosis-signaling pathways. The number of mitochondria in a cell is decided by its energy requirements (Alberts et al., 1989; Beattie, 2002; Voet and Voet, 1995). Cells that is metabolically more active, such as those in cardiac and skeletal muscles, the brain and the liver have the most mitochondria. All human cells, other than mature erythrocytes, have mitochondria. We believe strongly that medications targeting the mitochondria address the same issues that holistic medicine focuses on, because healthy mitochondria contribute substantially to the physical, mental, and emotional elements needed to complement the allopathic or modern medicine. Mitochondria are ubiquitous, and taking care of mitochondria is similar to taking care of all the parts leading to greater achievements than the sum of the parts. This is essentially the true slogan of holistic medicine.

A recent focus of research has been on a group of agents with anticancer activity, mitocans that induce apoptosis (Galluzzi et al., 2006) by way of mitochondrial destabilization (Biasutto et al., 2010). Natural compounds including fruits and vegetables that preferentially kill cancer cells with mitochondrial dysfunction are receiving closer scrutiny to understand the underlying mechanisms and therapeutic implications for cancer treatment and prevention (Aggarwal and Shishodia, 2006; Chen et al., 2010; Sarkar et al., 2009).

We have tried to establish a symbiotic relationship with modern medicine as well as holistic medicine by selecting a metal complex, palladium α-lipoic acid, which is active in mitochondrial cellular metabolism as well as in cancer cell death.

A substantial fraction of the cytoplasm in almost all eukaryotic cells is occupied by mitochondria (Alberts et al., 1989). Mitochondria were first identified at the end of the 19th century. The energy-converting organelles of eukaryotes were generally believed to be evolved from prokaryotes that were engulfed by primitive eukaryotic cells or aerobic bacteria. This symbiotic relationship started more than 1.5 billion years ago allowed the evolution of multicellular organisms with aerobic respiration (Alberts et al., 1989). Since, the development of procedures for isolation of intact mitochondria in 1948, extensive studies have been carried out to understand their role in energy metabolism (Voet and Voet, 1995).

An animal cell without mitochondria would be dependent on anaerobic glycolysis to make adenosine triphosphate (ATP). The conversion of glucose to pyruvate by glycolysis produces only two molecules of ATP compared to 36 molecules of ATP produced by glucose oxidation. The pyruvate produced in the cytosol by glycolysis and the fatty acids are selectively transported into the mitochondrial matrix where they are broken down into the acetyl group on acetyl coenzyme A (acetyl-CoA or acetyl-SCoA) before being fed into the tricarboxylic acid cycle or citric acid cycle or Krebs cycle.

The ATP in a cell is being continuously hydrolyzed and regenerated, with a half-life from seconds to minutes depending on the cell. An average person at rest consumes and regenerates ATP at a rate of ~ 3 mol (1.5 kg) hr^{-1} and as much as an order of magnitude faster during strenuous activity (Voet and Voet, 1995). The rapid deterioration of brain tissue by oxygen deprivation is due to the fact that brain cells have only a few seconds of ATP available (Voet and Voet, 1995). It is clear that the cellular role of ATP is as a free energy transmitter rather than as a free energy reservoir. Phosphocreatine acts as a reservoir of ATP in muscles and nerve cells that have high ATP turnover rates.

$$ATP + Creatine = Phosphocreatine + ADP \qquad (1)$$

Even though this is an endergonic reaction under standard conditions, it is close to equilibrium due to the prevailing intracellular concentrations of its reactants and products. This allows the equilibrium to shift to the right at resting state because of high ATP concentration and shift to the left at high metabolic activity because of low ATP.

The glycolytic product pyruvate is the immediate precursor to acetyl-CoA from carbohydrate sources.

$$Glucose + 2NAD^+ + 2ADP + 2Pi \rightarrow 2NADH + 2Pyruvate + 2ATP + 2H_2O + 4H^+ \quad (2)$$

For glycolysis to continue, the NADH (nicotinamide adenine dinucleotide) produced must be reoxidized to NAD^+ because of its limited availability in cells. Under anaerobic conditions, this is achieved by oxidation of NADH by pyruvate to yield NAD^+ and lactate with the aid of lactate dehydrogenase. Under aerobic conditions, each NADH oxidized by the mitochondrial electron transport chain produces one NAD^+ and 3ATP. The pyruvate, under aerobic conditions, undergoes a series of five sequential reactions and produces NADH and acetyl-CoA with the aid of the enzyme, pyruvate dehydrogenase.

$$Pyruvate + CoA + NAD^+ \rightarrow acetyl\text{-}CoA + CO_2 + NADH \quad (3)$$

The acetyl group of the common intermediate acetyl-CoA, obtained from the breakdown of carbohydrates, lipids, and proteins, is then converted to CO_2 and H_2O through a series of consecutive enzymatic reactions of Krebs cycle, the electron transport chain, and oxidative phosphorylation.

Even though the role of mitochondrial defects had been recognized in the development of cancer, more than 80 years ago, mitochondrial dysfunction and its restoration have started gaining momentum only recently. Our emphasis is on restoration from mitochondrial dysfunction. To minimize toxic side effects or to avoid toxic effects completely, we have selected a ligand, α-lipoic acid that plays a key role in the mitochondria. The α-Lipoic acid is part of the multi enzyme complexes, pyruvate dehydrogenase as well as α-ketogluarate dehydrogenase, the latter being involved in the Krebs cycle. A third enzyme, also containing α-lipoic acid, is the branched-chain α-keto acid dehydrogenase. This enzyme participates in the degradation of isoleucine, leucine, and valine. The other unique properties of this ligand are discussed in a later section.

After selecting a ligand, α-lipoic acid, that plays a critical role in biological energy metabolism, we wanted to tweak the properties of the ligand by complexing it with a metal that has very high catalytic and electronic properties. After numerous investigations with a variety of metals, the final selection was made to use palladium, a transition metal. The properties of the resulting complex were remarkable in many ways. After a series of investigations over numerous years, we have established that palladium α-lipoic acid complex formulation

1. Has practically no toxic effects and its aqueous solution is safe up to at least 40 ml (0.037 M) per day.
2. Repairs DNA damage resulting from radiation.
3. Scavenges free radicals and lowers lipid peroxidation.
4. Increases the levels of glutathione and glutathione peroxidase(GPx).
5. Increases the levels of manganese superoxide dismutase, and catalase.
6. Enhances the Krebs cycle enzymes: isocitrate dehydrogenase, α-ketoglutarate dehydrogenase, succinate dehydrogenase, and malate dehydrogenase.
7. Enhances mitochondrial respiratory enzymes, complex I, complex II, complex III, and complex IV.

8. Promotes cell death in a variety of cancer cell lines such as skin melanoma, human (SKMel-5); liver, hepatocellular carcinoma, human (Hep G2); lung, malignant melanoma, human (malme-3M); mammary gland, ductal carcinoma, human (MDA-MB 435); prostate, left supraclavicular lymph node carcinoma, human (LNCaP); colon, colorectal adenocarcinoma, human (HT-29); human brain, glioblastoma; astrocytoma (U87); and glioblastoma (U251MG).

9. Acts as a prophylactic for neuronal protection from transient ischemic attack.

10. Acts as a prophylactic for protection from radiation.

11. Exhibits unique electronic properties corresponding to diode or tunnel diode behavior.

The influence of protein structure on the rate of electron transfer is beyond the scope of this chapter. It is known that reduced hemes in the mitochondria can transfer electrons at physiologically significant rates over a distance of 100–200 nm (Voet and Voet, 1995). The electron transfer taking place through space or through bonds and the role of protein structure are all active areas of current research. To understand mitochondria related electron transfer, we have taken a few, but new, small steps to elucidate the electronic character of some components of the proteins involved in the electron transfer process. Apart from our ligand and our complex we have also investigated cysteine, lysine, histidine, and flavin adenine dinucleotide (FAD). Since, reactive oxygen species (ROS) is also a source of mitochondrial dysfunction, we have also looked at the electronic properties of H_2O_2.

The technique we have utilized to investigate the electronic properties of these small molecules is impedance spectroscopy, a field with high potential for drug discovery, but used only to a limited extent by researchers in the pharmaceutical industry.

To obtain a fairly complete picture of this complex, we have included, briefly at least, other topics such as platinum(II) complexes, mitochondria and its dysfunction or oxidative stress, free radicals, common antioxidants, diode or tunnel diode behavior of some enzymes, and electron spin coupling.

PLATINUM(II) AND PALLADIUM(II) COMPLEXES

Active platinum(II) compounds such as cisplatin, carboplatin, and oxaliplatin are the cornerstones of solid tumor chemotherapy. Cis-platin, cis-diamminedichloro platinum(II), is a square planar d^8 platinum(II) complex. Since, its approval in 1978 for clinical use, cisplatin has made significant contributions to the treatment of testicular and ovarian cancer (Sherman and Lippard, 1987). However, cisplatin and other platinum drugs suffer from serious side effects such as tissue toxicity, and resistance to the treatment (Dabrowiak, 2009; Fricker, 2007; Sherman and Lippard, 1987). Cisplatin is highly toxic to kidneys, limiting its dose. The therapy gets complicated due to the nauseas and intense vomits, indicating gastrointestinal toxicity. Cisplatin is also not orally bioavailable. The molecular target for the platinum drugs is DNA. Recent advances have identified other molecular targets such as thiol-containing proteins and growth factor receptors (Fricker, 2007).

Cisplatin reacts with water to give several aqua species, replacing the chloride ligands. The rate constants for the hydrolysis of the first chloride from cis or trans-platins at 25°C are 2.5×10^{-5} and 9.8×10^{-5} s^{-1}, respectively (Sherman and Lippard, 1987).

$$[Pt(NH_3)_2Cl_2] + H_2O = [Pt(NH_3)_2Cl(OH_2)]^+ + Cl^- \tag{4}$$

$$[Pt(NH_3)_2Cl(OH_2)]^+ = [Pt(NH_3)_2Cl(OH)] + H^+ \tag{5}$$

$$[Pt(NH_3)_2Cl(OH_2)]^+ + H_2O = [Pt(NH_3)_2(OH_2)_2]^{2+} + Cl^- \tag{6}$$

$$[Pt(NH_3)_2(OH_2)_2]^{2+} = [Pt(NH_3)_2(OH_2)(OH)]^+ + H^+ \tag{7}$$

$$[Pt(NH_3)_2(OH_2)(OH)]^+ = [Pt(NH_3)_2(OH)_2] + H^+ \tag{8}$$

These reactions are dependent on pH and chloride concentrations. The higher ($\sim$0.1 M) Cl$^-$ concentration in the plasma facilitates the passage across cell membranes as the neutral cisplatin. The lower ($\sim$0.004 M) Cl$^-$ concentration inside the cell facilitates its hydrolysis. At the pH of the blood of 7.4, most of cisplatin is in the monohydroxo form. The pK$_a$ for the deprotonation reaction of the monoaqua species is 6.41 (Dabrowiak, 2009).

Cisplatin interacts with DNA to form inter- and intra-strand cross-links. The intra-strand cross-link between adjacent guanine bases on the DNA strand causes cancer cell death.

The coordination chemistry of palladium(II) and platinum(II) compounds being similar, the antitumor activity of several palladium(II) complexes had been explored (Abu-Surrah et al., 2008; Caires, 2007; Gao et al., 2009; Rau et al., 1998). Mononuclear palladium(II) complexes with aromatic N-containing ligands, amino acid ligands, S-donor ligands, and P-containing ligands have respective qualities and properties due to the different structures as well as properties of the ligands (Gao et al., 2009). It is interesting to note that the cisplatin analogue of palladium did not exhibit any antitumor activity probably due to its high reactivity and consequent inability to reach the DNA. Palladium(II) analogues of platinum(II) complexes are about 10^4–10^5 times more reactive (Gao et al., 2009). To minimize the high lability and fast hydrolysis of palladium(II) complexes in biological environments, chelating ligands were used to synthesize the antitumor agents. An interesting observation was that the trans palladium(II) complexes had better activity than the cispalladium(II) or cisplatinum(II) complexes (Caires, 2007). Advances involving palladium complexes mainly for cancer therapy have recently been reviewed (Abu-Surrah et al., 2008; Caires, 2007; Gao et al., 2009). Even though there are structural and thermodynamic similarities between platinum(II) and palladium(II) complexes, palladium(II) complexes seem to exhibit biological action very different from those of the toxic platinum complexes. While the main target of platinum based drugs is DNA, palladium based drugs show preferential targets such as enzymes and lysosomes (Caires, 2007).

It has been found that the antitumor activity of a ligand or metal was much less than the metal-ligand complex because the binding affinity of metals to proteins or enzymes will change their interaction process with DNA thereby affecting the DNA replication and cell proliferation (Maloň et al., 2001). These conclusions were drawn from studies using cell lines, human malignant melanoma G-361, human osteogenic sarcoma HOS, human chronic myelogenous leukemia K-562, and human breast adenocarcinoma MCF7 and iron(III) and copper(II) complexes of N^6-benzylamino-purine derivatives. Similar results were also observed for palladium(II)–benzyl bis (thiosemicarbazonate) against cell lines, cervix epithelial human carcinoma (HeLa), transformed monkey kidney fibroblasts (Vero), normal murine keratinocytes (Pam 212), and murine keratinocytes transformed with the H-ras oncogene and resistant to cisplatin (Pam-ras) (Matesanz et al., 1999).

A recent review on palladium(II) complexes for the cancer therapy has lamented the lack of progress of palladium-based drugs. "In addition, it is important to note that, to the best of our knowledge, the palladium-based complex had not yet been tested in human beings due to the following factors: the success of platinum-based complexes in the cancer therapy, the enormous quantity of these complexes described in the literature, the high costs of the developmental phases in human clinical trials, the legal difficulties involving the drug assays in human beings and for the novelty of this subject" (Caires, 2007). We must add that the palladium α-lipoic acid complex formulation has been in the market for more than 15 years, without specifying any potential benefits for any cancer even though the cell line data presented here indicate its potential applications for a variety of cases.

GENE-BASED THERAPY

Still in its infancy, serious attempts are being made in drug discovery based on phar-macogenomics. It is based on the proteins, enzymes, and RNA molecules associated with genes and specific diseases and based on a patient's genetic profile. Sorting out a few single nucleotide polymorphisms (SNPs) responsible for the disease from the millions of SNPs and their response for each specific drug remain a Herculean challenge. For example, a recent sequencing of 20,661 protein coding genes in 22 human glio-blastoma multiforme (grade IV astrocytoma) samples revealed recurrent mutations in the active site of isocitrate dehydrogenase 1 (IDH1 gene on chromosome 2q33) (Parsons et al., 2008). The oxidative carboxylation of isocitrate to α-ketoglutarate re-sulting in the production of nicotinamide adenine dinucleotide phosphate (NADPH) is catalyzed by isocitrate dehydrogenase 1. These IDH1 mutations were found to occur preferentially in younger patients compared to the older patients with wild-type muta-tions in IDH1. A similar study of 20,661 protein-coding genes in 24 pancreatic cancers revealed 63 genetic alterations defining a core set of 12 cellular signaling pathways (Jones et al., 2008). The complexity of gene-based therapy can be recognized easily by knowing the enormous number of mutated genes in some tumors such as pancreas (1007), brain (685), and breast (1026) (Jones et al., 2008).

HALLMARKS OF CANCER

Self-sufficiency in growth signals, insensitivity to anti-growth signals, evading pro-grammed cell death or apoptosis, limitless replicative potential, sustained angiogen-esis, and tissue invasion and metastasis seem to characterize the cancer cells (Hanahan and Weinberg, 2000). The need for adding mitochondrial dysfunction to this list is sub-stantiated by a growing list of compelling evidence. Normal differentiated cells gener-ate their energy for cellular processes by mitochondrial oxidative phosphorylation. Cancer cells on the other hand produce their energy by glycolysis even under aerobic conditions (Heiden et al., 2009; McKnight, 2010; Vazquez et al., 2010; Warburg, 1956). The number of moles of ATP per mole of glucose produced by oxidative phosphorylation is ~ 36 and by glycolysis are 2. In a proliferative tissue, the number of moles of ATP produced per mole of glucose is ~4 (Heiden et al., 2009). The cancer cells' preference for the less efficient glycolytic pathway for energy production is still on a hot pursuit. A correlation is observed between glycolytic ATP production and aggressiveness of tumor cells (Simonnet et al., 2002). Numerous investigations have been carried out to understand this "Warburg effect" and the link between cellular metabolism and growth control. Several signaling pathways involved in cell proliferation have been linked to anabolic metabolism. These signaling pathways also regulate metabolic pathways that incorporate nutrients into production of nucleotides, amino acids, and lipids for accelerating cell proliferation instead of efficient energy production (Heiden et al., 2009).

The recent special section of "Science" on "Metabolism" has highlighted "the control of the metabolic switch in cancers by oncogenes and tumor suppressor genes" (Levine and Puzio-Kuter, 2010), "circadian integration of metabolism and energetics" and its consequences for treatment of obesity and diabetes (Bass and Takahashi, 2010), the role of "autophagy in metabolism" and its implications for treatment of cancer and degenerative diseases (Rabinowitz and White, 2010), and manufacturing molecules through metabolic engineering (Keasling, 2010).

Most anticancer drug development strategies are based on recent advances in the discovery of oncogenes and tumor suppressor genes. Recent studies on the role of mitochondria in signaling pathways for cell death and regulation of calcium homeostasis have generated renewed interest in investigating the role of antioxidants and nutraceutical supplements for induction of apoptosis and anticancer treatment (Aggarwal and Shishodia, 2006; Biasutto et al., 2010; Chen et al., 2010; Kroemer et al., 2007; Singh, 2006; Sarkar et al., 2009).

MITOCHONDRIA

Mitochondria or the "powerhouse of the cell", are about 0.5–1 μm in diameter and 7 μm in length (Voet and Voet, 1995). Mitochondria exist in a variety of different shapes depending on the source from which they are derived. In electron micrographs they appear as spheres, rods or filamentous bodies. Twenty percent by volume of a typical eukaryotic cell is occupied by about 2,000 mitochondria. These semi-autonomous, highly dynamic organelles, containing a double membrane structure, are involved in cellular respiration (aerobic metabolism), regulation of calcium homeostasis and cell death. Two membranes that have different sets of enzymes and biochemical functions surround the internal matrix. The matrix contains the enzymes of the Krebs cycle except succinate dehydrogenase (SDH). The SDH is bound to the inner membrane. To increase the surface area, nature has cleverly convoluted or invaginated the inner membrane into the matrix of the mitochondrion to form cristae, its number varying with the respiratory activity of the type of cell. The components of the respiratory chain and the mechanism for ATP synthesis are part of the inner membrane. While the outer membrane is relatively permeable or porous to metabolites and solutes smaller than ~5 kD, the inner membrane is highly selective. This makes the contents of the intermembrane space and the matrix different. The enzymatic composition of the various mitochondrial sub compartments, outer membrane, intermembrane space, inner membrane and matrix, are easily available (Alberts et al., 1989; Beattie, 2002; Voet and Voet, 1995).

The transport of electrons through respiratory chain complexes I–IV in the inner mitochondrial membrane requires a series of coupled redox reactions. Within the inner mitochondrial membrane, these complexes are all laterally mobile. The redox enzymes involved in the electron transfer process play a major part in the bioenergetic metabolism. The fate of the reducing equivalents from catabolic processes entering the respiratory chain as NADH and $FADH_2$ is briefly described (Beattie, 2002; Voet and Voet, 1995).

Complex I (NADH-ubiquinone oxidoreductase or NADH-CoQ reductase) catalyzes oxidation of NADH by coenzyme Q (also known as CoQ_{10} in mammals).

$$NADH + \text{oxidized CoQ} \rightarrow NAD^+ + \text{reduced CoQ or } CoQH_2, \Delta E^{o\prime} = 0.360V \quad (9)$$

Complex II (succinate-ubiquinone oxidoreductase or succinate-CoQ reductase) catalyzes oxidation of $FADH_2$ by coenzyme Q. This reaction does not produce enough energy to synthesize ATP. It serves as a conduit to inject electrons from $FADH_2$ to the electron transport chain.

$$FADH_2 + \text{oxidized CoQ} \rightarrow FAD + CoQH_2, \Delta E^{o\prime} = 0.015V \quad (10)$$

Complex III (coenzyme Q-cytochrome c reductase) catalyzes oxidation of $CoQH_2$ by cytochrome c

$$CoQH_2 + \text{oxidized cytochrome c} \rightarrow \text{oxidized CoQ} + \text{reduced cytochrome c}, \Delta E^{o\prime} = 0.190V \quad (11)$$

Complex IV (cytochrome c oxidase) catalyzes oxidation of reduced cytochrome c by O_2.

$$\text{Reduced cytochrome c} + \tfrac{1}{2} O_2 \rightarrow \text{oxidized cytochrome c} + H_2O. \Delta E^{o\prime} = 0.580V \quad (12)$$

Complex V (proton translocating ATP synthase) carries out energy coupling or energy transduction. The electron transport and ATP synthesis are coupled.

$$2H^+ + \tfrac{1}{2} O_2 \rightarrow H_2O, \Delta E^{o\prime} = 0.815V \quad (13)$$

Even though NADH can participate in a 2e transfer process only, the coenzymes FMN and CoQ of complex I are capable of receiving or donating one or 2e because of their stable semiquinone radical forms. Cytochromes, on the other hand, allow passage of only 1e.

Part of the energy released during this passage of "high energy" electrons along a series of electron carriers embedded in the ion-impermeable membrane is harnessed to pump protons from one side to the other side of the membrane. Complexes I, III, and IV pump protons. This movement of protons from the mitochondrial matrix to the intermembrane space creates an electrochemical gradient. The redox enzymes in the respiratory chain build this proton gradient or pH gradient in a stepwise fashion. The ATP-synthase, a non-redox enzyme, is responsible for keeping the ATP ratio far from equilibrium by catalyzing the phosphorylation of ADP. The ATP-synthase uses the gradient of the electrochemical potential of the proton as a source of free energy.

The electronic properties (bias or rectifier or "ratchet") of some of these redox enzymes and the group responsible for these activities are described later in this chapter.

Research in molecular biology during the 1950s and early 1960s focused on finding out the reasons for the deviations from Mendelian rules for the transmission of some mitochondrial characteristics and instead following the cytoplasmic inheritance patterns led to the discovery of mitochondrial DNA. Mitochondria contain their own genome with their own transcription, translation, and machinery for protein synthesis. Two genetic systems, the mitochondrial DNA (mtDNA) and the nuclear DNA (nDNA) encode the mitochondrial electron transport chain complexes. The mtDNA codes for 13 different complexes are given in Table 1. The codes for nDNA are 36, 4, 10, 10, and 14 protein subunits for Complexes I, II, III, IV, and V respectively (Carew and Huang, 2002). Complex II is encoded by nDNA only. Mitochondrial DNA also contains genes encoding 2 ribosomal RNAs (12S rRNA and 16S rRNA) and all the necessary 22 transfer RNAs that are required for protein synthesis in mitochondria. The human mtDNA is a supercoiled, double-stranded molecule containing 16,569 base pairs. It is also known that the frequency of mtDNA migration to nDNA is much greater than nDNA migration to mtDNA (Carew and Huang, 2002).

Table 1. Subunits of Electron Transport Chain Complexes Encoded by Human Mitochondrial DNA (Carew and Huang, 2002).

Complex Subunits	Number of Subunits	Encoded by mtDNA
I	NADH dehydrogenase	7
II	Succinate dehydrogenase	0
III	Cytochrome b	1
IV	Cytochrome c oxidase	3
V	ATP synthase	2

Mitochondria are not self-replicating organelles in spite of their ability to transcribe their own DNA and translate the resulting mRNAs. Most of the mitochondrial proteins (more than 90%), synthesized in cytosol and imported into mitochondria, are encoded in nDNA.

Apart from respiration, a second crucial function of mitochondria is the control of apoptosis or programmed cell death. An early activation of pro-apoptotic protein disrupts the mitochondrial membrane permeabilization and results in the formation of pores. Consequently, the electron transport chain protein, cytochrome c, is released into the cytosol, along with the release of pro-caspase 9.

Another important function of mitochondrion is the distribution/redistribution of Ca^{2+} pools within cells. Uptake of high concentrations of Ca^{2+} into mitochondria opens the pore of the outer membrane and consequently releases cytochrome c.

MITOCHONDRIAL DYSFUNCTION

Apart from ATP production, mitochondria also produce ROS. Some electrons escaping or leaking from the electron transport complexes, mainly from complexes I and III, during respiration react with oxygen to form superoxide radicals. Oxygen undergoes a series of progressive reduction reactions producing superoxide anion (O_2^-), hydrogen peroxide (H_2O_2), and finally hydroxyl radical (HO) along with hydroxide ion (OH^-). The cause of this leakage of electrons is not clearly understood. However, it may be possible for mtDNA mutations to disrupt the normal electron flow and seriously affect energy production. Oxidative damage and the resulting serious consequences have been extensively reviewed recently (Singh, 2006). Compared to nDNA, mtDNA is far more susceptible to mutations due to a lack of histone protection and limited repair capacity (Carew and Huang, 2002; Singh, 2006).

During the production of ATP in the cell, about 85% of oxygen is consumed by the mitochondria. Superoxide radical, O_2^-, may be produced from about 4% of all oxygen consumed (Singh, 2006). Enzymes such as NADPH oxidases, xanthine oxidase, cyclooxygenases, and lipooxygenases also produce ROS. The iron-sulfur cluster in the aconitase enzyme, localized to the matrix space of mitochondria, is oxidized by superoxide and the exposed iron reacts with the peroxide to produce hydroxyl radicals (Singh, 2006). Also the NO produced within mitochondria by mitochondrial NO synthase produces peroxynitrite radical ($ONOO^-$) by reaction with O_2^-. Superoxide and peroxinitrite radicals contribute to substantial mitochondrial damage.

Enzymes such as super oxide dismutase, GPx, catalase, peroxoredoxin, and thioredoxin can inactivate some of the ROS. Manganese superoxide dismutase or copper/zinc superoxide dismutase converts the superoxide radical into hydrogen peroxide. The active site of cytosolic and extracelllar forms of superoxide dismutase contain copper/zinc and the mitochondrial form contains manganese (Beattie, 2002). Oxidative damage is due to the inadequacy of these detoxifying processes.

Lipid peroxidation by the hydroxyl radical can alter the structural integrity of membranes. In patients with Parkinson's disease, the excess Fe^{2+} can reduce peroxide and produce HO. These radicals and their reactions cause oxidative stress and consequent mitochondrial damage resulting in mutations and probably cancer.

Table 2. Mutated Genes in Different Cancers (Carew and Huang, 2002).

Type of Cancer	Mutated Gene/Region	Affected Respiratory Complex
Breast	16S rRNA	None
	ND1	Complex I
	ND2	Complex I
	ND4	Complex I
	ND5	Complex I
	Cyt b	Complex III
	ATPase 6	Complex V
Ovarian	12S rRNA	None

Table 2. *(Continued)*

Type of Cancer	Mutated Gene/Region	Affected Respiratory Complex
	16S rRNA	None
	Cyt b	Complex III
Pancreatic	12S rRNA	None
	16S rRNA	None
	ND1	Complex I
	ND2	Complex I
	ND4	Complex I
	ND4L	Complex I
	ND5	Complex I
	ND6	Complex I
	Cyt b	Complex III
	COXI	Complex IV
	COXII	Complex IV
	COXIII	Complex IV
	ATPase 6	Complex V
Prostate	16S rRNA	None
	ND4	Complex I
	ND4L	Complex I

Since, each cell contains many mitochondria with multiple copies of mtDNA, it is possible for wild-type and mutant mtDNA to coexist in a state called heteroplasmy. After numerous cell divisions over time, this status may change to predominantly wild-type or mutant, a state called homoplasmy (Chatterjee et al., 2006). Since, tumors have mostly homoplasmic mtDNA mutations their cells carry the same mtDNA mutation (Carew and Huang, 2002).

Mitochondrial DNA depletion and deletion to cancer progression has been reviewed recently (Higuchi, 2007). The mitochondrial function and energy metabolism in cancer cells as well as mitochondrial genetics have also been reviewed (Kroemer and Pouyssegur, 2008; Mayevsky, 2009; Wallace and Fan, 2010).

The Warburg effect or aerobic glycolysis in cancer cells and its potential benefits for cancer cells have been examined in detail (Carew and Huang, 2002; Frezza and Gottlieb, 2009; Gogvadze et al., 2008; Hsu and Sabatini, 2008; Kroemer and Pouyssegur, 2008). Both glucose and glutamine are consumed heavily by cancer cells and may be the source of increased lactate production in cancer cells. In most cancer cells about 60% of ATP is produced by glycolysis (Frezza and Gottlieb, 2009). The linkage between aerobic glycolysis and apoptosis resistance remains higly elusive. The link between aerobic glycolysis and mitochondrial outermembrane permeabilization (which mediates the intrinsic pathway of apoptosis) resistance, is also not clearly established. Attempts are being made to counteract aerobic glycolysis and to induce mitochondrial outermembrane permeabilization and consequent apoptosis for therapeutic purposes (Kroemer, 2006).

Direct evidence of tumorogenesis from mitochondrial dysfunction was obtained when mutations in succinate dehydrogenase or fumarate hydratase were found to initiate familial paraganglioma and of papillary renal cell cancer respectively. A general feature of malignant cells seems to be alterations in respiratory chain activity and mtDNA abnormalities. Many tumors have somatic mutations in mtDNA (Chatterjee et al., 2006). Gene mutations observed in some common cancers are briefly included in Table 2.

Glioblastoma Multiforme (GBM) and Type I Meningioma (transitional meningioma, TM)

It has been found that mtDNA was highly amplified in most of the malignant glioma specimens (Carew and Huang, 2002). The comparative amplification of nDNA was very low. The membrane phospholipids of the brain containing high amounts of unsaturated fatty acids are likely to be damaged by oxidation by oxygen radicals. The formation of these lipid peroxides affects the integrity and function of the membranes proteins and DNA The natural defense mechanism against this adverse effect is by GPx, glutathione reductase (GRx), and superoxide dismutase.

Table 3. Comparison of glutathione peroxidase, glutathione reductase and proteinoxidation levels in Glioblastoma, transitional meningioma, and normal brain tissues (Tanriverdi et al., 2007).

Parameters	GPx (U/g wet tissue)	GRx (U/g wet tissue)	Pox (nmol/g wet tissue)
Glioblastoma	17.72±3.9	5.11±0.9	599.6±56
Transitional Meningioma	19.04±2.0	5.66±0.9	588.3±49
Normal Brain tissue	45.26±6.9	10.08±1.2	439.1±31

Superoxide dismutase converts O_2^- into H_2O_2, which is eliminated by the actions of catalases and peroxidases. An analysis, given in Table 3, of 48 brain tumors obtained during surgery and 15 normal brain tissues collected during autopsy for GPx, GRx, and protein oxidation (POx) revealed that GPx and GRx activities were significantly lower in GBM and TM when compared to the controls (Tanriverdi et al., 2007). The decrease in GPx and GRx were more obvious in GBM than in TM. Also the POx levels were much higher in both GBM and TM compared to controls.

Breast Cancer

The bulk of the mutations were identified in the D-loop region, the main non-coding area of the mtDNA. The others are given in Table 2. Lipid peroxidation, coenzyme Q10 levels and antioxidant status of breast cancer patients have been investigated (Portakal et al., 2000; Punnonen et al., 1994; Rajneesh et al., 2008; Sinha et al., 2009). It was observed that coenzyme Q10 concentrations were significantly less in tumor tissues compared to normal surrounding tissues (Portakal et al., 2000). Also higher levels of malondialdehyde (MDA) (a measure of lipid peroxidation) were observed in tumor tissues.

Table 4. Comparison of lipid peroxidation, catalase and superoxide dismutase levels innormal and breast cancer blood and tissue (Sinha et al., 2009).

Parameters in blood	Control	Patients
Malondialdehyde		
(nmol/ml plasma)	2.27±0.36	4.52±0.78
Catalase (U/ml red blood cell)	15.42±0.59	10.60±0.99
Superoxide dismutase (U/ml red blood cell)	10.52±0.37	7.36±0.55
Parameters in tissue		
Malondialdehyde		
(nmol/ml plasma)	2.20±0.22	4.73±0.69
Catalase (U/ml red blood cell)	15.61±0.72	10.37±1.16
Superoxide dismutase (U/ml red blood cell)	10.61±0.36	7.24±0.26

Table 5. Comparison of lipid peroxidation, catalase and superoxide dismutase levels in different stages of breast carcinoma in blood and tissue (Sinha et al., 2009).

Parameters in blood plasma	Stage I	Stage II	Stage III	Stage IV
Malondialdehyde				
(nmol/ml plasma)	3.38±0.44	3.99±0.60	4.52±0.58	5.12±0.49
Catalase				
(U/ml red blood cell)	10.76±0.95	11.23±1.24	11.03±0.55	9.90±0.65
Superoxide dismutase				
(U/ml red blood cell)	8.15 ±0.90	7.58±0.55	7.22 ±0.22	7.13±0.39
Parameters in tissue				
Malondialdehyde				
(nmol/ml plasma)	3.86±0.63	4.60±0.71	4.57±0.41	5.12±0.63
Catalase				
(U/ml red blood cell)	12.21±1.02	10.85±1.07	9.82±0.72	9.99±0.97
Superoxide dismutase				
(U/ml red blood cell)	7.08 ±0.32	7.43±0.26	7.23 ±0.21	7.19±0.32

However, the activities of manganese superoxide dismutase, total superoxide dismutase, glutathione peroxidase, and catalase levels were also higher in tumor tissues compared to normal tissues (Portakal et al., 2000; Rajneesh et al., 2008). On the other hand, the superoxide dismutase and catalase levels, given in Table 4 and Table 5, reported in another recent study (Sinha et al., 2009) indicate a trend that is consistent with data for other cancers. This discrepancy is attributed probably to the differences in the stage of the tumor selected for different studies. It was suggested, from a study of free radicals and antioxidants in stages I–IV of carcinoma breast in blood and tissue that at the early stages of cancer, the antioxidant levels may be higher to meet the challenge of carcinogenesis (Sinha et al., 2009).

Ovarian Cancer
Somatic mutations were mostly observed in 4 regions of the mitochondrial genome (Table 2), D-loop, 12S rRNA, 16S rRNA, and cytochrome b (Carew and Huang, 2002). The levels of lipid peroxidation and conjugated dienes were much higher in ovarian cancer patients compared to controls (Senthil et al., 2004). The catalase and superoxide dismutase levels were lower in the ovarian cancer patients. The levels of antioxidant vitamins C and E were also lower in the ovarian cancer patients.

Table 6. Comparison of lipid peroxidation, conjugated dienes, catalase, superoxide dismutase, vitamin C and vitamin E levels in blood in normal and ovarian cancer patients (Senthil et al., 2004).

Parameters in blood	Control	Patients
Malondialdehyde		
(nmol/ml plasma)	2.13±0.18	5.64±0.52
Conjugated dienes		
(μmol/ml plasma)	0.71±0.06	1.71±0.13
Catalase (U/mg hemoglobin)	5.71±0.61	4.4±0.39
Superoxide dismutase		
(U/mg hemoglobin)	1.91 ±0.29	0.9±0.11
Vitamin C (mg/dl of plasma)	1.05 ±0.09	0.40±0.03
Vitamin E (mg/dl of plasma)	2.82 ±0.20	1.36±0.10

Prostate Cancer
Incidence of mutations in mitochondrial DNA of prostate cancer was infrequent (Carew and Huang, 2002). A recent study of lipid peroxidation and antioxidant status in prostate cancer patients, shown in Table 7, revealed elevated levels of lipid peroxidation and decreased levels of vitamin C, vitamin E, reduced glutathione, glutathione peroxides, and superoxide dismutase in plasma, erythrocytes and erythrocyte membranes when compared with normal patients (Sandhya et al., 2010).

Table 7. Comparison of lipid peroxidation, catalase, reduced glutathione, glutathione peroxidase, vitamin C and vitamin E levels in plasma, in erythrocytes and erythrocyte membranes of normal and prostate cancer patients (Sandhya et al., 2010).

Parameters in plasma	Control	Patients
Malondialdehyde		
(nmol/ml plasma)	3.8±0.2	6.9±0.52
Conjugated dienes		
(µmol/ml plasma)	0.71±0.06	1.71±0.13
Catalase (U/ml plasma)	0.76±0.07	0.56±0.04
Vitamin C (mg/dl of plasma)	1.39 ±0.007	1.29±0.06
Vitamin E (mg/dl of plasma)	1.4 ±0.06	1.28±0.09
Reduced glutathione		
(mg/dl plasma)	52.7 ±4.2	42.8±2.9
Glutathione peroxidase		
(U/l)	189.8±23.4	160.1±12.7
Parameters in Erythrocyte		
Malondialdehyde		
(nmol/mg protein)	0.33±0.04	5.7±0.42
Reduced glutathione		
(mg/dl plasma)	54.9 ±3.8	44.8±2.7
Vitamin E (µg/mg protein)	2.31 ±0.09	1.76±0.09
Parameters in Erythrocyte Membrane		
Superoxide dismutase		
(U/mg hemoglobin)	4.71±0.52	4.32±0.34
Catalase (U/mg hemoglobin)	1.7±0.09	1.3±0.07
Glutathione peroxidase		
(U/g hemoglobin)	22.2 ±1.7	20.6±1.7

It is obvious from the examples given above that the main gateway for electrons to enter the respiratory chain, complex I, is affected in all these cancers.

FREE RADICALS AND ANTIOXIDANTS

The appearance of oxygen in the atmosphere is associated with a great expansion of the varieties and numbers of higher living forms. Oxygen is the source for the emergence of respiratory metabolism and energy efficiency. It is also the source of free radicals such as hydroxyl and superoxide.

A free radical is a highly reactive species with an unpaired electron. It can be a neutral species such as hydroxyl, HO, or a charged negative ion (anion) such as superoxide, O_2^-, or a charged positive ion (cation) such as guanine radical. An unpaired electron is shown as a dot after the symbol (example: HO). Free radicals are, in general, good oxidizing agents. They can remove an electron from other materials and in that process the unpaired electron gets paired. They can also participate in chain reactions to produce new free radicals.

The free radicals produced during phagocytosis are beneficial (Singh, 2006; Voet and Voet, 1995). The primary purpose of leukocytes is phagocytosis, which is the engulfing and destruction of particulate matter and bacteria. Leukocytes contain the enzymes of the hexose-monophosphate shunt, glycolysis, citric acid cycle, and respiratory enzymes. Phagocytosis requires a lot of energy, which is obtained from glucose by glycolysis and also by the hexose-monophosphate shunt. The role of this shunt is to produce hydrogen peroxide from superoxide free radical, which is used in the phagocytotic process.

The beneficial aspect of hydrogen peroxide in cell signaling is emerging. Neurons and brain macrophages produce superoxide ions in pathological situations and the hydrogen peroxide produced from superoxide increases gap junctional communication in astrocytes (Rouach et al., 2004). Examples of signaling processes include the over oxidation of the cysteine in peroxiredoxins from the cysteine sulfenic acid to cysteine sulfinic acid, and the over oxidation of methionine residues in proteins to methionine sulfoxide (Wood et al., 2003).

The need for a certain amount of oxidative stress and the role of redox for embryonic and fetal growth have been exemplified recently (Dennery, 2010). It details the level of oxygen levels and antioxidant status at the first, second and third trimester of pregnancy. It is also interesting to note that low levels of H_2O_2 and superoxide produced by human sperm are important for the capacitation process that allows the sperm to penetrate the zona pellucida of the ovum. It has also been observed that at low, moderate, and highly oxidative state, proliferation, differentiation, and apoptosis or necrosis respectively are favored.

Free radicals are also a liability because they produce DNA damage by easily oxidizing the guanine base in DNA. The altered form of guanine, 8-oxoguanine, has been the subject of much study. Another liability of free radicals is that oxyradicals allow lipid peroxidation.

Antioxidants are physiologic reducing agents. They donate electrons to free radicals and in that process become oxidized. Their specific reactions are a function of their redox potential, measured in volts.

Reduction or redox potentials predict the direction of a reaction. They cannot predict how fast the reaction will take place. Each oxidized species of a redox couple having a higher positive voltage is capable of extracting an electron from a reduced species of a redox couple having a less positive or higher negative voltage. Some examples of 1e reduction potentials and 2e reduction potentials of reactions of biological interest are given in Table 8 (Buettner, 1993) and Table 9 (Voet and Voet, 1995). Depending on the position of the redox couple in the redox table of potentials, free radicals can act as both oxidizing and reducing agents and produce other free radicals.

Table 8. 1e reduction potentials at pH 7.0, 1 atm, and 1.0 M (Buettner, 1993).

Couple	E/mV
HO, H^+/H_2O	2310
O_3^-, $2H^+$/$H_2O + O_2$	1800
HOO, H^+/H_2O_2	1060
PUFA, H^+/PUFAH	600
(Polyunsaturated fatty acid, bis-allylic-H)	
α-Tocopheroxyl, H^+/α-tocopherol	500
(Vitamin E)	
H_2O_2, H^+/H_2O, HO	320
Ascorbate⁻, H^+/ascorbate monoanion	282
(Vitamin C)	
Ferricytochrome c/Ferrocytochrome c	260
Semiubiquinone, H^+/ubiquinol	200
(CoQ⁻, $2H^+$/CoQH$_2$)	
Ubiquinone, H^+/semiubiquinone	−36
(CoQ/CoQ⁻)	
Dehydroascorbic/ascorbate⁻	−174
O_2/$O_2^=$	−330
O_2, H^+/HO_2	−460
GSSG/GSSG⁻ (Glutathione disulfide and its radical ion)	−1500

Enzymes such as superoxide dismutase, catalase, and glutathione peroxidase are known as preventive antioxidants because they eliminate the species involved in the initiation of free radical chain reactions. Hydrogen peroxide and organic hydroperoxides in the cytosol are destroyed by a selenium (a cofactor) containing metalloenzyme glutathione peroxidase. Superoxide dismutases exist in several varieties with copper, zinc, and manganese in the active center. The dismutation yields hydrogen peroxide, which can be removed by catalase and glutathione peroxidase to oxygen and water by different mechanisms. The highest concentration of catalase is present in peroxisomes and to a lesser extent in cytosol and mitochondria (Beattie, 2002).

Table 9. 2e reduction potentials at pH 7.0, 1 atm, and 1.0 M (Voet and Voet, 1995).

Reaction	E/mV
$2H^+ + 2e^- = H_2$	−421
Cystine + $2H^+ + 2e^-$ = Cysteine	−340
$NAD^+ + H^+ + 2e^-$ = NADH	−315
$NADP^+ + H^+ + 2e^-$ = NADPH	−320
Lipoic acid + $2H^+ + 2e^-$ = Dihydrolipoic acid	−290
FAD + $2H^+ + 2e^-$ = FADH$_2$ (free coenzyme)	−219

Table 9. *(Continued)*

Pyruvate + 2H$^+$ + 2e$^-$ = Lactate	−190
FAD + 2H$^+$ + 2e$^-$ = FADH$_2$ (in flavoproteins)	~ 0.
Ubiquinone + 2H$^+$ + 2e$^-$ = Ubiquinol	45
½ O$_2$ + 2H$^+$ + 2e$^-$ = H$_2$O	820

Food industry uses butylated hydroxyl toluene and butylated hydroxyl anisole for preservation. However their metabolic fate is not clearly understood.

Small molecules such as ascorbate (vitamin C), tocopherols (vitamin E), reduced coenzyme Q10 (CoQH$_2$), glutathione (γ-glutamylcysteinylglycine), and α-lipoic acid "repair" oxidizing radicals directly and are known as chain breaking antioxidants.

The criteria often used to evaluate the antioxidant potential as well as preventive or therapeutic applications of a compound are (1) specificity of free radical quenching, (2) metal chelating ability, (3) interaction with other antioxidants, (4) effects on gene expression, (5) absorption and bioavailability, (6) concentration in tissues, cells, and extracellular fluid, and (7) location (in aqueous or membrane domains or in both) (Packer et.al., 1995).

FREE RADICAL PRODUCTION AND CHAIN REACTIONS

Normal (triplet state) oxygen, O$_2$, has two single parallel (spin) electrons in separate orbitals. A 2e interaction is not possible because it will result in parallel spins in the same orbital, which is not allowed. Thus the preferable interaction is reduction of oxygen by addition of 1e at a time. This process leads to the production of oxygen radicals that can cause cellular damage. The high energy singlet oxygen with 2e and opposite spins in the two orbitals is capable of 2e interactions.

Progressive 1e reduction of O$_2$ produces O$_2^-$, H$_2$O$_2$, and finally HO· along with OH .

$$O_2 + e^- \rightarrow O_2^- \text{ (superoxide anion)} \tag{14}$$
$$O_2^- + e^- + 2H^+ \rightarrow H_2O_2 \text{ (hydrogen peroxide)} \tag{15}$$
$$H_2O_2 + e^- \rightarrow OH^- + HO \text{ (hydroxyl radical)} \tag{16}$$
$$HO + e^- + H^+ \rightarrow H_2O \tag{17}$$

The hydroxyl radical is undoubtedly the most dangerous. It is involved in lipid peroxidation and generation of other toxic radicals. While there is no enzyme to destroy it, there is enzymatic transfer of hydroxyl to the proline in procollagen. Because of its high reactivity, hydroxyl radical has a short life.

The superoxide ion can act both as a reductant (for Fe^{3+}) and as an oxidant for catecholamines. Free iron and copper present under physiological conditions are sequestered by proteins (iron as transferrin and ferritin and copper by ceruloplasmin) to minimize production of free radical chain reactions such as reactions (18) and (19).

$$O_2^- + Fe^{3+} \rightarrow O_2 + Fe^{2+} \tag{18}$$

$$H_2O_2 + Fe^{2+} + H^+ \rightarrow HO\cdot + Fe^{3+} + H_2O \text{ (classical Fenton reaction)} \qquad (19)$$

Adding reactions (18) and (19) gives the Haber-Weiss reaction (20) which is catalyzed by metal ions.

$$H_2O_2 + O_2^- + H^+ \rightarrow HO + O_2 + H_2O \qquad (20)$$

The superoxide anion shown in reaction (14) is often released by mitochondria. Dismutation of superoxide anion, shown in reaction (21) produces hydrogen peroxide.

$$2H^+ + O_2^- + O_2^- \rightarrow H_2O_2 + O_2 \qquad (21)$$

Damage to both mtDNA and nDNA may result in mutations. Nonspecific binding of Fe^{2+} to DNA may result in the formation of HO·(Reaction 19) that attack individual bases and cause strand breaks.

An example of a polyunsaturated fatty acid (PUFAH) peroxidation chain reaction is the following.

Initiation reaction:	PUFAH $\rightarrow$ PUFA + H·	(22)
Propagation reaction:	PUFA + O_2 $\rightarrow$ PUFAOO	(23)
Propagation reaction:	PUFAOO + PUFAH $\rightarrow$ PUFAOOH + PUFA	(24)

Tocopherol (vitamin E) can break the propagation chain reaction by reacting with lipid peroxyl radical, PUFAOO.

The most reactive hydroxyl radical, HO·, is produced in biological systems by reductive cleavage of H_2O_2 by a reduced metal complex. The source of iron (II) complex may be ferrocytochrome c, iron(II) citrate, iron(II) transferrin, and iron(II) ADP. The source of H_2O_2 may be a direct 2e reduction of O_2 or a 1e reduction of O_2 to produce superoxide ion.

$$\text{Iron (II) complex} + H_2O_2 \rightarrow \text{Iron (III) complex} + OH^- + HO \qquad (25)$$
$$HO_2 \text{ (the perhydroxyl radical)} + O_2^- (+ H^+) \rightarrow H_2O_2 + O_2 \qquad (26)$$

The dangerous superoxide ion converts the iron (III) complex directly to the iron (II) complex.

$$O_2^- + \text{iron(III) complex} \rightarrow \text{iron(II) complex} + O_2 \qquad (27)$$

Production of O_2^- is from the use of stronger reductants. Thus O_2^- can produce both hydrogen peroxide and the iron (II) complex needed for the Fenton reaction.

VITAMIN C, L-ASCORBIC ACID

Ascorbic acid is in the form of ascorbate anion at biological pH because it has pK values of 4.17 and 11.57. It is a cofactor in several biosynthetic pathways. It is also an antioxidant. Humans do not synthesize it due to lack of the enzyme L-gulono-γ-lactone oxidase. This enzyme mediates the last step in the ascorbate biosynthetic pathway originating from glucose.

Ascorbic acid is a cofactor for the enzyme prolylhydroxylase, which modifies the polypeptide collagen precursor to facilitate the formation of collagen fibers. It also plays important roles in carnitine synthesis, catabolism of tyrosine, synthesis of norepinephrine by dopamine β-monooxygenase or dopamine β-hydroxylase, and the amidation of peptides with C-terminal glycine to activate hormone precursors.

Due to resonance, the ascorbate radical has a long half life of 1 second. Ascorbate can be oxidized in two successive 1e steps to ascorbate free radical and dehydroascorbic acid respectively.

$$\text{Ascorbate anion} - e^- \rightarrow \text{Ascorbate free radical} \tag{28}$$

$$\text{Ascorbate free radical} - e^- \rightarrow \text{dehydroascorbic acid} \tag{29}$$

The unpaired electron in the ascorbate free radical is distributed over its ring structure. This electron distribution stabilizes the molecule. Ascorbate radical disproportionates to give ascorbate anion and dehydroascorbic acid. This acid is a strained molecule and is not stable. The strain is relieved by hydration and subsequent bicyclic structure formation, which is hydrolyzed to form a linear molecule 2,3-diketo-L-gulonic acid. This ring opening reaction is biologically irreversible and results in the loss of the vitamin. However the oxidation of ascorbate to the radical and dehydroascorbic acid can easily be reversed. Both ascorbate radical anion and dehydroascorbic acid can be reduced by enzyme systems that use NADH or NADPH as sources of reducing equivalents.

The redox chemistry of ascorbate is pH dependent. The ascorbate radical has pK values of 1.10 and 4.25 and is an anion at physiological pH.

Dehydroascorbic acid imported into the mitochondria via facilitative glucose transporter 1, GLUT1, is reduced by glutathione and protects the mitochondrial genome and membrane (Nualart et al., 2003).

VITAMIN E

Vitamin E includes eight different related homologues. Of these, α-tocopherol is the most abundant and active form *in vivo*. The dynamics of antioxidant action of vitamin E have been recently reviewed (Niki and Noguchi, 2004). Vitamin E acts only in membrane or lipid domains. It quenches lipid peroxyl radicals. It has no activity in the aqueous phase.

Vitamin E, the primary lipid soluble small molecule antioxidant and vitamin C, the terminal water soluble small molecule antioxidant cooperate to protect lipids and lipid structures against peroxidation. Although vitamin E is located in membranes and vitamin C is located in aqueous phases, vitamin C is able to recycle vitamin E (See Table 8 and reaction (31). That is, vitamin C repairs the tocopheroxyl (chromanoxyl) radical of vitamin E thereby permitting vitamin E to function again as a free radical chain breaking antioxidant.

α-Tocopheroxyl + ascorbate monoanion → ascorbate⁻ + α-tocopherol,

$$E = +218 \text{ mV} \tag{30}$$

(Vitamin E)   (Vitamin C)

The concentration of vitamin E is less than 0.1 nmol per mg of membrane protein which corresponds to about one molecule for every 1000–2000 membrane phospholipids molecules that are the target of oxidation (Buettner, 1993). Lipid peroxyl radicals are generated at the rate 1–5 nmol per mg of membrane protein per minute (Packer et.al., 1995). Since, vitamin E is recycled by other antioxidants such as vitamin C, ubiquinols and glutathione, the membrane is not degraded and the vitamin E levels stay nearly the same. Recycling of vitamin E by dihydrolipoic acid seems weak. However, dihydrolipoic acid prevents lipid peroxidation by regenerating glutathione. Dihydrolipoic acid can recycle vitamin E *via* glutathione, vitamin C, ubiquinol, NADPH and NADH (Packer et al., 1995).

Each α-tocopherol (vitamin E) can donate 2e as a chain breaking antioxidant.

GLUTATHIONE

Glutathione or γ-glutamylcysteinylglycine, GSH, one of the body's major antioxidants, can react with various highly oxidizing species such as HO, RO, or ROO and make, H_2O, ROH, or ROOH and GS·which is glutathiyl radical. This is less oxidizing. However, GS can react rapidly with GSH, most efficiently *via* GS⁻ to make GSSG⁻, which is a very strong reducing species. It can produce O_2^- and glutathione disulfide, GSSG, by reaction with oxygen.

$$GSSG^- + O_2 \rightarrow O_2^- + GSSG \tag{31}$$

Selenium (as selenocysteine) is a cofactor of glutathione peroxidase (Beattie, 2002). One can see that superoxide dismutase and glutathione providing an excellent natural combination for cellular antioxidant defense by removing O_2 and HO· respectively.

The GS reacts with oxygen to form GSOO and other free radicals such as GS⁻ sulfonylperoxyl radical (GSO$_2$OO), GS-sulfonyl radical (GSO$_2$), and GS-sulfinyl radical (GSO). The stable end products of glutathione oxidation are glutathione disulfide, glutathione sulfinic acid (GSOOH), and glutathione sulfonic acid (GSO$_3$H).

The intracellular concentration of GSH is about 1 mM while the mitochondrial respiration keeps O_2 about 0–10 μM in the cell. Therefore, 99% of GS·formed should react with GSH to make GSSG and O_2^-. Thus the importance of superoxide dismutase is obvious. The normal GSH to GSSG ratio in erythrocytes is 100:1 (Beattie, 2002).

Glutathione is involved in reactions such as peroxide detoxification by glutathione peroxidase, NADPH dependent reduction of GSSG to GSH by GRx, thiol transferase modulation of protein disulfide balance and leukotriene biosynthesis by glutathione-S-transferase (Voet and Voet, 1995). It is also involved in the transport of amino acids across cell membranes. GRx contains an electron-transfer prosthetic group FAD. The electronic properties of the cysteine and FAD groups are discussed in a later section.

HYDROGEN PEROXIDE (H$_2$O$_2$)

Pure hydrogen peroxide is a pale blue syrupy liquid with a boiling point of 152.1°C and a freezing point of –0.89°C. The dielectric constant of 93 at 25°C for the pure liquid increases to 120 for a 65% aqueous solution (Cotton and Wilkinson, 1972). In the pure liquid state, the hydrogen peroxide is more strongly associated by hydrogen bonding than pure water. The dipole moment of hydrogen peroxide is 2.1 Debye units compared to 1.84 Debye units for water. Thus ion-dipole interactions are stronger with hydrogen peroxide than with water. Its influence on ion solvation is discussed in a later section.

Hydrogen peroxide has a skew, chain structure. The O-H bond distance is 97 pm and O-O bond distance is 149 pm. A dilute aqueous solution of hydrogen peroxide is more acidic than water (Cotton and Wilkinson, 1972).

$$H_2O_2 = H^+ + HO_2^- \quad K_{20}°C = 1.5 \times 10^{-12} \tag{32}$$

The potential given by the following equations indicate that hydrogen peroxide is a strong oxidizing agent in both acidic and basic solutions.

$$H_2O_2 + 2H^+ + 2e^- = 2H_2O, \ E° = 1.77V \tag{33}$$
$$O_2 + 2H^+ + 2e^- = H_2O_2, \ E° = 0.68V \tag{34}$$
$$HO_2^- + H_2O + 2e^- = 3OH^-, \ E° = 0.87V \tag{35}$$

Hydrogen peroxide behaves as a reducing agent only in the presence of stronger oxidizing agents such as permanganate.

The enzymes, monoamine oxidases, located in the outer mitochondrial membrane of mammalian tissues catalyze the oxidation of biogenic amines and produce H_2O_2.

Hydrogen peroxide plays a dual role (Lázaro, 2007). Cancer cells produce high amounts of H_2O_2. These increased levels of H_2O_2 result in DNA alterations, cell proliferation, apoptosis resistance, metastasis, angiogenesis, and hypoxia inducible factor 1(HIF-1) activation. Activation of HIF-1 plays crucial roles in apoptosis resistance, invasion/metastasis and angiogenesis. Many human cancers have over expressed HIF-1. On the other hand, hydrogen peroxide also induces apoptosis in cancer cells selectively and the activity of many anticancer drugs is mediated, at least in part by H_2O_2.

With increasing concentrations of cellular H_2O_2, its function gradually changes from cell signaling to cell malignant transformation to cell death (Lázaro, 2007). The mystery surrounding the different roles of hydrogen peroxide may be solved, at least partially, by looking at its electronic properties, which is described in a later section. Our impedance data suggest that the electronic properties (and consequent circuits) of H_2O_2 are dependent on its concentration. Our data also suggest that one has to take a serious look at another important contribution of H_2O_2, the preferential solvation of ions such as sodium and its consequences.

The direct administration of H_2O_2 for cancer treatment is controversial. However treatments using H_2O_2 generating systems such as high-dose intravenous vitamin C are less controversial. Since, with increasing concentrations of H_2O_2, its effect changes gradually from chemopreventive effects to carcinogenic effects to chemotherapeutic effects, the choice of antioxidant/prooxidant agents and their concentrations should be evaluated very carefully for use as chemopreventive and chemotherapeutic agents (Lázaro, 2007).

Oxyradical reactions catalyze the mitochondrial electron transfer chain to oxygen. While the energy advantage of oxygen metabolism favors selection of such developments, we have studied the contribution of periodic oscillation which peroxide brings to hydrated physico-chemical systems. Hydrogen peroxide exhibits a variety of oscillations (Koper, 1996; Mukouyama et al., 2001) under potentiostatic conditions.

Spatiotemporal oscillation in a system allows the far reaching electronics of alternating current circuits, long range signals, and oscillation amplifier behavior. Peroxide may allow these reactions to occur in the thin film hydration double layers throughout the cell and organism.

To highlight the importance of mitochondrial dysfunction in other major diseases, other than cancer, we have included two brief sections, Parkinson's disease and Alzheimer's disease,

Parkinson's Disease

Oxidative stress is implicated in the pathogenesis of Parkinson's disease (Olanow and Lieberman, 1992; Weiner et al., 2007). Reduced activity of Complex I of the electron transport chain and the gene mutations in Parkinson's disease have been discussed in great detail (Greenamyre et al., 1999; Parker et al., 1989; Schapira, 2004; Winklhofer and Haass, 2010). The hydroxyl radical can lead to lipid peroxidation and alter the structural integrity of neural membranes. Excess Fe^{2+}, also found in patients with Parkinson's disease, can reduce peroxide and produce HO. Dopamine undergoes autooxidation, producing HO, H_2O_2, semiquinone radical and finally a quinone (Olanow and Lieberman, 1992). Enzymatic metabolism of dopamine also produces H_2O_2.

$$Dopamine + O_2 \rightarrow Semiquinone + O_2^- + H^+ \tag{36}$$
$$Dopamine + O_2^- + 2H^+ \rightarrow Semiquinone + H_2O_2 \tag{37}$$
$$Semiquinone + O_2 \rightarrow Quinone + O_2^- + H^+ \tag{38}$$

Hydrogen peroxide is also produced when dopamine is metabolized enzymatically by monoamine oxidase (Olanow and Lieberman, 1992).

$$Dopamine + O_2 + H_2O ® 3,4 \ Dihydroxyphenylacetaldehyde + NH_3 + H_2O_2 \tag{39}$$

Alzheimer's Disease

Oxidative damage to both mtDNA and nDNA has been examined in several studies (Bubber et al., 2005; Castellani et al., 2002; Gibson et al., 2000; Mecocci et al., 1994). Significant 3-fold increase in the amount of 8-hydroxy-2'-deoxyguanosine in parietal cortex of Alzheimer's patients in mtDNA and a small significant increase in oxidative damage to nDNA have been observed (Mecocci et al., 1994). A deficiency in cytochrome c oxidase has been reported in Alzheimer's disease (Castellani et al., 2002). Significant decreases were observed in the activities of pyruvate dehydrogenase complex (−41%), isocitrate dehydrogenase (−27%), α-ketoglutarate dehydrogenase complex (−57%). There were good correlations between the diminished activity of these enzymes and the Clinical Dementia Rating (Bubber et al., 2005; Gibson et al., 2000). On the other hand the activities of succinate dehdrogenase (complex II) (+44%) and malate dehydrogenase (+54%) were increased. The activities of the other 4 Krebs cycle enzymes, citrate synthase, aconitase, succinate thiokinase, and fumarase were unchanged.

α-LIPOIC ACID

Lipoic acid, shown in Figure 1, is a very unique biological molecule. It has a carboxylic acid (pK_a 4.7) which is ionized at biological pH, and it has a cyclic disulfide or dithiolane ring (Baumgartner et al., 1996; Patel and Packer, 2008). It exists intracel-lularly as the reduced form, dihydrolipoic acid. The redox property, the antioxidant capacity and the fatty acid properties of lipoic acid account for its biological effects. We will describe its electronic contributions later in this chapter.

The dihydrolipoic acid can regenerate or recycle the antioxidants CoQ (ubiquinol), vitamins C and E, and glutathione. Both lipoic acid and its reduced form are known to scavenge reactive oxygen and nitrogen species such as H_2O_2, HO·, hypochlorous acid (HOCl), and peroxynitrite (ONOO⁻) (Packer et al., 1995; Patel and Packer, 2008).

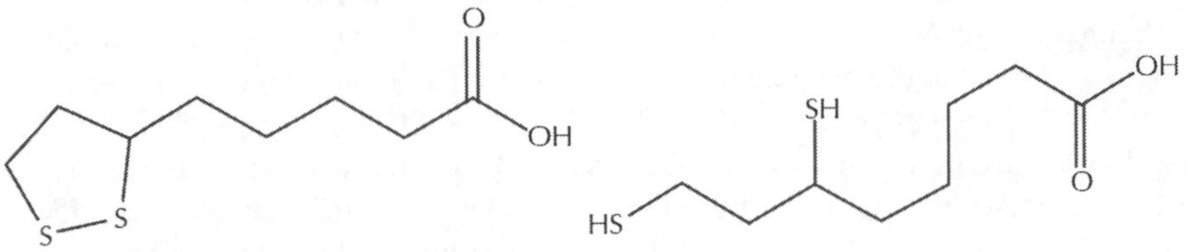

Figure 1. Alpha lipoic acid in its oxidized and reduced forms.

Compared to the inefficient transport of disulfides such as cystine that is needed in modulating GSH levels in cells, the efficient transport of lipoic acid and dihydrolipoic acid in and out of the both mitochondria and cells as well as mitochondrial β-oxidation have been attributed to its fatty acid properties, similar to that of octanoic acid (Patel and Packer, 2008). Lipoic acid can also cross the blood-brain barrier. The β-oxidation products of lipoic acid, the oxidized and reduced forms of bisnorlipoic acid and tetra-norlipoic acid may also have important redox and antioxidant biological effects.

The α-lipoic acid/dihydrolipoic acid couple is called a "universal antioxidant" be-cause it fulfills all the criteria mentioned earlier (Packer et al., 1995). The α-lipoic acid absorbed from the diet is readily converted into dihydrolipoic acid in many tissues. There is ample evidence to indicate the usefulness of this redox couple as a therapeu-tic agent for diabetes, ischemia-reperfusion injury, and heavy metal poisoning. The α-lipoic acid was found to protect hematopoietic tissues in mice from radiation dam-age (Ramakrishnan et al., 1992). It was also found that α-lipoic acid offered protection from radiation for children affected by the Chernobyl nuclear accident (Korkina et al., 1993), neurodegeneration, and HIV infection (packer et al., 1995; Patel and Packer, 2008). The α-lipoic acid scavenges hydroxyl radicals but is not effective against hy-drogen peroxide and superoxide radical. The reduction potential for the α-lipoic acid/ dihydrolipoic acid couple of –320 mV (Packer et al., 1995) or –290 mV (Voet and Voet, 1995) and the GSSG/GSH) couple of –240 mV indicate that dihydrolipoic acid can react with glutathione disulfide and regenerate glutathione (Packer et al., 1995). Thus lipoic acid helps to maintain GSH/GSSG ratio (about 100–10,000 times greater than other redox couples such as NAD⁺/NADH, and NADP⁺/NADPH), an estimate of redox state, in cells (Patel and Packer, 2008).

Treatment with lipoic acid increases the GSH levels in cells. This is explained by (1) facile transport of lipoic acid into cells, where it is reduced by NADH or NADPH dependent pathways to dihydrolipoic acid. (2) Dihydrolipoic acid is transported back into the extracellular media where it is oxidized by cystine regenerating lipoic acid and producing cysteine. (3) Compared to cystine, cysteine is more easily transported into the cell which aids the synthesis of GSH (Patel and Packer, 2008).

The pharmacokinetics of R-lipoic acid, reviewed recently, revealed a plasma level concentration, C_{max}, of 1.154 µg/ml from 1 g R-lipoic acid compared to the proposed therapeutic range of 10–20 µg/ml or 50–100 µM (Carlson et al., 2008). A dose of 600–800 mg sodium R-lipoate gave plasma levels of 8–18 µg/ml, which is within the therapeutic range. The upper limit suggested for therapeutic action of 45 µg/ml or 225 µM is reached by a dose of about 1.2 g of racemic-α-lipoic acid. The no adverse observed effect level (NOAEL) of racemic lipoic acid is considered to be 60 mg/kg body mass/day.

The oxidized form α-lipoic acid can undergo further oxidation at sulfur or get reduced. Therapeutic and energy production applications of this powerful antioxidant have also been explored extensively (Patel and Packer, 2008).

Located within the mitochondrial matrix is lipoic acid requiring enzymes: three α-keto acid dehydrogenase complexes, that catalyze the oxidative decarboxylation of α-keto acids such as pyruvate, α-ketoglutarate, and branched chain α-ketoacids (Voet and Voet, 1995). In organisms, hydrogen atom transfer and acyl group transfer take place in the oxidative decarboxylation of α-ketoacids with the aid of α-lipoic acid. The reversible redox reaction between α-lipoic acid and dihydrolipoic acid is thus a very important biochemical reaction. The reversible reduction to dihydrolipoic acid is favored by the presence of the ring strain in the 1,2-dithiolane ring of about 15 25 kJmol^{-1} (Patel and Packer, 2008).

The multienzyme complex, pyruvate dehydrogenase, consists of three enzymes, pyruvate dehydrogenase (E1), dihydrolipoyl transacetylase (E2), and dihydrolipoyl dehydrogenase (E3) (Voet and Voet, 1995). This enzyme complex participates in five sequential reactions during the conversion of pyruvate to acetyl-CoA. The lipoic acid is covalently linked to a ε-amino group of lysine residue via an amide linkage. These lipoic acid containing enzymes participate in four out of the five reactions.

The multienzyme complex, α-ketoglutarate dehydrogenase, also consists of three enzymes, α-ketoglutarate dehydrogenase (E1), dihydrolipoyl transsuccinylase (E2), and dihydrolipoyl dehydrogenase (E3) (Voet and Voet, 1995).

The branched chain α-ketoacid dehydrogenase is also a multienzyme complex resembling the other two enzymes mentioned above. These three enzymes have the same dihydrolipoyl dehydrogenase and employ the coenzymes thiamine pyrophosphate, lipoamide, FAD and the terminal oxidizing agent NAD$^+$ (Voet and Voet, 1995). The importance of lipoic acid in the energy metabolism is illustrated by these three enzymes.

SYNTHESIS OF PALLADIUM α-LIPOIC ACID COMPLEX

The synthesis of copper, zinc, and arsenic complexes of α-lipoic acid have been reported (Baumgartner et al., 1996; Strasdeit et al., 1995). Palladium α-lipoic acid complexes with (1:2) (Strasdeit et al., 1995) and 1:1 (Garnett, 1995a) stoichiometry have also been reported. Details of synthesis of palladium α-lipoic acid complex (1:1) using alkaline sodium lipoate and H_2PdCl_4 in basic conditions and its possible applications for treatment of tumors and psoriasis are also available (Garnett, 1995b; 1997; 1998).

INVESTIGATIONS USING PALLADIUM α-LIPOIC ACID COMPLEX FORMULATION

The different characteristics of this complex in comparison with that of the ligand are described in this section. These include *in vitro* cell lines studies, animal mitochondria, radiation protection, animal glioblastoma studies, human safety studies, voltammetry, and impedance spectroscopic studies.

Voltammetric Studies of Palladium α-Lipoic Acid Complex Formulation

The anodic oxidation of α-lipoic acid at a glassy carbon electrode and palladium α-lipoic acid complex interaction with double stranded DNA have been investigated using atomic force microscopy and voltammetry at highly oriented pyrolytic graphite electrode (Corduneanu et al., 2007; 2009). An important observation was the dissociation of the palladium α-lipoic acid complex at negative potentials and deposition of Pd(0) nanoparticle deposition. The application of a positive potential induced the oxidation of the palladium α-lipoic acid complex and the formation of a mixed layer of lipoic acid and palladium oxides.

Oxygen Radical Absorbance Capacity or ORAC analysis of Palladium α-Lipoic Acid Complex Formulation

The ORAC assay measures the oxygen radical absorbance capacity of a compound as compared to Trolox (vitamin E). These analyses carried out by Brunswick Labs, Inc., Wareham, Massachusetts gave the following normalized values as Trolox equivalent per gram: Vitamin A 1.6; Vitamin C 1.12; Vitamin E 1.0; α-Lipoic acid 1.4; and Palladium α-lipoic acid complex formulation 5.65. Thus the superior free radical scavenging capacity of the palladium α-lipoic acid complex formulation is obvious. This radical scavenging superiority of the metal complex compared to that of the ligand is similar to the antitumor activities observed for metal complexes (Maloň et al., 2001; Matesanz et al., 1999).

In vitro Cell line Studies using Palladium α-Lipoic Acid Complex Formulation

The effects of the palladium α-lipoic acid complex formulation on the following 8 different cell lines were examined at K.G.K. Synergize Inc, Canada. (1) Skin melanoma, human (SKMel-5); (2) Liver, hepatocellular carcinoma, human (Hep G2); (3) Lung, malignant melanoma, human (malme-3M); (4) Mammary gland, ductal carcinoma, human (MDA-MB 435); (5) Prostate, left supraclavicular lymph node carcinoma, human (LNCaP or lymph node carcinoma of the prostate): (6) Colon, colorectal adenocarcinoma, human (HT-29); (7) Human brain, glioblastoma; astrocytoma (U87); (8) Glioblastoma (U-251MG). Palladium α-lipoic acid formulation was administered at 3 different dosages and the cell growth was measured using [^{3}H] thymidine uptake after 24, 48, and 72 hr of culture. The data shown in Figure 2 is 48 hr after exposure. Palladium α-lipoic acid formulation was effective to varying degrees of cell death (statistically significant level of cell death), on the entire group of cell lines tested. The varying effectiveness appears to be a consequence of the particular cell lines used and their associated degree of anaplasia.

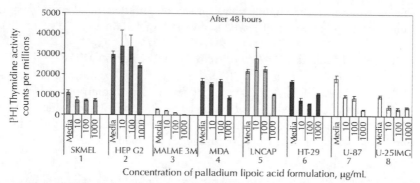

Figure 2. Effect of palladium α-lipoic acid complex formulation, after 48 hr, on (1) Skin melanoma, human (SKMel-5); (2) Liver, hepatocellular carcinoma, human (Hep G2); (3) Lung, malignant melanoma, human (malme-3M); (4) Mammary gland, ductal carcinoma, human (MDA-MB 435); (5) Prostate, left supraclavicular lymph node carcinoma, human (LNCaP): (6) Colon, colorectal adenocarcinoma, human (HT-29); (7) Human brain, glioblastoma; astrocytoma (U87); (8) Glioblastoma (U-251MG).

The effect of palladium lipoic acid complex formulation on the growth of canine osteosarcoma (CCL-183, D17) cells was also examined *in vitro* by a similar procedure. While the lowest dose did not have any significant effect, the higher doses of 100 and 1000 µg/ml inhibited the growth of the cells after 48 and 72 hr of culture.

We have examined the effects of palladium α-lipoic acid complex formulation on different cell lines from National Cancer Institute's (NCI) repository, breast cancer (adenocarcinoma, MCF-7), brain tumor (stage IV glioblastoma multiform, U-251Mg), lung (non-small cell carcinoma, A-549), and brain (astrocytoma, H-4), ovarian cancer (OVCAR-5) using NCI's cell screening protocol, sulforhodamine B assay. The results shown in Figure 3 indicate significant cell death.

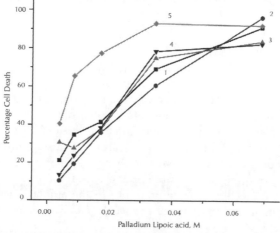

Figure 3. Effect of palladium α-lipoic acid complex formulation on (1) Breast cancer (adenocarcinoma, MCF-7), (2) brain tumor (stage IV glioblastoma multiform, U-251MG), (3) lung (non-small cell carcinoma, A-549), (4) brain (astrocytoma, H-4), and (5) ovarian cancer (OVCAR-5).

Whether we use [³H] thymidine uptake assay or suforhodamine B assay, significant reduction in cell growth is observed in a variety of cell lines.

In vivo Studies of Palladium α-Lipoic Acid Complex Formulation

These studies were carried out at Calvert Labs (previously known as Pharmakon USA), PA. The Ames/Salmonella Plate incorporation assay confirmed that the complex formulation is free of mutagenicity. Also acute oral toxicological studies showed no accumulation in or damage to any tissues. The median lethal dose, LD_{50}, in mice was found to be greater than the highest dosage tested, 5000 mg kg⁻¹.

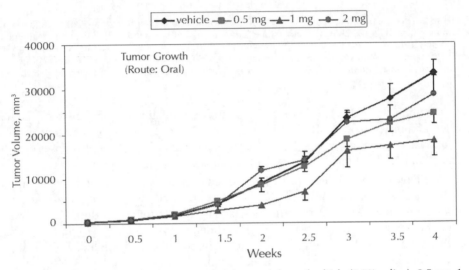

Figure 4. Glioblastoma tumor volume in nude mice, oral dose of vehicle (0.9% saline), 0.5 mg, 1 mg, and 2 mg palladium lipoic acid formulation per mouse daily for 4 weeks. To reduce clutter only one half of the error bar is shown.

The effectiveness of palladium lipoic acid formulation in halting the growth of glioblastoma cells *in vivo* was studied using nude mice. On day zero, 10 million U-87 MG tumor cells (glioblastoma-astrocytoma, human) from American Type Culture Collection (ATCC) were injected subcutaneously in the scruff of the neck of female Swiss nude mice (11 weeks old). When the tumors reached 200–400 mm³ in volume, the mice were divided into 8 groups of 10 mice. Four groups of mice were given daily intravenous (i.v.) doses of this formulation or placebo (0.9% saline); four groups were given orally by gavage (p.o.) doses of 0.5, 1.0, or 2.0 mg palladium lipoic acid complex per mouse for a total of 4 weeks or until the tumors became too large for the viability of the animal. Tumor volume was measured throughout the study, twice per week. The results are given in Figures 4 and 5.

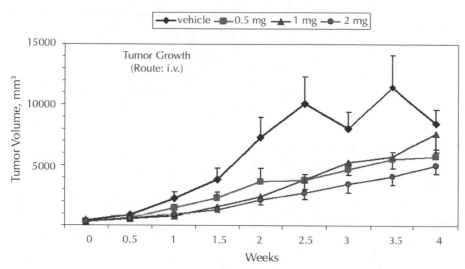

Figure 5. Glioblastoma tumor volume in nude mice, intravenous dose of vehicle (0.9% saline), 0.5 mg, 1 mg, and 2 mg palladium lipoic acid formulation per mouse daily for 4 weeks. To reduce clutter only one half of the error bar is shown.

A reduction in tumor size compared to the placebo treated group was seen in all groups of mice treated orally with the palladium lipoic acid complex. However the only statistically significant reduction was in the group treated with 1 mg/mouse.

When mice were treated intravenously with the palladium lipoic acid complex, a statistically significant reduction was observed in all treatment groups compared to the placebo group.

Clinical Veterinary Studies

The largest integrative cancer investigation of palladium lipoic acid complex formulation was an open-label, veterinary oncology program at CVS Angel Care Cancer Center, San Diego, CA, USA, with over 900 dogs enrolled. The dogs received palladium lipoic acid complex formulation as part of their chemotherapy, radiation and/ or surgical protocol at a dosage of 1ml/2.3kg. p.o. twice daily (equivalent human dose of approximately 40 ml per 70 kg.). The palladium lipoic acid formulation seemed most effective in the cases of solid tumors (such as soft tissue sarcoma, hemangiosarcoma, mast cell, transition cell carcinoma, lung, anal sac carcinoma, renal carcinoma, squamous cell carcinoma, fibrosarcoma, melanoma, meningioma, neuroblastoma, and mammary adenocarcinoma). Some of the most effective findings were apparent in the dogs suffering from osteosarcoma. The etiology of osteosarcoma in large dogs is considered identical to the disease progression in humans. While in canines the "standard of care" is limb amputation followed by chemotherapy, in human patients, limb–sparing surgery following tumor excision is performed (Ogilvie and Moore, 2000). The results summarized in Table 10 suggest the following. In this open labeled study, integrative palladium lipoic acid complex formulation support improved the animals' median survival time 62% (103 days more) compared to surgery alone (n = 11 and 162 respectively).

Table 10. Open label veterinary oncology study using Palladium α-Lipoic acid complex formulation.

Study	Median Survival, days
Amputation alone (n = 162)	165
Amputation with palladium lipoic acid complex formulation (n = 11)	268
Amputation with chemotherapy (n = 32)	288
Amputation with chemotherapy + palladium lipoic acid complex formulation (n = 17)	367

When the palladium lipoic acid complex formulation was added to the chemotherapeutic regimen (carboplatin + doxorubicin) the dogs exhibited a 27% longer median survival (79 days more). Furthermore, there was no significant difference (p = 0.30) in median survival time between dogs treated with amputation + palladium lipoic acid complex formulation versus those that were treated with amputation + the "standard of care" chemotherapy.

It was observed that following palladium α-lipoic acid complex formulation complementary support, chemotherapeutic animals' demonstrated improvements in various objective parameters (i.e., weight, anemia, liver and kidney function). In addition to these enhanced clinical parameters, a subjective owner quality of life survey resulted in an 86% improvement following the addition of palladium α-lipoic acid complex formulation adjunctive support.

Transient Ischemia Studies with Gerbils

Animal studies, carried out at Stony Brook University using adult male Mongolian gerbils (Charles River, Inc., New York), used as controls or treatment group, demonstrated that acute, post ischemic and prophylactic administration of palladium α-lipoic acid complex formulation limits ischemic damage. The animals were sacrificed after 72 hr after transient ischemia surgery (n = 6 per surgical group; n = 6 per sham group, each trial in triplicate) (Antonawich et al., 2004). The palladium α-lipoic acid complex formulation was administered intraperitoneally (IP) immediately after surgery, then once daily for 3 days. The control group received saline while the treatment group received 30, 50 or 70 mg/kg of palladium lipoic acid formulation.

Selective neural damage to hippocampal cornus ammon's field 1 (CA1) of the hippocampus neurons takes place after transient ischemic attack. An activation of the pro-apoptotic protein, bax, results in a shift in the dimerization ratio between the anti-apoptotic protein bcl-x1 and bax. The increase in bax results in the formation of pores in the mitochondrial membrane and these pores facilitate the passage of the electron transport chain protein, cytochrome c, into the cytosol along with the release of the pro-caspase 9. The initiator caspase 9 activates the caspase family of cysteine proteases and results in the destruction of the cell.

Following bilateral carotid artery occlusion in the Mongolian gerbil, palladium lipoic acid complex formulation treatment significantly protected CA1 hippocampal pyramidal cells from transient global ischemia at 30 ($p < 0.05$), 50 ($p < 0.01$), and 70 ($p < 0.05$) mg/kg per 24 hr.

A delayed application of the palladium α-lipoic acid complex formulation after 48 hr of ischemic attack had no significant effect in protecting CA1 cells. On the other hand, a delayed administration of palladium α-lipoic acid complex formulation after 6 hr of ischemic attack was as good as giving it immediately after ischemic attack in minimizing cell death.

Nesting behavior is an inherent behavior in Mongolian gerbils. Five minutes of carotid artery occlusion was sufficient to hinder or impair nesting behavior for approximately 3 days. The nesting behavior of gerbils was observed to improve significantly after treatment with palladium lipoic acid complex formulation (50 mg/kg every 24 hr ($P < 0.05$) and 30 mg/kg/24 hr at 24 and 72 hr after ischemia. There were no significant differences after the 70 mg/kg/24 hr treatment (n = 6 per group, each experiment was conducted in triplicate). The 70 mg/kg treated animals demonstrated excessive energy, thus ignoring the nesting material.

It was observed that preventive or prophylactic treatment with 10 mg/kg gerbil (based on allometric scaling from rodent to human, 10 ml human dosage) offered significant behavioral and morphological improvement from transient global ischemia. While behavioral improvement was apparent with 3 days of pretreatment, approximately one week of pre-treatment was necessary for morphological rescue.

In summary, treatment with palladium α-lipoic acid complex formulation after a transient ischemic attack offers behavioral improvement as well as morphological protection of CA1 hippocampal pyramidal cells.

Clinical Human Studies

A Phase I, palladium α-lipoic acid complex formulation "dose escalation safety study in normal individuals" (DESSTINI) was carried out at Stony Brook University, New York, USA. This study was divided into three tiers, each consisting of five subjects. Tier I, Tier II, and Tier III received oral dosages of the formulation, 10, 20, and 40 ml/day respectively for a period of 6 weeks. Subjects were monitored for the washout of palladium by examining the concentration of palladium in both blood serum and urine. Washout periods ranged from three to 17 weeks after cessation of the formulation. However, the washout period did not appear to be related to dosage.

No serious adverse effects occurred. The 15 subjects experienced a total of 24 AE (Adverse Events) during the study that was considered potentially, possibly or probably related to the study formulation. The events included: fatigue after cessation of oral dosage, diarrhea, worsening leg cramps, headache, increased urination, light-headedness, difficulty sleeping, and increased excitement. All AEs were adjudicated by the Data Safety and Monitoring Board (DSMB), with approximately 66% being anticipated or considered mild. Overall, the tolerability of all three tiers was 93.3% and the DSMB deemed the formulation to be safe. In addition, DSMB gave consent to continue with a subsequent, ongoing glioblastoma trial.

Mitochondrial Studies using Palladium α-Lipoic Acid Complex Formulation

The results with the transient ischemia studies with gerbils prompted us to investigate the influence of palladium lipoic acid complex on the activities of enzymes involved in energy production. In eukaryotes and prokaryotes, the most common mode of oxidative degradation of carbohydrates, fatty acids, and amino acids is by the citric acid cycle or the tricarboxylic acid cycle or Krebs cycle. The net reaction is

$$3NAD+ + FAD + GDP + Pi + acetyl\text{-}CoA \rightarrow 3NADH + FADH_2$$
$$+GTP + CoA + 2CO_2 \tag{40}$$

The liberated energy is used for ATP generation. The influence of palladium lipoic acid complex formulation has been investigated on the activities of four Krebs cycle enzymes, isocitrate dehydrogenase (ICDH), α-ketoglutarate dehydrogenase (α-KGDH), 6) succinate dehydrogenase (SDH), and 8) malate dehydrogenase (MDH). The other 4 enzymes of the Krebs cycle, citrate synthase, aconitase, succinyl-CoA synthetase, and fumarase as well as the enzyme, pyruvate dehydrogenase were not investigated. These investigations were carried out Amala Cancer Research Centre, Kerala, India (Sudheesh et al., 2009; 2010).

Table 11. Effect of Palladium Lipoic Acid Complex on the Activity of Krebs cycle Enzymes (Sudheesh et al., 2009).

Groups	ICDH	α-KGDH	SDH	MDH
Aged control	702.8±133.4	63.0±15.1	42.4±14.2	260.9±26.1
DL-α-lipoic acid (5 mg/kg body mass)	3428.2±348.9	189.0±50.4	73.4±21.2	386.1±265.5
Palladium lipoic acid complex, (0.38 mg/kg body mass)	3483.1±388.9	145.0±50.6	98.6±7.4	1305.7±56.4

Units: ICDH–μ moles of NAD + reduced/min/mg protein; α-KGDH–μ moles of NAD + reduced /min/mg protein; SDH–μ moles of 2,6-dichlorophenol indophenol sodium salt (DCPIP) reduced /min/mg protein; MDH–μ moles of NADH oxidized/min/mg protein

Table 12. Effect of Palladium Lipoic Acid Complex on the Activity of Respiratory Complexes (Sudheesh et al., 2009).

Groups	Complex I	Complex II	Complex III	Complex IV
Aged control	23.34±2.12	26.75±2.09	13.57±3.89	30.85±1.31
DL-α-lipoic acid (5 mg/kg body mass)	62.04±11.90	45.55±28.25	21.16±8.36	47.36±7.54
Palladium lipoic acid complex, (0.38 mg/kg body mass)	58.76±31.11	83.37±28.46	21.34 ±3.31	48.13±7.32

Units: Complex I–μ moles of DCPIP reduced/min/mg protein; complex II–μ moles of DCPIP reduced/min/mg protein; Complex III–μ moles of ferricytochrome-C reduced/min/mg protein; Complex IV–μ moles of ferrocytochrome-C oxidized/min/mg protein.

Male albino rats of Wistar strain and 24–26 months old were used to study their hearts. Each group had six rats and the animals were sacrificed at the end of 30 days of oral administration. The results for the Krebs cycle enzymes are given in Table 11.

The activities of ICDH, α-KGDH, SDH, and MDH, when compared to the aged control animals, indicate that administration of palladium lipoic acid complex formulation significantly increased the Krebs cycle enzyme activities. Both the α-lipoic acid and palladium lipoic acid complex increased the activities of the enzymes.

The results for the respiratory complexes I, II, III, and IV in aged rats is given in Table 11. The enhanced activities of complexes I, III, and IV were very similar for both the palladium α-lipoic acid formulation and the α-lipoic acid administered groups. The average values indicate a ~2.5-, 1.6-, and 1.6-fold increase for the activities of the complexes I, III, and IV when compared to the aged control group. In the case of complex II, the palladium α-lipoic acid complex formulation group had ~1.8-fold increases in the activity compared to the α-lipoic acid administered group. Sice the actual α-lipoic acid equivalent in the metal complex used for the oral administration is 13.2 times less than that of the ligand, we are tempted to conclude that the palladium α-lipoic acid complex is far superior to α-lipoic acid.

The major question which is a still an unsolved puzzle is the source of the superiority of the metal complex compared to that of the ligand. Since, we know from the pharmacokinetics of α-lipoic acid that the oral dose and the available plasma concentration are completely different, it is possible that the available plasma concentration for therapeutic effect in the presence of the palladium α-lipoic acid complex may be much higher than that of the α-lipoic acid only. Or somehow the chemistry of the transition metal is playing a dominant role in the enzymatic activity. It is interesting to note that the 2010 Noble Prize in chemistry was awarded to three palladium chemists, Richard F. Heck, Ei-ichi Negishi, and Akira Suzuki for "palladium-catalyzed cross-couplings in organic synthesis". While their methods are used by pharmaceutical industry for the synthesis of at least 25% of drugs, it is ironic that no palladium-based drugs are available in the market today. However, a palladium α-lipoic acid complex formulation had been available in the market for more than 15 years as a dietary supplement. The starting material in the synthesis of the palladium α-lipoic acid complex is palladium(II). If the final complex is also palladium(II), the chances are it has no paramagnetism because almost all palladium(II) complexes are diamagnetic. An ESR/EPR spectrum would help solve this puzzle. It is also possible, that under physiological conditions, if dihydrolipoic acid is produced through 1e reduction processes, then it is possible to have reactive intermediates with unpaired electrons. In such a case the electron spin may be involved in the enzymatic process. The impedance characteristics of the palladium α-lipoic acid as well as that of the α-lipoic acid, described later in this review, strongly suggest this possibility.

Male albino Wistar strain rats, both young and old, were also used to examine the declined mitochondrial antioxidant status in the myocardium of aged rats. The animals were administered orally for 30 days 0.38 mg lipoic acid and an equivalent dose of lipoic acid from the palladium lipoic acid complex formulation. The results for Mn SOD, CAT, and GPx are given in Table 13. As expected the young group had higher levels of all the three enzymes than that of the aged control group. Also the levels of Mn SOD, CAT, and GPx were higher with the palladium lipoic acid treated group than with the α-lipoic acid group.

Table 13. Effect of Palladium Lipoic Acid Complex on the Activities of Enzymes in the Heart Mitochondria of Rats (Sudheesh et al., 2010).

Groups	Mn SOD, U/mg protein	CAT U/mg protein	GP$_x$ U/mg protein
Aged control	12.23±2.33	4.05±0.82	22.70±4.24
Young control	16.34±1.17	9.61±1.17	73.24±20.65
DL-α-lipoic acid (0.38mg/kg body mass)	15.59±5.31	8.26±1.48	168.58±63.74
Palladium lipoic acid complex, 0.38 mg/kg body mass)	12.72±5.94	4.81±1.34	64.19±15.50

Mn SOD = manganese superoxide dismutase; CAT = catalase; and GPx = glutathione peroxidase

The results of the lipid peroxidation levels measured as thiobarbituric acid reacting substance (TBARS) and expressed as equivalents of MDA and the glutathione levels are given in Table 14.

Table 14. Lipid Peroxidation and GSH Level in the Heart Mitochondria of Aged Rats (Sudheesh et al., 2009).

Groups	Lipid peroxidation, n moles of MDA	GSH (moles/mg protein) formed/mg protein
Aged control	1.94±0.27	5.08±0.39
Young control	0.88±0.06	6.78±0.45
DL-α-lipoic acid (0.38mg/kg body mass)	1.68±0.19	5.20+0.18
Palladium lipoic acid complex, (0.38 mg/kg body mass)	1.17±0.09	6.42±0.35

As expected, the lipid peroxidation level was less and the glutathione level was higher in the young control compared to that of the aged control. There was no significant different difference between the aged control group and the α-lipoic acid group for both the lipoic peroxidation level and glutathione level. However, the lipid peroxidation was less and glutathione levels were higher with the palladium lipoic acid complex formulation group when compared to the aged control group.

The Krebs cycle and mitochondrial respiratory chain enzymatic studies data also indicate that the palladium lipoic acid complex is catalytically more active than that of the ligand, α-lipoic acid. This is similar to the observations of antitumor activity of iron (III) and copper (II) complexes of N[6]-benzylaminopurine derivatives and palladium (II) –benzyl bis (thiosemicarbazonate) where the complex had more activity than the ligand (Maloň et al., 2001; Matesanz et al., 1999).

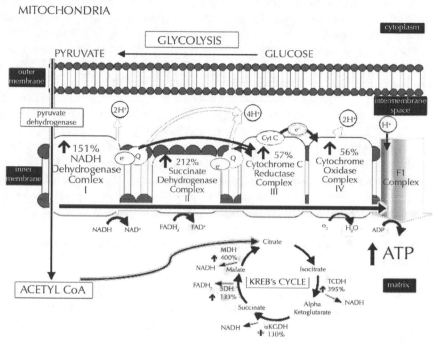

Figure 6. Influence of palladium α-lipoic acid complex formulation on Krebs cycle enzymes and mitochondrial electron transport chain complexes.

The influence of palladium α-lipoic acid complex formulation on the activities of some of the Krebs cycle enzymes and mitochondrial respiratory enzymes are summarized in Figure 6. The percentage increase in enzymatic activities are indicated by an upward arrow. The CoQ is pictorially shown twice for convenience to show that the electron transfer from complex I and complex II are to CoQ and then to complex III.

It is not clear at this time whether the antioxidant properties of the palladium *α-lipoic acid* complex formulation has anything to do with its enhancement of Krebs cycle and mitochondrial enzyme activities. Since, *α-lipoic acid* also enhances the activities of these enzymes but to a much less extent than palladium *α-lipoic acid* complex formulation, we are tempted to assume an interconnection between the two. It suggests that scavenging some free radicals by either *α-lipoic acid or palladium α-lipoic acid* complex formulation results in better performance of Krebs cycle and mitochondrial enzymatic activities.

It should be mentioned that succinate dehydrogenase which is part of the Krebs cycle as well as Complex II is known to be a tumor suppressor (Frezza and Gottlieb, 2009). The enhanced activity of this enzyme in the present studies correlates well with the inhibition of the growth of tumor cell lines studied. It is also suggested that the inhibitory effects of increased succinate due to mutated succinate dehydrogenase can be overcome by increased α-ketoglutarate. The activity of α-ketoglutarate is also increased substantially by palladium α-lipoic acid formulation.

In cancer cells lactate dehydrogenase and pyruvate dehydrogenase kinase are over expressed. Inhibition of lactate dehydrogenase by oxamate as well as suppression of pyruvate dehydrogenase kinase by dichloroacetate have been found to stimulate mitochondrial ATP production. Stimulation of mitochondrial oxidative metabolism has also been found to inhibit growth of cancer cell lines (Gogvadze et al., 2008). Even though the upregulation of rate limiting steps of glycolysis, the accumulation of mutations in in the mitochondrial genome, the hypoxia induced switch from mitochondrial respiration to glycolysis and the metabolic reprogramming resulting from the loss of function of fumarate hydratase, succinate and isocitrate dehydrogenases (Kroemer, 2006; McKnight, 2010) are not yet well understood, our Krebs cycle and mitochondrial enzyme activities data as well as the *in vitro* and *in vivo* cancer cell death data with palladium α-lipoic acid complex formulation support the notion that promotion of Krebs cycle and mitochondrial oxidative phosphorylation is a good approach for inhibiting cancer cell growth promoting wellness.

Protection from Radiation using Palladium α-Lipoic Acid Complex Formulation

These studies were also carried out at Amala Cancer Research Centre, Kerala, India (Menon et al., 2009; Ramachandran et al., 2010). *In vivo* radioprotection of cellular DNA was investigated using 6–8 weeks old Swiss albino mice exposed to 8 Gy radiation from ^{60}Co at a dose rate of 1.88 Gy per min. The palladium lipoic acid complex formulation dose (oral), administered 1 hr prior to radiation exposure, was 1ml/kg and 2 ml/kg body mass for two different groups. After 1 hr, the animals were sacrificed and their blood leukocytes and bone marrow were examined for DNA damage using alkaline single cell gel electrophoresis (alkaline comet assay) and compared with those with sham irradiation and with distilled water as control. The comet parameters, DNA in tail, tail length, tail moment and olive tail moment were analyzed. All the comet parameters were significantly reduced in animals administered with the palladium lipoic acid complex formulation 1 hr prior to the radiation exposure. This significant reduction in DNA damage in mice receiving palladium lipoic acid complex formulation with doses of 1ml/kg and 2 ml/kg body mass demonstrates the *in vivo* radioprotection ability of the palladium lipoic acid complex.

Antioxidant Activity, Prophylactic Effects of Palladium α-Lipoic Acid Complex Formulation Determined from Radiation Experiments

The antioxidant activity of palladium lipoic acid formulation was examined using 4 groups of Swiss albino mice, 6–8 weeks old, one group receiving distilled water and the other group palladium lipoic acid complex formulation, 2 ml/kg body mass. Two other groups similar to the earlier ones received radiation exposure, 6 Gy at the rate of 1.88 Gy per minute. The animals were sacrificed after 7 days of administration, and then radiation to two groups. Liver, kidney and brain were examined for lipid peroxidation, glutathione, super oxide dismutase, and glutathione peroxidase.

Table 15. Antioxidant Activity of Palladium α-Lipoic Acid Complex Formulation in Liver, Kidney and Brain of Mice (Menon et al., 2009).

Groups	Lipid peroxidation, nano moles of MDA formed/mg protein	GSH (nanomoles/ mg protein	Super oxide dismutase U/mg protein	Gutathione Peroxidase U/mg protein
(1) Liver				
With radiation	4.65±0.86	15.28± 1.73	8.36±0.63	14.07±2.87
With complex and with radiation	1.82± 0.36	21.46±3.30	10.90±0.50	22.44± 2.40
(2) Kidney				
With radiation	8.62±0.76	21.19±7.25	0.45±0.09	24.48±2.30
With complex and with radiation	5.44±0.98	42.61±4.61	0.98±0.29	39.28⊥10.28
(3) Brain				
With radiation	16.94±2.04	55.60±14.58	0.68±0.10	32.68±2.90
With complex and with radiation	11.42±0.79	126.81±9.43	1.08±0.09	44.10±2.90

6 Gy radiation, 7 days palladium lipoic acid complex formulation dose before irradiation, 2 ml/kg body mass

The differences between the distilled water group and the palladium lipoic acid treated group were not statistically significant for all the enzymes studied. On the other hand the data given in table for the group that received water and the group that received 2ml/kg body mass palladium lipoic acid complex formulation for 7 days prior to 6 Gy irradiation indicate remarkable differences in each case. The glutathione, glutathione peroxidase, and superoxide dismutase levels were higher and the lipid peroxidation levels measured as TBARS and expressed as equivalents of MDA were lower in liver, kidney and brain for the group that received palladium lipoic acid complex formulation for 7 days prior to 6 Gy irradiation. This clearly indicates the prophylactic protective effect of palladium lipoic acid complex formulation from radiation. It was also observed that 6 Gy radiation significantly reduced GSH, GPx, and SOD levels and increased the lipid peroxidation levels compared to the controls that received no radiation.

It should also be mentioned that the over expression of superoxide dismutases in tumor cells has been found to reduce malignant features of cancer cells such as tumor cell growth and metastasis (Lázaro, 2007). It is not clear whether these anticancer effects are due to the catalytic conversion of O_2^- to H_2O_2 or due to the increased concentration of H_2O_2. The reversal of this effect by over expression of catalase and glutathione peroxidase supports the concept of increased levels of H_2O_2.

Radiation induced significant lowering of antioxidant levels. Administration of palladium lipoic acid complex formulation for 7 days, at a dose rate of 2 ml/kg body mass, kept nearly the same levels of antioxidants as the ones that received no radiation. It is not clear at this time whether this observation is the due to the ability of the tissues to counteract the ROS generated from radiation injury or the ability of the tissue to regenerate the cellular antioxidants in response to radiation injury.

Oral administration of palladium lipoic acid complex formulation to male Balb/C mice, 6–8 weeks old, exposed to sub lethal 6 Gy γ-radiation enhanced endogenous spleen colony formation. Also alkaline comet assay showed that nuclear DNA comet parameters such as percent DNA tail, tail length, tail moment, and olive tail moment of the bone marrow and spleen cells increased after the whole body radiation of 8 Gy. These DNA damages as well as mortality rates were reduced by the administration of palladium lipoic acid complex formulation. Also it aided in the recovery from radiation induced weight loss in mice surviving after 8 Gy radiations.

These studies, carried out at Amala Cancer Centre coupled with the toxicity and cell line studies suggest the following. Unlike toxic platinum chemotherapy agents, the commercially available palladium α-lipoic acid complex formulation is safe and nontoxic. Its oral administration can be continued indefinitely. It is specially designed to provide energy for compromised body systems and promote overall health. It facilitates aerobic metabolism much more than that of α-lipoic acid, by significantly enhancing enzymatic activity of isocitrate dehydrogenase, α-ketoglutarate dehydrogenase, succinate dehydrogenase and malate dehydrogenase at the Krebs cycle and mitochondrial complexes I, II, III, and IV of the electron transport chain in the heart of aged rats (Sudheesh et al., 2009). It also enhances the activities of catalase and glutathione peroxidase more than that of α-lipoic acid. The level of glutathione also was significantly improved and the level of lipid peroxidation was decreased in the heart mitochondria of aged rats (Sudheesh et al., 2010). It also protects DNA from radiation.

It must be pointed out that preventive or prophylactic effects observed in these radiation experiments are consistent with the observations of similar effects in gerbils after induction of transient global ischemia (Antonawich et al., 2004).

DIODE OR TUNNEL-DIODE BEHAVIOR IN BIOLOGICAL SYSTEMS

To gain an understanding of the electronic aspects of biological functions such as cell signaling, long-range electron transfer, and biochemical oscillations in ATP production (Field and Gyorgyi, 1993), one needs at least a rudimentary knowledge of the solid state electronics. A very brief attempt is made here to introduce the concepts.

A diode material is normally doped with one impurity atom per 10 million semiconductor atoms. This results in a relatively wide depletion region. When the potential applied is large enough to overcome the potential barrier of the junction, conduction takes place (Fink, 1975). In a tunnel diode, on the other hand, the doping level is about thousand impurity atoms per ten million semiconductor atoms. This results in an extremely narrow depletion region. Compared to a normal junction diode, the tunnel diode exhibits an unusual current-voltage characteristic curve, a negative differential resistance (NDR) region (Fink, 1975).

Protein film voltammetry data (Ackrell et al., 1993; Elliot et al., 2002; Gwyer et al., 2005; Hurst et al., 1996; Léger and Bertrand, 2008; Pershad et al., 1999; Sucheta et al., 1992; Van Hellemond et al., 1995) have indicated that the catalytic activity of enzymes, especially electron transport enzymes involved in the respiratory chains, may be optimized at certain electrochemical potentials as well as pH. This technique allows the rate of catalysis to be measured accurately as a function of the applied potential (the driving force). Interesting current-potential curves were observed for several enzymes in which the optimum rate occurs at a particular potential and the rate thereafter drops in spite of the increase in the thermodynamic driving force. We must keep in mind that the active site, such as in flavins and Mo-bismolybdopterin guanine dinucleotide cofactors, may be the oxidized state, intermediate state or reduced state and these states may have their own characteristic affinities for the substrate before the reaction and for the product after the reaction. This offers the possibility for catalytic pathway by several different routes (Léger and Bertrand, 2008). The electrochemical potential controls the rate and thermodynamics of electron supply for the different states. A unique current-potential curve, often observed for respiratory enzymes such as succinate:ubiquinone oxidoreductase (complex II of mitochondria, with active site FAD and three Fe-S clusters)) and molybdoenzyme nitrate reductases, is interpreted in terms of a "potential dependent gate that bars catalysis of the reverse process" (Léger and Bertrand, 2008). This intrinsic property of the enzyme is similar to the behavior of a tunnel diode with a characteristic NDR region observed in the current potential curves. In SDH, the group responsible for this behavior is attributed to the active site FAD. Similar to the electrochemical potential, the membrane provides a variable potential in the form of the ratio of quinone to hydroquinol (Q/QH_2). This potential can be further tuned depending on the nature of the quinone present. At least three different quinones (ubiquinone being the dominant redox carrier during aerobic growth and menaquinone and demethylmenaquinone dominating under anaerobic conditions) are synthesized depending on the aerobicity.

An attenuation of the reductive activity at low potential was also observed for the mitochondrial enzyme, the "Fp" subcomplex of Complex I. This is understandable because, mitochondrial complex I (NADH-Ubiquinone oxidoreductase) also houses a flavin at the site of NADH oxidation and nine iron-sulfur clusters.

Our reason for including this section on tunnel diode behavior in biological systems is to indicate the "ratchet" or biased nature of enzymes systems depending on the potential and pH allowing possible feedback fine control of respiratory rates. We have demonstrated the ability of an enzyme to "rectify" electron flow at potentials close to electrochemical reversibility by studying impedance characteristics of simple biological molecules that are an integral part of the enzyme. For example, some of these enzymes have FAD, and Mo and we had shown in impedance studies the NDR characteristics of FAD as well as Mo-peroxo complexes (Krishnan and Garnett, 2006).

IMPEDANCE SPECTROSCOPY

We have utilized the technique of impedance spectroscopy for understanding solute-solvent interactions, 'π–way' conduction, ion pair formation, water-structure enforced ion pair formation, potential induced and solvent mediated ion pair formation at the double layer, and semiconduction characteristics of simple biological molecules (Krishnan and Garnett, 2006; Krishnan et al., 2007a, 2007b; 2008a, 2008b, 2008c, 2008d; 2009a, 2009b). Simple molecules such as arginine, histidine, lysine, FAD, riboflavin, cysteine, lidocaine hydrochloride, α-lipoic acid, and hydrogen peroxide exhibit negative differential resistance, which is a characteristic of diode or tunnel diode behavior. This technique has not been utilized extensively for discovery of drug molecules. Our technique of exploring drug discovery is based on impedance characteristics and self assembly and differs from the conventional drug discovery techniques. A brief outline of this technique (Lasia, 1999; Macdonald and Johnson, 2005) is given below.

In impedance measurements, a perturbing sinusoidal voltage $E = E_0 \sin(\omega t)$ is applied at angular frequency ω (2π f, where f in the conventional frequency in Hz) to the electrode system. The response is analyzed in terms of the resultant current $I = I_0 \sin(\omega t + \Phi)$, where Φ represents a characteristic phase angle shift. The corresponding complex impedance spectrum $Z(\omega)$, obtained by varying the signal frequency ω, is expressed in terms of the displacement of the vector $Z(\omega)$. In the plane of Cartesian coordinates, an impedance is expressed by its real (Z') and imaginary (Z'') parts, that is $Z(\omega) = Z' - jZ''$. The modulus $|Z|$ and phase angle Φ of $Z(\omega)$ can be obtained from $|Z| = [Z'^2 + Z''^2]^{1/2}$ and $\Phi = \tan^{-1}[Z''/Z']$, respectively. Over a frequency bandwidth of interest, the impedance spectrum can be represented in various ways; typically in the well known Nyquist or Cole-Cole plot (Z'' as the Y-axis and Z' as the X-axis for the range of frequencies explored at a fixed potential) or Bode plots ($|Z|$ and Φ vs. $\log\omega$). The impedance spectrum reflects dialectic behavior, oxidation-reduction reactions and mass migration across the electrochemical interfaces, that are determined by the electrical and chemical properties of the corrosive medium, and the electrode materials. The impedance spectrum can also be considered as a "fingerprint", which is related to the transient behavior of a specific electrochemical interface. In simple terms, impedance is like a frequency dependent generalized resistance. In electrochemistry, the imaginary impedance is almost always capacitive and therefore negative. Phase angle is a balance between capacitive and resistive components. For a pure resistance $\Phi = 0$ and for pure capacitance $\Phi = \pi/2$.

The electrochemical impedance measurements reported in this chapter were made using and EG & G PARC Model 303A SMDE trielectrode system (mercury working electrode, platinum counter electrode and Ag/AgCl saturated KCl reference electrode) along with Autolab ecochemie. The measurements were carried out in the range 1,000 Hz to 30 mHz. The amplitude of the sinusoidal perturbation was 10 mV.

In our present studies we have explored the behavior of mercury in both the negative and positive range of potentials because in natural biochemical systems we have both positively and negatively charged surfaces at close distances where water molecules will be subjected to competing influences from the electric field of these charged centers as well as the charges from the electrolytes. We have used mercury as the working electrode because it allows us to get reproducible surface for our studies by using a fresh drop each time. Compared to using any other metal, fresh mercury drops allow repetitions and reproducibility better and easy. For example if we corrode a metal, it is not easy to clean and get the noncorroded surface again and again for each experiment.

Electronic Properties of H_2O_2

All living systems exhibit dynamical spatio-temporal periodicities (Field and Gyorgyi, 1993). The dynamical oscillations observed in the electrochemical passivation of metals and used as models for biological oscillations are attributed to the negative Faradaic impedance of the electrode (Koper, 1996).

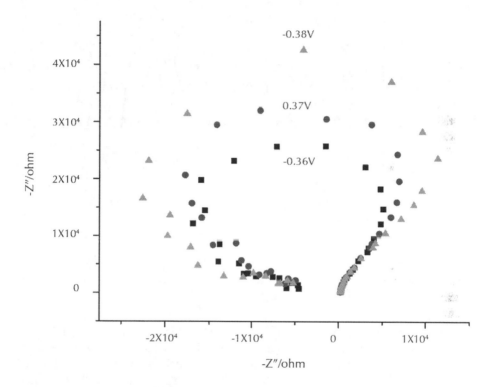

Figure 7. Nyquist plot for 0.10 M KCl, 88 mM hydrogen peroxide at pH 4.5.

Potential or current oscillations of different types have been observed in hydrogen peroxide systems at high concentrations and high acidities (Mukouyama et al., 1999; 2001). The coupling of two or more chemical oscillations occurring at different locations, an important aspect for signal transport or communication in biological systems has also been duplicated in an electrochemical system involving hydrogen peroxide (300–400 mM in 0.5 M H_2SO_4) (Fukushima et al., 2005). To simulate biological systems, we had focused our studies on oscillatory behavior at low concentrations of peroxide and at low acidities. We had established and reported (Krishnan et al., 2008d) the concentration range needed to exhibit oscillations in the presence of NaCl.

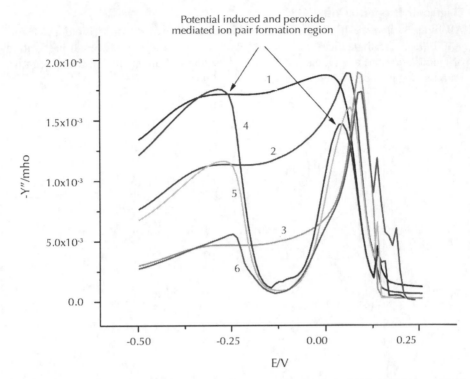

Figure 8. Admittance comparison of 0.10 M NaCl, pH 5.25 1) 500 Hz 2) 250 Hz 3) 100 Hz and 0.10 M NaCl and 88 mM H_2O_2, pH ~ 6.0 4) 500 Hz 5) 250 Hz 6) 100 Hz.

Here we report, as an example, the impedance behavior of 88 mM H_2O_2 in 0.10 M KCl at pH 4.5. It is obvious that negative differential resistance (NDR), a characteristic of tunnel diode behavior is observed at the potentials shown in Figure 7. It was observed that NDR occurred at 3.72 Hz, 2.90 Hz, and 2.24 Hz at potentials of –0.36 V, –0.37 V, and –0.38 V.

We had carried out detailed cyclic voltammetric and impedance investigations of aqueous solutions of H_2O_2 in the presence of NaCl to understand Parkinson's disease (Krishnan et al., 2008c, 2008d). Some relevant points from these studies of hydrogen peroxide in aqueous sodium chloride are illustrated here

The negative impedance observed in Figure 7 is also seen at hydrogen peroxide concentrations as small as 10 mM and is sensitive to pH. At higher acidities, the potential at which NDR occurred shifted to more anodic potentials. Also, as the hydrogen peroxide concentration is decreased, the potential at which NDR occurred shifted to more anodic potentials. The frequency at which NDR occurred also depended on the potential and concentration of hydrogen peroxide. We have also observed sensitivity for chloride.

The importance of impedance measurements in understanding solute-solvent interactions is vividly illustrated in Figure 8. By comparing the admittance measurements of NaCl in the presence and absence of H_2O_2 at 3 different frequencies, it is obvious that the sodium and chloride ions are forming ion pairs under the influence of H_2O_2 at potentials in the range –0.25 to 0.0V. This results in a decrease in admittance.

To understand the admittance behavior of small amounts of H_2O_2 in 100 mM NaCl, it is worthwhile to look at its relevant aqueous solution properties. The activity coefficient of hydrogen peroxide in sodium chloride and sodium sulfate solutions, determined using partition experiments with iso-amyl alcohol (Livingston, 1928), was found to be less than unity. This salting in effect was later confirmed for several electrolytes (Gorin, 1935). These results suggest that water molecules surrounding the sodium ions were displaced by peroxide. This was attributed to the higher dipole moment of hydrogen peroxide compared to that of water. On the other hand, it was concluded from solubility measurements in hydrogen peroxide-water mixtures that smaller ions such as Li^+ and Na^+ were solvated by water and K^+, Rb^+, and Cs^+ were preferentially solvated by hydrogen peroxide (Everhard et al., 1962).

The properties such as (1) deviations from Raoult's law, (2) finite heat of mixing and (3) finite volume changes on mixing for hydrogen peroxide-water mixtures indicate an enhancement of either the number or the force of attractions between the two molecules on forming the solutions (Everhard et al., 1962). The decrease in conductance of alkali chlorides in hydrogen peroxide-water mixtures correlated well with the changes in viscosity. These results could not give any indication as to when the solvation of an ion changes from water to hydrogen peroxide (Thomas and Maass, 1958).

It should be mentioned that the studies mentioned above were not at low hydrogen peroxide concentrations. The low concentrations employed in admittance measurements are comparatively low and closer to biological concentrations. However, the data are more complicated because of the double layer and changing potentials as well as frequencies. The results do suggest an ion-dipole interaction with peroxide preferentially, especially when the applied potential is about to change from negative to positive. We had explained these results using the concept of "potential induced and peroxide mediated ion pair formation" (Krishnan et al., 2008d).

These indicate the role of peroxide not only in neuron degeneration but also in controlling of electronic circuits involved in neuronal communications. The role of the stimulator implants seems to be to counteract the role of the new circuits caused by neuronal degeneration. Also the variability of the electronic circuit or signaling produced by hydrogen peroxide depending on the concentration, the ion-dipole interaction with water and/or peroxide, and the potential available may partially explain the multiple roles of hydrogen peroxide in biological systems.

Before closing this section, we want to add a comment on another related topic, "mechanisms for DNA charge transport". This hot subject has been investigated extensively during the last 15–20 years (Genereux and Barton, 2010). Numerous arguments regarding the nature of DNA as to whether it is a wire, a semiconductor or an insulator have been proposed and discussed. The role of the π-stacked base pairs in DNA has also been investigated in detail. In our impedance measurements with aqueous lidocaine hydrochloride, we could see the influence of "π-way" conduction (Krishnan et al., 2009a). This technique has not been explored in detail in the case of DNA. More importantly our results with H_2O_2 indicate its unique electronic properties. These properties are very sensitive to its concentration, electrolyte, frequency and available potential. Our results along with that of salting in effect of peroxide by electrolytes suggest a mechanism by which an electrolyte can pass though membranes as an ion pair solvated by peroxide. The solvation effect of peroxide on DNA bases and the DNA charge transport in the presence of small amounts of peroxide need to be investigated to get a deeper understanding of this important field. Unfortunately the varying and tremendous influences of peroxide on these processes such as ion pair formation, preferential solvation by peroxide and its unique electronic properties have been ignored or neglected so far. We hope physicists, chemists and biologists will take a serious look at these properties of hydrogen peroxide in relation to their investigations.

Modulation of Electronic Properties of Simple Molecules by Transition Metals

The target of most metal based drugs is DNA (Dabrowiak, 2009; Sherman and Lippard, 1987). Targets other than DNA that have recently been reviewed include a gold(I) carbene complex interacting with mitochondrial membrane (Fricker, 2007). However, the focus of our work was to improve mitochondrial enzyme activity by selecting a simple molecule involved heavily in mitochondrial enzyme activities and modulate its enzymatic activity by complexing with the metal palladium. Palladium (II), Platinum(II), and gold(III) have the same number of d^8 electrons. We believe strongly that by improving the mitochondrial enzyme activities, we can improve the quality of life, can induce apoptosis, and thus ward off many diseases including cancer.

The technique we have utilized to investigate the modulation of properties of simple molecules by transition metals is the electrochemical impedance technique. While we have investigated many molecules using this technique (Krishnan and Garnett, 2006; Krishnan et al., 2007a, 2007b; 2008a, 2008b, 2008c, 2008d; 2009a, 2008b) the electronic properties of hydrogen peroxide are briefly included in this chapter because of its unique electronic properties and importance in biological systems.

Figure 9(a) gives the Nyquist plot for differing concentrations of H_2O_2 in 0.10 M NaCl at –0.28 V. This may be compared with that in Figure 7 for 88 mM H_2O_2 in 0.10 M KCl. The results are similar in that they both are characterized by NDR. However, the electronic circuits are subtly different because of their own unique shapes. The data for 88 mM H_2O_2 in 0.10 M NaCl shown as almost a dot in Figure 9(a) are shown in the expanded scale in Figure 9(b). Also the frequencies at which the NDR takes place as well the potentials are slightly different. The data at for 8.8 mM H_2O_2 indicate double capacitance and are different from the NDR for other concentrations. Even 8.8 mM H_2O_2 exhibits NDR behavior by changing the potential. It is shown here to show the sensivity of NDR to the applied potential as well as to the concentration of H_2O_2. The modulation by molybdenum in the peroxo complex at a higher acidity is impressive (Figure 9(c)). We had discussed earlier the diode like behavior of the molybdoenzyme nitrate reductases (Sucheta et al., 1992).

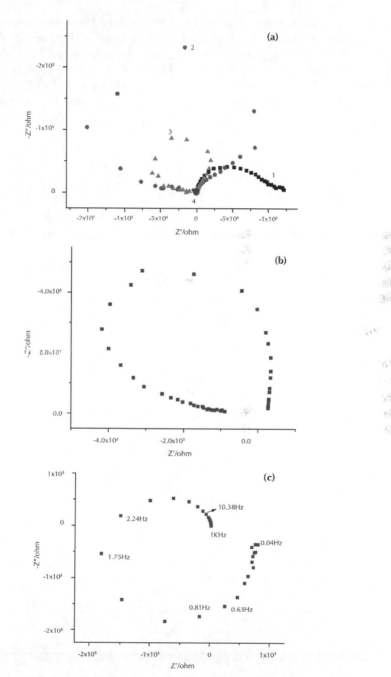

Figure 9. (a) Nyquist plot in 0.10M NaCl, pH 5.2, for different H_2O_2 concentrations, mM (1) 8.8 (2) 26.4 (3) 35.2 (4) 88 and (b) Expanded curve 4 for 88mM H_2O_2 in 0.10M NaCl; Potential applied is –0.28 V for and b. (c) Modulation of peroxide impedance by molybdenum. Nyquist plot for 0.005M $H_2Mo_2O_3(O_2)_4$ (obtained by dissolving Mo metal in peroxide), pH 1.87, 0.15V.

Similarly the impedance spectra for α-lipoic acid and its modulation by complexing with palladium are shown in Figure 10. While α-lipoic acid exhibits NDR and shows impedance in only 3 quadrants, it is extended to 4 quadrants and much more smoothly by complexation with palladium. Of course the NDR behavior can be optimized by slightly tweaking the applied potential. This enhancement in NDR behavior may be compared to the similar enhanced Krebs cycle and mitochondrial respiratory chain enzymatic activities of the palladium α-lipoic acid compared to that of the ligand.

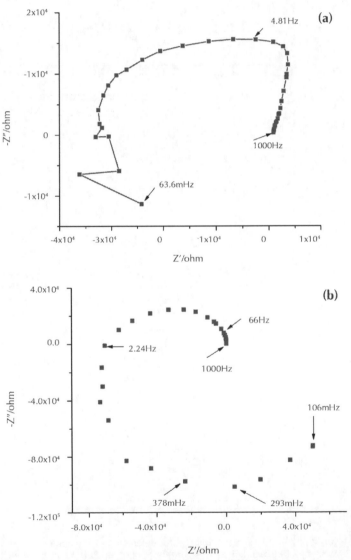

Figure 10. (a) Nyquist plot for 0.0373 M sodium lipoate, −1.15V, pH 7.79, NDR at 4.81Hz. (b) Modulation of lipoate impedance by palladium in 0.0373M palladium α-lipoic acid (1:1 complex) in 0.1792 M NaCl, −1.18V, pH 7.78, NDR at 66Hz.

Before concluding this chapter, we want to include the electronic properties of a few other simple biological molecules such as lysine, FAD, cysteine, and histidine. Their involvement in the mitochondrial electron transport chain is included in a later section of this chapter. The data in Figures 9–12 are intended to demonstrate the usefulness of the impedance technique to understand the electronic character of simple biological molecules. These also illustrate the sensitivity of the electronic character for concentration, pH, surface area, applied potential, and the frequency at which the NDR is observed.

The Nyquist plots for L-lysine as well its modulation by molybdenum are shown in Figure 11.

L-lysine, a dibasic amino acid with a butyl ammonium side chain has pK_1(α-COOH), pK_2(α-NH_3^+, and pK_3(ϵ-NH_3^+) values of 2.16, 9.06, and 10.54 respectively so that it is positively charged at physiological pH. Elevated levels of lysine in blood and urine have been linked to mental and physical retardation. Histones have a large number of lysine residues and its positive charge promotes interaction with negatively charged phosphodiester linkages of DNA. Acetylation of lysine weakens this electrostatic interaction and loosens the chromatin structure allowing gene expression. The reversible histone acetylation and deacetylation reactions control the activation and inactivation of gene expression.

Another important aspect of this system is the fact α-lipoic acid is linked to lysine by an amide bond in the multienzyme complexes of pyruvate dehydrogenase, α-ketoglutarate dehydrogenase and branched chain α-ketoglutarate dehydrogenase. Thus both α-lipoic acid and lysine have heavy involvement in the electronic aspects of the enzymatic process.

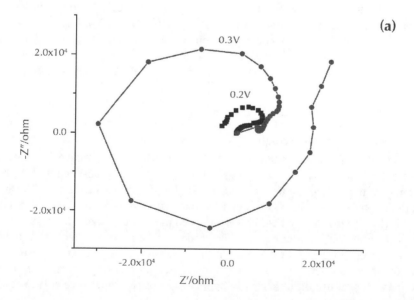

Figure 11. *(Continued)*

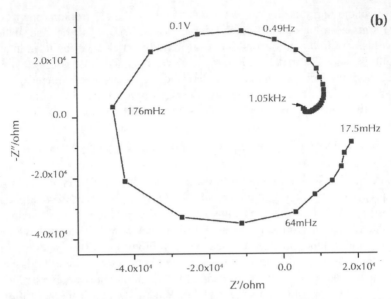

Figure 11. Nyquist plot for (a) 0.10 M lysine, 0.021 M HCl, pH 9.6; (b) 0.095 M Na_2MoO_4, 0.19M lysine, 0.12 M HCl, pH 8.9.

The impedance data on the interaction between sodium molybdate and FAD are shown in Figure 12. The FAD, a cofactor in a number of enzymes, when bound to a protein can exist as it's fully oxidized flavoquinone form, its 1e reduced flavosemiquinone form or its 2e reduced flavohydroquinone form.

It is well known that the orientation of the flavin and adenine groups at the electrode surface depends on the concentration of FAD (Roscoe, 1996). The cyclic voltammogram of FAD is highly concentration dependent. The same behavior is reflected in the impedance data shown in Figure 12(a). The data in Figure 12(b) indicate the potential dependence of its electronic character. The NDR is observed only at select potentials.

Another important aspect of this system is the fact FAD is also an integral part of the multienzyme complexes of pyruvate dehydrogenase, α-ketoglutarate dehydrogenase and branched chain α-ketoglutarate dehydrogenase.

An important group present in complex I, II, and III is the cysteine group. We have carried out extensive investigation of this in the presence and absence of molybdate (Krishnan et al., 2008a, 2008b). A typical example is shown in Figure 13. The pH dependence on the observed NDR is vividly demonstrated in Figure 13(a). The data in Figure 13(b) demonstrate that either the adsorbed molecule is regenerated for a repeat cycle or that the double layer near the electrode surface remains intact. In all our experiments a fresh mercury drop is used at the start of every impedance measurement. One of our major concerns was that the applied potential was very near the passivation of mercury. Repeat use of mercury giving nearly identical impedance curve seems to validate the procedure.

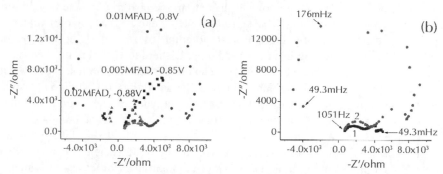

Figure 12. Nyquist plot for (a) molybdate-FAD system, 0.02 M molybdate, pH 6.5 and (b) 0.02 M Na_2MoO_4, 0.01 M FAD, (1) –0.7 V, (2) –0.8V.

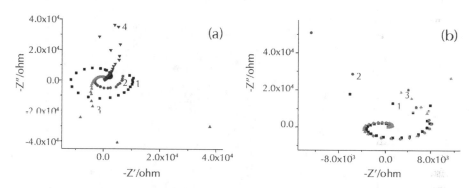

Figure 13. Nyquist plot for 0.1M cysteine-sodium molybdate, (a) 0.3 V, pH (1) 5.22 (2) 5.79 (3) 6.91 (4) 9.34 and (b) 0.25 V (1) Fresh Hg drop (2) Repeat with the used Hg drop (3) Repeat second time with the used Hg drop.

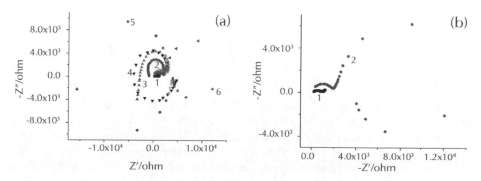

Figure 14. Nyquist plot for 0.177 M histidine-sodium molybdate, 0.067 M NaOH, pH 9.60, (a) (1) –0.1 V (2) 0.0V (3) 0.03 V (4) 0.05 V (5) 0.07 V (6) 0.09 V and (b) expanded scale for (1) –0.1 V (2) 0.09 V

L-Histidine, an essential amino acid, has an aromatic nitrogen-heterocyclic im-idazole side chain with $pK_1(\alpha\text{-COOH})$, $pK_2(\alpha\text{-NH}_3^+)$, and $pK_3(\text{imidazole})$ values of 1.78, 8.97, and 5.97 respectively. Its isoelectric point (pH) is 7.47. Decarboxylation of histidine yields the neurotransmitter histamine. Histamine occurs in mast cells and basophils of blood. Histamine binds to H_1 receptors of the smooth muscle of bronchi which contracts leading to breathing difficulties (as in Asthma). Histidine is also an important component of enzymes such as carbonic anhydrase. The histidine residues in cytochromes a, b, c stretch both on the cytosolic side as well as on the matrix side. The electronic character of this important molecule is exemplified in Figures 14 and 15. The influence of the surface is exemplified in Figure 15. It is clear the NDR or diode or tunnel diode characterisitic is sensitive to potential as well as surface area.

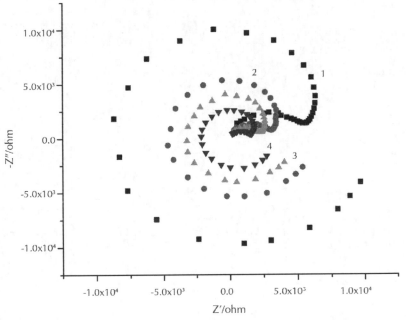

Figure 15. Nyquist plot for 0.177 M histidine-sodium molybdate, 0.067 M NaOH, pH 9.60, 0.05 V, influence of surface area of mercury drop, mm^2 (1) 0.011 (2) 0.017 (3) 0.022 (4) 0.031.

These impedance data provide information on the instabilities or bifurcations and distinguish between saddle-node and Hopf bifurcations. However these aspects are not included in this chapter. Only the importance of the electronic properties of these mol-ecules and its modulation by molybdenum to demonstrate the diode or tunnel diode characteristics of this system. The unique impedance behavior reflects periodicities and suggest global electronic coupling. Our data suggest that we have to include the electronic properties of these molecules to complement the enzymatic process.

Thus we have made a brief attempt to demonstrate the resourcefulness of the im-pedance technique as illustrated in Figures 7–15, to understand the electronic properties of biological molecules. The negative differential resistance characteristics are demonstrated vividly and support the conclusions drawn from protein film voltammetry regarding the tunnel diode characteristics of some enzymes. Our data presented here raise the possibility that some of these simple molecules that are present in the enzymes may be the ones that are exhibiting the unique electronic properties in biological systems.

SELF-ASSEMBLY OF PALLADIUM α-LIPOIC ACID COMPLEX

The phase microscopy pictures (300X) of 1.34×10^{-2} M and 2.7×10^{-4} M palladium α-lipoic acid complex (1:1) are shown in Figure 16. The self-assembly of the complex even at very dilute solutions is remarkable. No self-assembly was observed for sodium lipoate even at concentrations as high as 0.20 M.

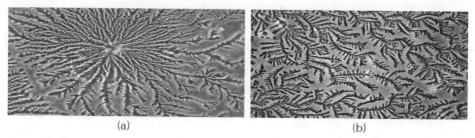

(a)   (b)

Figure 16. Phase microscopy 300X (a) 1.34×10^{-2} M and (b) 2.7×10^{-4} M palladium α-lipoic acid complex.

A long flexible arm that can oscillate a distance of ~200 Å produced by the binding of a lysine residue in the protein to the lipoyl group of E2 in 2-oxoacid dehydrogenases is utilized during the catalytic cycle (Patel and Packer, 2008). It is obvious that the self assembled palladium α-lipoic acid complex can make this process more facile.

It must be pointed out that in homogeneous systems, autocatalytic reactions and diffusion resulting from chemical instabilities lead to the formation of spiral waves and other concentration patterns of spatiotemporal phenomena. Our data suggest that the propagation of electrical signaling among the packing units and extending to long distances is viable by such self-assembled systems. Thus the self-assembly of biological molecules facilitates local disturbances to be felt at long distances by global coupling.

The physics and chemistry of non-equilibrium systems have been utilized to understand some of the spatial patterns and temporal patterning observed in biological processes such as bacterial colonies shaped by diffusive instabilities and calcium waves governed by nonlinear amplification during intracellular signaling (Levine and Jacob, 2004). We believe that the self assembled patterns of palladium lipoic acid may help electron transfer processes by extending it into the bulk from the membrane. In other words it may provide a spatial extension of the membrane with much more surface area with much less need for a bulky multi enzyme complex.

This is similar to the coupling that takes places in large multi-enzyme systems such as complex I where the Fe-S clusters help the signaling process during electron transfer.

SPIN COUPLING IN ELECTRON TRANSFER

Numerous electron paramagnetic resonance (EPR) or electron spin resonance (ESR) measurements have been carried out in biological systems (Berliner et al., 2000). This technique allows detection of unpaired electrons in any phase and the large magnetic dipole of the electron results in very-long range effects on the line shapes on responses to pulses and electron-electron spin relaxation times. It also allows to measure distances between spins based on the dipolar interactions.

The most complicated mitochondrial complex I, with a molar mass greater than 850 kD and at least 26 subunits, has been studied thoroughly by this technique to understand its structural aspects, the location of the NADH binding site, flavin, and most of the iron-sulfur clusters located in the hydrophilic electron entry domain of complex I. Also from spin-spin coupling interactions, it has been possible to identify the locations of cluster $[4Fe-4S]_{N2}$ and two complexes I associated species of semiquinone (Ohnishi, 1998). The nature of spin and orbitals states in $[4Fe-4S]$ complexes have been reviewed recently (Noodleman et al., 1995). Vectorial translocation of 4 or 5 protons across the mitochondrial inner membrane is coupled to this electron transfer process from NADH to quinone.

$$NADH + CoQ + H^+ + n(H^+)_{matrix} \rightarrow NAD^+ + CoQH_2 + n(H^+)_{intermembrane\ space} \qquad (41)$$

The electron transfer takes place from NADH to Complex I by passing through flavin mononucleotide, FMN, to a series of redox active iron-sulfur clusters such as $[2Fe-2S]_{N1a}$, $[2Fe-2S]_{N1b}$, $[4Fe-4S]_{N3}$, $[4Fe-4S]_{N4}$, $[4Fe-4S]_{N5}$, and $[4Fe-4S]_{N2}$, and two protein bound species of quinone, Q_{Nf} and Q_{Ns}.

Complex II, which is much less complicated than Complex I has a molar mass of about 127 kD and 5 subunits. The electrons pass through FAD to iron-sulfur clusters, $[2Fe-2S]_{S1}$, $[4Fe-4S]_{S2}$, and $[3Fe-4S]_{S3}$ as well as cytochrome b_{560}.

Complex III has a molar mass of about 280 kD and 10 subunits. The electrons pass through cytochrome b_L (b_{566}), cytochrome b_H (b_{562}), $[2Fe-2S]$, and cytochrome c_1.

Complex IV with a molar mass of about 200 kD has 6–13 subunits. The electrons pass through cytochrome a, Cu_A, Cu_B and cytochrome a_3.

The iron-sulfur clusters as well as semiquinone radicals in complex I are all EPR detectable. The oxidized forms of these clusters are diamagnetic and reduced forms are paramagnetic. The iron atoms are bridged by acid-labile inorganic sulfides. Each iron-sulfur cluster has four protein cysteinyl sulfur bonds. The iron, with oxidation state varying between +2 and +3, in each cluster is tetrahedrally bonded to the sulfur.

Cytochromes a, b, and c have heme proteins compared to the nonheme proteins in the above mentioned iron-sulfur clusters. The heme group of c cytochromes has added cysteinyl sulfhydryl groups across their double bonds to forming thioether linkages to the protein. The heme iron of the cytochromes a, b, and c also have one or two histidine residues as axial ligands. The histidine residues are on the cytoplasmic side as well as the matrix side. Cytochrome c also has several invariant lysine residues that lie in a ring around the exposed edge of it's otherwise buried heme group (Voet and Voet, 1995).

Apart from understanding the electron transfer pathways, topology of iron-sulfur clusters, and site of coupling in NADH-ubiquinone reductase, Complex I investigations have also been instrumental in understanding the mechanism of superoxide generation at the flavin site of Complex I (Berrisford and Sazanov, 2009; Galkin and Brandt, 2005; Kussmaul and Hirst, 2006).

Since, complex I dysfunction is implicated in many human neurodegenerative diseases as well as cancer, it is critical to understand its function thoroughly. We must point out a missing link here. We have briefly indicated the contributions from the electronic character of cysteine from our impedance studies. Since, it is bonded to the iron in the iron-sulfur clusters, it is important to investigate its electronic contributions to the electron transfer process. A recent X-ray investigation confirms our suggestion. "Cluster N2 is the electron donor to quinone and is coordinated by unique motif involving two consecutive (tandem) cysteines. An unprecedented "on/off switch" (disconnection) of coordinating bonds between the tandem cysteines was observed upon reduction" (Noodelman et al., 1995). This is also true of FAD and histidine in Complex II. Since, the palladium lipoic acid complex formulation enhances the Complex I and Complex II activities by 151 and 212% more than that α-lipoic acid, we have reason to believe that the self-assembled structure of the complex, by providing a spatial extension of the membrane with much more surface area, may be catalyzing the electron transfer process by enhancing the spin coupling.

Some supporting evidence for the probable electron spin coupling, even though not directly from the data of palladium α-lipoic acid complex, is given by the free radical reaction mechanism for the reaction of dihydrolipoyl dehydrogenase (Massey et al., 1960), studies on the 1e reduction of the disulfide linkages (Hoffman and Hayon, 1972) and studies on the lipoic acid free radical (Chan et al., 1974). Sulfhydryl free radicals of monothiol compounds tend to interact with their parent compounds.

$$R\text{-}S + RS^- \rightarrow [R\text{-}S\text{-}S\text{-}R]^- \tag{42}$$

There was no similar reaction between the lipoic acid radical and dihydrolipoic acid. The pK_a of lipoyl radical ($RS\cdot S(H)R$ of 5.85 compared to 4.7 of the carboxyl group implied that the negative charge is on the sulfur of the radical (Chan et al., 1974; Hoffman and Hayon, 1972). A direct electron transfer from the lipoic acid radical to FAD forming FADH was suggested (Massey et al., 1960) and confirmed by pulse radiolysis studies (Chan et al., 1974).

$$[RS\text{-}SR]^- + FAD + H^+ \rightarrow RS\text{-}SR + FADH\cdot \tag{43}$$

The FADH radicals disproportionate eventually forming FAD and $FADH_2$. Similar radical formation with the lone electron in the sulfur or palladium or an oscillation between the two can couple the electron transfer process and enhance the catalytic process.

OXIDATIVE STRESS IN HIV INFECTION

The HIV infected patients were found to have lower level of intracellular glutathione, plasma cystine, and cysteine (Dröge, 2006). Increased lipid peroxidation was also evident from the increased plasma MDA and plasma lipid peroxides. Plasma concentrations of vitamin C and β-carotene/vitamin A were also significantly reduced. Increased levels of oxidized 8-hydroxyguanine in DNA as well as TBARS along with decreases in the levels of superoxide dismutase and catalase in HIV infected patients have also been reported (Dröge, 2006; Packer et al., 1995). Supplementation for 6 months with vitamin A or vitamin C or vitamin E decreased the level of DNA damage, along with a reduction of TBARS and restoration of the activity of the enzymes (Jaruga et al., 2002). The α-lipoic acid supplementation study, 150 mg of lipoate three times daily for a period of 14 days, of HIV positive (classified CDC IV) patients showed increased levels of plasma ascorbate and glutathione and decreased plasma MDA in most patients. Also in a majority of patients, the T-helper cells increased and the T-helper/T-suppressor ratio improved (Packer et al., 1995).

A small study to probe the effectiveness of palladium α-lipoic acid complex formulation was also carried out with 5 HIV/AIDS patients suffering from chronic fatigue. This work was done at CIRCLE Medical LLC, Norwalk, CT, USA. It was observed that the palladium α-lipoic acid complex formulation was generally well-tolerated in all subjects; 4/5 patients reported sustained improvements in energy/fatigue through week 4 (1/5 patients noted improvements through week 2 with "decrease" by week 4); all subjects reported decrease energy/increased fatigue during the 2 week "wash-out" period; mean MOS-HIV Energy/Fatigue scores increased significantly through week 4, with a significant decrease in scores during the "wash-out" period; decreases were observed in TC, TC/HDL, and TG throughout the study period; and increased CD4%, decreased CD8%, and increased CD4:CD8 were observed. Of course these results are only preliminary and a comparative study with α-lipoic acid and many patients have to be carried out to arrive at meaningful conclusions. But the preliminary results are very promising.

AMELIORATION OF DRUG INDUCED TOXICITY

A recent review has detailed the medication-induced mitochondrial damage and disease and suggested mitochondrial toxicity testing as part of the pre-approval process for medications to protect the public by identifying the most toxic medications before they are allowed to reach the market (Neustadt and Pieczenik, 2008). Recent studies indicate effectiveness of, natural antioxidants against adriamycin-induced toxicity in cancer patients (Principal et al., 2010), lipoic acid against methotrexate-induced oxidative stress when treating leukemia and autoimmune diseases (Tabassum et al., 2010), and lipoic acid against isoniazid-rifampicin-induced hepatotoxicity when treating tuberculosis (Saad et al., 2010). Since, all studies with palladium lipoic acid formulation have indicated that it is much more effective than lipoic acid, there is no reason to doubt its effectiveness in using it as an adjuvant for treating tuberculosis, leukemia, other cancers and autoimmune diseases. Of course confirmation of these statements needs experimental verification.

CONCLUSION

We have suggested a new way of looking at the holistic medicine or alternative medicine. Mitochondria are ubiquitous. By developing new ways of treating mitochondrial dysfunction, a symbiotic or bridging relationship between modern medicine and a generally neglected part in modern medicine, the mitochondria, can be generated for improving the mental, emotional, and spiritual elements of the body. Medications targeting the mitochondria are much closer to a real holistic medicine because if you have healthy mitochondria, they will contribute substantially to the physical, mental, and emotional clements needed to complement the modern medicine.

Unlike toxic platinum chemotherapy agents, palladium α-lipoic acid complex formulation is safe and nontoxic. Its oral administration can be continued indefinitely. Palladium α-lipoic acid complex formulation is designed to provide energy for compromised body systems and promote overall health. It facilitates aerobic metabolism much more than that of α-lipoic acid, by significantly enhancing the enzymatic activity of isocitrate dehydrogenase, α-ketoglutarate dehydrogenase, succinate dehydrogenase, and malate dehydrogenase at the Krebs cycle and mitochondrial complexes I, II, III, and IV of the electron transport chain. Of course further investigations are needed to understand the mechanism of action of palladium α-lipoic acid complex formulation on some of these activities because the enzymes containing lipoamide are not direct participants in some of these activities.

Prior ischemia studies in gerbils demonstrated this energy benefit provided by palladium α-lipoic acid complex formulation to maintain the integrity of the electron transport chain following an ischemic insult.

Preliminary studies of HIV/AIDS patients under various cocktail treatment protocols demonstrated an almost immediate improvement in patient quality of life. Benefits included less depression and lethargy, more daily energy and increased appetite. Patients demonstrated significantly improved MOS-HIV Energy/Fatigue scores, increases in CD4, decreases in CD8, as well as improved lipid levels.

The unique electronic properties of palladium modulating the properties of α-lipoic acid appear to be a key to this physiological effectiveness. This is exemplified in our electrochemical impedance spectroscopic studies of α-lipoic acid and palladium α-lipoic acid.

The electronic properties of palladium also appear to modulate the antioxidant properties of α-lipoic acid in that palladium α-lipoic acid complex formulation enhances the activities of catalase and glutathione peroxidase more than that of α-lipoic acid. The level of glutathione also was significantly improved and the level of lipid peroxidation was decreased in the heart mitochondria of aged rats. Oral administration of palladium α-lipoic acid complex formulation showed an increase in glutathione and glutathione peroxidase levels and a decrease in MDA (a secondary product of lipid peroxidation) in the kidney and liver. Also palladium α-lipoic acid complex formulation offered protection to cellular DNA from whole body radiation (8 Gy). It decreased the radiation–induced hematopoietic injury as revealed by the bone marrow cellularity, hemoglobin level, and endogenous spleen colony formation in irradiated animals.

Palladium α-lipoic acid complex formulation is similar to a multi-spectrum drug in that it carries out several functions such as combating age related as well as disease associated fatigue, and minimizes the effects of ischemic injury. It acts as a prophylactic for neuronal regeneration from transient ischemic attack and also for protection from radiation. Apart from being a powerful free radical scavenger, it is also highly effective against various cancer cells such as glioblastoma, breast, ovarian, osteosarcoma, and lung.

Finally, we believe that the aim of the slogan for holistic medicine or alternative medicine, "the whole is much more than the sum of the parts", is accomplished readily by targeting mitochondria, a ubiquitous organelle in the human body. This is achieved with the judicious choice of a naturally present ligand in the human body, α-lipoic acid, that plays a crucial role in the mitochondrial energy metabolism because of its unique chemical structure and consequent redox properties, and complexing it with a metal with very high catalytic and electronic properties, palladium. What we lack in its continuing saga is many more challenging investigations to probe more deeply to understand the underlying mechanisms of some of the impressive or remarkable observations.

KEYWORDS

- **Adenosine triphosphate**
- **Antioxidants**
- **Chemotherapy**
- **Cisplatin**
- **Flavin adenine dinucleotide**
- **Glutathione**
- **Glutathione peroxidase**
- **Glutathione reductase**
- **Hypoxia inducible factor 1**
- **Malondialdehyde**
- **Mitochondria**
- **Polyunsaturated fatty acid**
- **Reactive oxygen species**
- **Succinate dehydrogenase**

ACKNOWLEDGMENT

The authors wish to express their sincere thanks and gratitude for many fruitful discussions and collaborations in various aspects of the work presented in this chapter: B.Chu, C. J. Perkins, G. Blick, G.K. Ogilvie, P. Valane, K. K. Janardhanan, T.A. Ajith, C.K.K. Nair, N.P. Sudheesh, A. Menon, L. Ramachandran, Calvert Labs, Brunswick Labs, Inc., and K.G.K. Synergize Inc.

Chapter 8

Unity of Mind and Body: The Concept of Life Purpose Dominant

Bukhtoyarov Oleg Viktorovich and Samarin Denis Mikhaylovich

INTRODUCTION

Problems of links between mind and body, ideal and material always attracted attention of the scientists and philosophers and within the framework of medicine there has always been a clear understanding of necessity in holistic perception of the patients, however actual approach to the patients appears to be determinative. Unobviousness of influence of mind on body and lack of a system view on psychosomatic links continuity have made modern practical medicine somatically focused both in diagnostics of diseases and in their treatment and preventive maintenance. The scientific search is also mainly focused on study of somatic parameters of organism without the account of mind influences on them. The appearance of new research technology still carries scientists even more in depths of organism. The huge piles of fragmented facts are taken on a surface which are difficult to give the system analysis to. At the same time, the huge amount of scientific data has kept showing extensive damaging influences of chronic psycho-emotional stress (CPS) on organism of animals in experiment and on human being in daily life (Gidron et. al., 2006; McEwen, 2007; Ostrander et. al., 2006; Simon et al., 2006; Spinelli et al., 2009). It is possible to state that CPS is an important an etiological and pathogenetic factor in development of many somatic diseases including "diseases of civilization": atherosclerosis, cardiovascular disease (Dimsdale, 2008; Nemeroff, 2008; Knox, 2001; Roy-Byrne et al., 2008; Shpagina et. al., 2008) and cancer (Adamekova et al., 2003; Mravec et. al., 2008; Reiche et. al., 2005) about that has been stated earlier in a hypothesis of psychogenic carcinogenesis. Psychogenic factor has always been and still remains essential component which mainly defines occurrence, development and outcome of diseases in human beings, however in view of its idealness and unobviousness it is latent behind a facade of a clinical disease picture and as a rule is left untouched by pathogenetic treatment. In connection with above stated, there is one large, difficult and, at first sight, unsolved question: "How to see mind, biological, personal and social aspects of a healthy human and a patient in dynamic unity instead of considering only separate pathological process?"

THE CONCEPT OF LIFE PURPOSE DOMINANT

The answer to this raised question would allow bringing in the proved and purposeful corrective amendments to scientific researches, diagnostic, medical and preventive measures in work with the patients. We offer the concept of life purpose dominant (LPD) which opens a system view on health of a human and process of any serious chronic disease formation with participation of mind and shows a possibility to control this pathological condition. On the basis of this offer by us, LPDs concept lays inter-subject doctrine of a dominant as universal, biological principle of work of the nervous centers and vital functions of all living systems, general law of the intercentral relations in living organism (Ukhtomsky, 1927; 1966). The doctrine of a dominant was created by the academician A. A. Ukhtomsky (1884, 1942), who is the largest thinker and ingenious scientist of the twentieth century. However, his doctrine has not received a due estimation and recognition neither during life of the author nor after his death. His scientific school existed simultaneously and in parallel with a school of the Nobel winner academician I. P. Pavlov that was recognized by the Soviet power as "sole correct scientific idea", therefore discovery of the ingenious scientist remained unnoticed for a long time. For the sake of justice it is necessary to tell that the basic rules of the doctrine of a dominant and a term "dominant" used in the works of scientists which have created a lot of the well-known theories: theory of human being motivation (Maslow, 1943), theory of installation (Uznadze, 1997), psychological theory of activity (Leont'ev, 1978), theory of movement behavior (Bernstein, 1967), theory of dynamic localization of mental functions (Luria, 1970), theory of the functional system (Anokhin, 1970), search activity concept (Rotenberg, 2009) and even a lot in Pavlov's doctrine of conditioned reflex appear to be component of the doctrine of a dominant. Really, uncountable set of reflexes in complete sense would blow up organism in the first instant of the existence if submission to their principle of a dominant when all reflexes work under the slogan "everybody for one, one for everybody". By the way, the formation of each conditional reflex under influence of conditional irritant is nothing else as the process of a dominant formation in which preservation directly depends on supporting influences of conditional irritant.

BRIEFLY ABOUT THE DOCTRINE OF A DOMINANT OF THE ACADEMICIAN A. A. UKHTOMSKY

Dominant, according to A. A. Ukhtomsky, is not any one topographic certain center of excitation in the central nervous system. It is a certain constellation of the nervous centers with increased excitability in various departments of a brain and spinal marrow, in vegetative nervous system as well as it is a temporary association of the nervous centers for the solution of the certain task (Ukhtomsky, 1966). Spiral marrow and brain stem, conditional reflexes, processes of association, integrated images are equally subordinate to a principle of work of dominant reflexes of a spinal marrow where the environment as well as high nervous activity is perceived. The dominant is characterized with the following four features: (1) high excitability, (2) stability of the excitation, (3) ability to sum (accumulate) coming excitations and also (4) inertia (the dominant "insists on itself"). The condition of a dominant is not super excitation which would by all means be finished by braking and more or less long persistence of excitation "in one place and connected braking in the other". The dominant is capable to pull external irritants together that are not related to it, and do not prevent its development but strengthen it. The dominant represents prevailing need, motivation, and aim and is the powerful activator of activity. However, any dominant is always temporary and stops in the following cases: complete spontaneous end of dominant condition (for example, any of the biological acts), complete termination of reinforcement by adequate irritant and suppression by a more powerful competing dominant. It is necessary to pay special attention that at incomplete cancellation of adequate irritant, the dominant amplifies, aspires to keep itself. We shall return to this situation while considering treatment of human diseases.

A. A. Ukhtomsky paid special attention to cortical dominant—dominants of the high order which are the latent factors of psychological activity. All vital functions of a human being are dominant in their sense; they consist of a set of uncountable functional conditions of organism consistently changing each other—current dominants. However, there is the main dominant of a human to which all current dominants (more precisely subdominants) are subordinated, which holds in its power a whole field of spiritual life, defines "spiritual anatomy" and a vector of human existence. We dared to name it the LPD.

LIFE PURPOSE DOMINANT IN A HUMAN

The LPD is a non-material construction with material expression, which is formed in mental sphere and is shown by the maximal integration of mental and somatic processes, subordination of the current subdominants of a human being, maximal sanogenetic and adaptive possibilities of organism that allows him to resist to constant pressure of the environmental factors successfully. The LPD is formed extremely under influence of a complex of verbal and not verbal suggestive irritants (processes of education and training, skills development, models of other people behavior etc.) which defines the life purpose that a human being aspires to achieve. A vivid example of an exclusive role suggestive irritants play in formation of life aims and personality is the well known phenomenon of Homo ferus ("Mowgli Syndrome") (Yousef, 2008) when children who have been brought up by animals completely acquire all behavior stereotypes of animals. In view of suggestive basis of LPD, life purpose and its loss can not be clearly realized by a human. For achievement of long-term, instead of momentary goal, whole organism appears in subordination to its main conductor—LPD. The LPD provides coordination of asynchronous work of organs and systems, mental and somatic processes, defines a vector of apparent chaos of numerous reflexes of organism, current subdominants (biological, mental, social etc.) and trajectory of everyday behavior of a human being. The LPD has certain similarity to work of ants carrying construction material in an anthill when the vectors of movement of separate ants are multidirectional and even opposite, but the resulting vector of their movement allows moving construction material in an anthill (Perelman, 2008). The LPD defines not only functional condition of the central nervous system, high nervous activity and vector of behavior of a human being, it defines a functional condition of a whole organism at all its levels—from subcellular up to organismic. Let us notice, that at the adult human LPD has the most various contents but in a fetus, neonatus and a child, LPD is shown by aspiration to safety. However, in process of development of a personality which represents a set of already holding suggestions, LPD is filled with other suggestive by the contents, that stability of LPD depends on.

INTERRELATIONS BETWEEN A LIFE PURPOSE DOMINANT AND CURRENT SUBDOMINANTS OF A HUMAN

The LPD has supporting influences from numerous current subdominants, which do not have any direct attitude to it at all. However, there are basic subdominants among numerous LPD subdominants—"subdominants of health", its reinforcement and strengthening, which are actively created only by human being despite of constant action of external irritants (unfavorable environmental factors), competing subdominants, menacing formation and capable to occupy a place of LPD or even to destroy it. For example, a scientist is overcoming inconceivable number of obstacles in search of the truth or an actor is constantly aspiring to improve himself to be in demand, to feel love of the spectators and to receive the worthy fee. If these people terminate to create basic subdominants, their dominants of life purpose by all means will disappear that threatens with heavy mental and somatic consequences, we shall speak below about. Restriction of possibilities to create supporting basic subdominants is observed among refugees, disabled, prisoners and other people who lost life prospect. At the same time, use of the minimal possibilities to reinforce LPD allows a human to keep his/her health even in conditions of massive chronic psycho emotional stress. For example, during the Second World war, some war prisoners in concentration camps died quickly and others planned their lives after concentration camps, they washed, had a shave, cared for others every day and being in inhuman conditions of existence they did not even catch colds at all (Rotenberg and Arshavsky, 1984). There is a great variety of examples of huge LPD force in a world history, in daily life and in clinical practice.

We have to mention numerous situations connected with achievement of life purpose, the termination of basic subdominants formation and natural LPD loss. A good example is the people with the most favorable financial, economic and social status who have achieved the life purpose and any possible well-being but imperceptibly appeared in "without dominant" condition—condition of CPS with the subsequent development of heavy diseases.

LIFE PURPOSE DOMINANT AT AN ANIMAL

Proceeding from universality of the doctrine about a dominant for all living systems LPD should exist at an animal too. We consider that unlike a human being, LPD at an animal is biologically predetermined, formed in the central nervous system, constant at any age and is the dominant of safety—filled with aspiration to safety. Unlike human being, the animal practically is unable to show own activity in creation of strengthening basic LPDs subdominants. At wild animals, the strengthening LPD occurs by a natural image under action of short-term subdominants—functional condition of an organism arising as a result of reactions on acute stressful irritants. At domestication and training of an animal, human being becomes main irritant in formation of a unique basic subdominant strengthening an animal dominant of safety. This understanding is important, as it allows in experimental models on animals to simulate loss of LPD, similar to loss of LPD at a human.

ROLE OF SUGGESTIONS IN OCCURRENCE AND LOSS OF A HUMAN'S LIFE PURPOSE DOMINANT

From above stated, there is a clear exclusive role of suggestions in life of a human, as LPD and personality are a product of systematic suggestive influences. From all variety of irritants influencing a human being during his life suggestive influences are capable to destroy LPD directly and to become a lead though invisible pathogenic part in development of many diseases. In contrast to animals at which the acute stress always strengthens LPD, at a human depends on various results of intrapsychic processing of suggestive information of acute stress. For example, if the threat to life of an animal is finished with flight and LPD reinforcement, the threat to life of a human can both support LPD and be finished with its loss and development of disease, for example, post traumatic stress disorder. Besides, suggestive influence can in some minutes deprive a human being of life purpose and result in his death; how an academician V. M. Bekhterev informed in the work describing experiment on a criminal sentenced to a death penalty (Bekhterev, 1998).

DISEASES AS DOMINANT CONDITIONS

Any disease of a human being contains all features of a dominant therefore it can be considered as pathological dominant condition which is formed under influence of somatogenic and/or psychogenic irritants–etiological factors. The dominant dies away and disappears according to the doctrine of dominant after termination of adequate irritant. However, human diseases as pathological dominant condition do not disappear at complete termination of etiological irritants, but become chronic, as are supported by others, already pathogenic irritants. In this connection, chronic diseases, as pathological dominant condition, have the supporting influences on the part of numerous current subdominants. Please note that there are pathological basic subdominants among them—"subdominants of disease" which are formed under the influence of hetero- and auto suggestive irritants. Actually, they are pathological reflexes, for example, bronchial asthma attack, spasm of colon, arrhythmia attack or more complex cascade of reflex disorders at a relapse of a multiple sclerosis or cancer generated in a result of psycho-emotional shocks. These basic pathological subdominants (pathological reflexes) become a basis psychogenic component of chronic diseases.

PSYCHOGENIC COMPONENT OF DISEASE AS THE BASIC PART OF PATHOGENESIS

Psychogenic component of disease is an indispensable reaction of the person to disease with a complex of emotional, intellectual and volitional disorders connected to comprehension, experience and attitude of the patient to the condition and also with vegetative component which naturally interweaves with a structure of clinical displays of disease that gives it qualitatively new features. We consider that namely psychogenic component in human being defines development and outcome of human diseases as its basic pathogenic role consists of a distortion or blocking of sanogenesis mechanisms. There are no human diseases without psychogenic component and this is the cardinal difference of human diseases from diseases of animals. It is possible to state that the body does not suffer at influence of the unfavorable environmental factors but the mind is always injured, that is psychogenic factor cannot be etiological but it becomes pathogenic. Psychogenic component cannot be missed, deliberately ignored and waved away from it. On the contrary, it is necessary to see psychogenic component of disease to reveal pathological basic subdominants that is to understand and control it to use successfully during treatment of the patients.

Thus, utter elimination of pathological dominant condition, that is the patient's recovery, assumes elimination of not only a set of known etiological and pathogenic irritants supporting a pathological dominant but also requires indispensable elimination of a psychogenic component of disease. Otherwise, the incomplete elimination of irritants will indeed strengthen a pathological dominant of disease, which becomes more active, progressing and/or resistant therapy. Unfortunately, this phenomenon is quite often observed in clinical practice.

THE CHARACTERISTIC OF BASIC INTEGRATED HUMAN FUNCTIONAL CONDITIONS

The basic integrated functional conditions of a human organism are defined by the contents of his main dominant that allows marking out 5 integrated functional conditions which replace each other during a whole life of a human in direct and opposite directions as a result of constant pressure of the various factors (irritants) of an environment:

1. "Ideal health dominant" is a functional organism condition which is characterized by LPD presence with its basic subdominants, maximum integration of psychosomatic processes, maximum and adaptive organism possibilities and lack of any chronic diseases.

2. "Relative health dominant" is a functional condition of organism which is characterized by LPD presence with basic subdominants, sufficient integration of psychosomatic processes, sufficient sanogenetic and adaptive organism resources, compensating any available chronic diseases.

3. "Without dominant condition" is a transitive functional condition of organism deprived of basic subdominants and LPD which is characterized by disintegration of brain systems, psychosomatic processes, progressing reduction of sanogenetic and adaptive organism resources, formation of any psychosomatic pathology or decompensation of already available chronic diseases.

4. "Disease dominant" is a pathological functional condition of organism which is characterized with occurrence of a dominant of any psychosomatic or soma psychic disease instead of LPD with formation of pathological basic subdominants supporting disease.

5. "Self-destruction dominant" is a pathological functional condition of organism which is characterized by occurrence of a dominant condition instead of LPD described by aspiration to death—a dominant of death with numerous pathological basic subdominants, maximal disintegration of brain systems and psychosomatic processes, failure of sanogenetic and adaptive of processes conducting to organism destruction.

DYNAMICS OF THE INTEGRATED HUMAN FUNCTIONAL CONDITIONS WITHIN A LIFE SPAN

The dynamic links and change of the basic integrated functional condition of a human organism on a background of constant pressure of the environmental factors (irritants) are presented in Figure 2. To visualize the dynamic presentation of complex psycho-somatic processes, each integrated condition of a human being is shown as "iceberg of psychosomatics" where the surface part—soma, underwater part—mind (psychogenic component) and central place in each condition is occupied with predominant dominant subordinating numerous current subdominants. All subdominants are formed in the central nervous system, in mental sphere, but have obligatory manifestations in soma and the speed of these manifestations depends on lag effect of somatic processes (nervous reactions, vascular reaction, hormone reaction, exchange processes in bones etc.). In Figure 1 the small black circles are various current subdominants (meals, dream, walking etc.), black triangles—basic LPD subdominants, black squares—pathological basic subdominants of disease.

"Ideal health dominant" (see Figure 2, I) which is met in a smaller part of the population and more often among young people, turns into "relative health dominant" condition (see Figure 2, II) under influence of the unfavorable (pathogenic) factors of an environment (trauma, infections, stresses etc.). Thus, pathogenic factors (irritants) do not destroy predominant dominant—LPD but result in occurrence of some chronic diseases (rather serious ones) which appear to be compensated because they become the current subdominants subordinate to LPD, and psychogenic component of these diseases carries out no pathogenic and sanogenic role. The people with disabilities participating in Paralympic Games or keen people living with HIV/AIDS, elderly people conducting an active lifestyle, that is actively creating and supporting basic "subdominants of health" can serve as an example. The reverse transition from condition II in a condition I seem to be difficult. In case of LPD (sense, life purpose), loss under pressure of the environmental factors, a human being appears in transitive "without dominant condition", in power of daily subdominants (see Figure 2, III) that is characterized by a condition of chronic consumptive psycho-emotional stress with its mental and somatic manifestations. For example, loss of the close person with whom the plans for the future are connected or loss of any life prospects as a result of social shocks (war, terrorism, financial and economic crisis, acts of nature etc.) and also others psycho-traumatic situations. A person can stay in a condition "without dominant" from several minutes up to several years. Under favorable conditions (the life purpose appearance), a person comes back in a condition of "relative health dominant" (see Figure 2, II) otherwise he/she stays in power of "disease dominant" (see Figure 2, IV) or "self-destruction dominant" (see Figure 2, V).

"Dominant of serious chronic disease" is represented in some serious chronic disease which has arisen in the period of "without dominant condition" (CPS), with formation of pathological basic subdominants which make a basis psychogenic component of disease. They are manifested both in mental sphere (anxiety, depression, phobias etc.), and in somatic sphere (vegetative, neuroendocrine, neuroimmune disorders, etc.) deforming psychosomatic relation and actively participating in pathogenesis of disease. There are numerous examples of occurrence of the most various diseases on a CPS background including development of malignant tumors (Levav et al., 2000) or multiple sclerosis (Li et al., 2004) after loss of the close person.

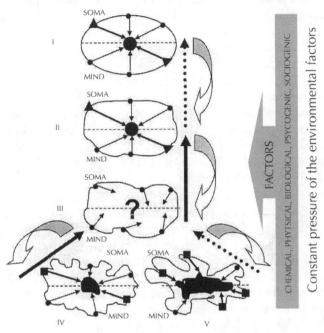

Figure 1. "Iceberg psychosomatics": dynamics of the basic integrated conditions of the human organism within the life span under constant pressure of the environmental factors. ● - dominant of life purpose (LPD); • - current subdominants; ▲ - basic subdominants LPD; ■ - pathological basic subdominants of illness; ◖ - dominant of serious chronic disease; ◤ - dominant of death. (I) Condition "ideal health dominant": LPD presence and its basic subdominants, orderliness of psychosomatic processes, absence of illnesses; (II) Condition "relative health dominant": LPD presence and its basic subdominants, equilibrium of psychosomatic processes ensuring remission of any chronic diseases; (III) "without dominant condition": LPD absence, disorder of subdominants, disintegration of psychosomatic processes, chronic psycho-emotional stress, possibility of transition into condition II; (IV) Condition "disease dominant": Occurrence instead of LPD dominant of serious chronic disease supported by pathological basic subdominants, deep disintegration of psychosomatic processes, opportunity of return into condition III. (V) Condition "self-destruction dominant": occurrence of death dominant instead of LPD with numerous pathological basic subdominants, practically irreversible disintegration of psychosomatic of processes, failure of sanogenesis mechanisms leading to death.

"Self-destruction dominant" (see Figure 2, V) always occurs from "without dominant condition" (see Figure 2, III) which in turn can arise from "disease dominant" (see Figure 2, transition IV in III). Psychogenic component "self-destruction dominant" contains a significant number of pathological basic subdominants that makes "self-destruction dominant" very strong and complicates reverse transition in "without dominant condition". Psychogenic component of "self-destruction dominant" is always brightly painted and clinically is shown through depressive symptomatology, phenomena of feebleness, hopelessness, down to catatonoid state with complete refusal of a human of the further life prospects and from the life itself, it is psychological capitulation (phenomenon "given-up/giving-up") under pressure of the environmental factors with active or passive aspiration to death. Somatogenic component "self-destruction dominant" is frequently shown through expressed somatic disorders connected mainly to heavy frustration, intimate—of vascular system (cardiac arrhythmias, weakness of cardiac activity etc.). A vivid example of "self-destruction dominant" is a known phenomenon "voodoo death" or psychogenic death (Lester, 2009), which was studied by us in oncological practice (Bukhtoyarov and Arkhangelsky, 2006). Psychological capitulation on a background of depression results in suicides precedes and accelerates approach of death of the patients with diseases of heart (Seymour and Benning, 2009; Surtees et al., 2008), cancer patients (Lloyd-Williams et al., 2009; Rodin et al., 2009) and patients with other diseases (Grossardt et al., 2009). By the way, self-liquidating behavior of some fans, sectarians or suicide attacker also is caused by "self-destruction dominant" arisen under influence of the external unfavorable mainly suggestive factors.

VIEW OF AN ANIMAL FROM POSITIONS OF A LIFE PURPOSE DOMINANT CONCEPT

The main differences between a human and an animal are the second signal system (speech) and ability to abstract thinking, which defines existence of psychogenic component at a human only. The set of integrated functional condition of animal's organism within a life span is sharply narrowed because of absence of a psychogenic component (see Figure 3).

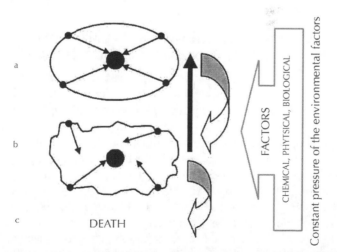

Figure 2. Dynamics of the basic integrated functional conditions of an animal organism within a life span on a background of constant pressure of the environmental factors. ● — safety dominant" (SD), • — current subdominants (CD). (a) Condition "dominant of life": presence SD, supported CD, integration nervous-somatic processes; (b) Condition "chronic stress dominant": presence of SD but CD mismatch, increasing but convertible disintegration of nervous-somatic processes; (c) Disappearance of SD on a background of irreversible disintegration nervous-somatic processes conducting to inevitable animal destruction.

A unique (sole) integrated functional condition with the maximum integration of nervous and somatic processes, maximum adaptive and sanogenetic resources is the condition when an animal LPD (safety dominant) is kept. We named this integrated condition of an animal organism "life dominant" where all current subdominants are subordinated to an animal LPD (see Figure 3a). For a wild animal, the acute stresses and for a pet, human being is the irritants, which strengthen their LPD. In situations of long influence of unfavorable irritants (chemical, physical, biological), there is a threat of LPD loss with chaos of the current subdominants, increasing disintegration of nervous and somatic processes, reduction of adaptive and sanogenic resources of organism. We named this integrated condition of an animal organism "chronic stress dominant" (see Figure 3b) that has a certain similarity with "without dominant condition" of a human described also by a CPS condition. The LPD does not disappear in this condition only at an animal as its disappearance is equivalent to death. "Chronic stress dominant" is supported only by external irritants and is capable to reverse transition in "a life dominant" only after the termination of exogenous influences. Otherwise, there will be irreversible disorders in organism with LPD loss and subsequent destruction of an animal (see Figure 2c).

The stated representations show that the experimental models on animals can not precisely correspond to real events in human organism and require very careful preparation of experiments. For example, it is incorrect to run experimental approbation of anti-cancer drugs on animals that are in an integrated condition of "life dominant" and/ or exposed to acute stress as organism of such animals has greatest sanogenetic and adaptive resources, which can not be basically present in cancer patients. It would be more correct to put animals into chronic stress condition on which background to test action of anti-cancer drugs.

EXAMPLE OF A SYSTEM VIEW OF CHRONIC DISEASE FROM POSITIONS OF THE CONCEPT LIFE PURPOSE DOMINANT--CANCER DISEASE

In the hypothesis of psychogenic carcinogenesis was shown the scheme of formation of basic pathogenic parts of carcinogenesis under CPS influence. Thus, term "CPS" has remained only general concept not reflecting all depth of its origin but from positions of the LPD concept CPS genesis with its known damaging influences on organism becomes clear. Our long-term researches have shown that up to an actual making out a cancer diagnosis, majority of the patients were in a condition of feebleness, hopelessness, helplessness despair (frequently not realized by the patients) which characterize LPD loss, appeared CPS. Statistic data prove dramatic increase in possibility of malignant tumors diseases with age (Jemal et al., 2008). It may be connected with loss of life prospects and plans for the future of an elderly person, in fact this is LPD loss with all ensuing negative psychosomatic consequences. Making out diagnosis of a cancer is in turn a powerful iatrogenic (suggestive) influence closing a vicious circle of carcinogenesis with formation of new additional pathological basic subdominants, supporting and strengthening the main pathological dominant—cancer dominant, which strongly occupies a LPD place. Modern somatic focused therapy of a cancer does not take into account and does not pay due influence to psychogenic component of cancer disease which defines development and outcome of a cancer in human. Somatic approach to cancer therapy is not capable to explain uncontrollability of carcinogenesis. The reasons for uncontrollability of cancer process during somatically focused therapy become clear from positions of the LPD concept (see Figure 3).

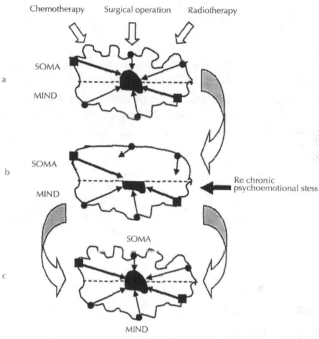

Figure 3. The "Iceberg psychosomatics": schema of psychogenic reproduction of a cancer disease (cancer relapse). ◖ — cancer dominant (CD), • —current subdominants, ■—pathological basic subdominant CD. (a) Influence of standard anticancer treatment on somatic component CD and in general "disease dominant"; (b) "Reconstructed soma" with previous psychogenic component (c) Complete reflex reproduction of CD and in general "disease dominant" (cancer relapse) during repeated reminding CPS.

The modern complex therapy of cancer (surgery, chemotherapy, radiotherapy) results in incomplete elimination of irritants supporting cancer dominant and on the whole pathologically integrated condition of organism "disease dominant", that is carries out correction of its somatic component only (see Figure 4b) that can even strengthen manifestations of cancer disease. Besides, maintenance of psychogenic component of cancer dominant and "disease dominant" on the whole creates sufficient conditions for complete reflex restoration of its somatic component that is occurrence of a recurrent cancer or occurrence of cancer of other tissue localizations at repeated reminding influence of psychogenic irritants (see Figure 4c) even after many years of the first cancer incident. In this connection, in pathogenically proved complex approach to cancer treatment the effective influences on psychogenic component of cancer disease should be stipulated.

CONCEPT IMPLICATIONS

1. The presented concept allows seeing close interaction of mind and body, to generate holistic view of vital functions of a human.
2. The concept proves complex pathogenetic approaches to prophylaxis and treatment of human diseases.
3. The concept states a special role of social medium as a source of suggestive flows of information in the personality development of a human and his/her life aims.
4. On the basis of this concept the processes occurring not only in separate human being but also in various people communities can be clarified.
5. From positions of this concept an opportunity appears to develop purposeful experimental models on animals that will become maximum adequate to the research problems.

CONCLUSION

The concept of a LPD gives an opportunity of new vision of interrelations between ideal and material, mind and body, dynamic unity of psychosomatic processes and also allows to understand and to predict the phenomena of human vital functions of healthy person and a patient.

KEYWORDS

- **Chronic psycho-emotional stress**
- **Ideal health dominant**
- **Life purpose dominant**
- **Psychogenic component**
- **Sanogenetic and adaptive**

Chapter 9

Thuja occidentalis and Breast Cancer Chemoprevention

B. K. Ojeswi, M. Khoobchandani, S. Medhe, D. K. Hazra, and M. M. Srivastava

INTRODUCTION

Breast cancer is the most common cancer affecting women throughout the world (Bryle et al., 2003). It accounts highest morbidity and mortality worldwide. Globally, 1.9 million new cases of breast cancer were diagnosed and 0.6 million deaths were caused in the year 2009 from this disease (DeSantis et al., 2009, 2010). In India, breast cancer is the second most common cancer, where 0.07 million new cases and 0.035 million deaths are reported every year (Ghumare and Cunningham, 2007). The present trend in the management of cancer development involves either reduction of the exposure of an individual to known carcinogen to the extent possible or seeking advantage of the inhibitors of carcinogenesis for their eventual application as anticancer agents. Since, exposure to the environmental carcinogens is often unavoidable, the latter field has been widely explored.

Owing to recently observed side effects and toxicity in various commonly used therapies for breast cancer, it has now become the need of the day to develop second generation drugs which are safe, effective, and non-resistant (Ojeswi et al., 2009). This search has brought about newly emerging term like come back to nature, grey to green chemistry, and various eco-friendly therapeutic remediation involving green chemicals from natural products (Khoobchandani et al., 2009; Werneke et al., 2004). Phytochemical prevention for severe health problems has recently gained scientific recognition worldwide. Studies on the pharmacological mechanisms and search for chemical structures of herbal extracts responsible for anticancer activity caught great interest. The present piece of work explains protective effects of the plant against 7, 12 dimethylbenz (a)anthracene (DMBA) induced mammary tumor in ICRC mice.

Thuja occidentalis Linn. is a plant of the family Cupressaceae, commonly known as Arbor-Vitae and a native tree of Europe. It has coniferous pyramidal features with flattened branches and twigs in one plane, bearing small scale-like leaves. The plant leaves were first identified as a remedy by native Indians in Canada during sixteenth century for the treatment of scurvy (Millspaugh, 1974). In folk medicine, *T. occidentalis* worked as an abortificiant, contraceptive, migraine remedy, antidiarrhoel, and hepatoprotective (Deb et al., 2007; Naser et al., 2009). As mother tincture, it is used to treat fever, warts, and piles (Dubey and Batra, 2008; Gupta, 2002). *T. occidentalis* leaves and twigs mainly contain flavonoids, terpenoids, steroids, and polysaccharides.

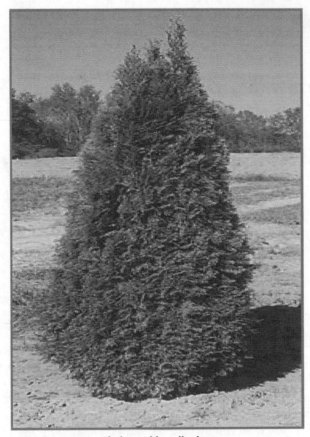

Thuja occidentalis plant

EXPERIMENTS AND PROTOCOL

The shade dried powdered leaves of the plant *T. occidentalis* were subjected to extraction, successively with solvents of increasing polarity (petroleum ether (Pt. ether), ethyl acetate (EtOAc), and methanol (MeOH)) to recover the wide range of compounds. The residual portions, obtained after removing the respective solvent (vacuum distillation Rota vapor) were dried by purging nitrogen, weighed, and refrigerated until further use.

The MCF-7 and MDA-MB-468 human breast cancer cell lines were procured from National Centre for Cell Sciences, Pune, India. Cells were grown in Nutrient mixture F-12, 82.5% supplemented with 2.5% FBS, 0.2% sodium bicarbonate, antibiotic, and antimycotic solution. The cells were grown in the following conditions: 5% CO_2, 95% atmosphere in high humidity at $37°C$ in a CO_2 incubator. Each batch of cells was assessed for cell cytotoxicity by Trypan blue exclusion (Frieauff et al., 2001) and Methyl thiazole tetrazolium cell viability assay (Lee et al., 2002). Cells for passage number between 18 and 25 were used in the study. The ICRC mice are inbred line of albino mouse of high breast-tumor incidence produce at Indian Cancer Research Centre,

India. This strain has high susceptibility for spontaneous mammary tumors (Kanekar, 1962). Female ICRC mice (20 ± 5 g body weight) were maintained in ventilated animal house at temperature 24 ± 2°C with a 12 hr light/dark cycle and 60 ± 5% humidity. They were provided with standard pellet diet and water *ad libitum*. The experiment was carried out as per the guidelines of Ethical Committee for the Purpose of Control and Supervision of Experiments on Animals (CPCSEA), New Delhi, India.

All ICRC mice were divided into seven groups of eight mice each. Group I: normal control animals were administered with 2% Dimethylsulphoxide (DMSO) (Yao et al., 2002). Group II: tumor induced cancerous control animals received a single dose of DMBA dissolved in olive oil. Group III and IV: animals received two doses of EtOAc extract (5 and 10 mg/kg body weight) after DMBA administration on 0 day. Group V and VI: animals received two doses of MeOH extract (5 and 10 mg/kg body weight) after DMBA administration on 0 day. Group VII: received doxorubicin (standard drug 5 mg/kg body weight) (*In vivo* cancer model (1976–1982)) after DMBA administration on 0 day. The DMBA is a carcinogen which induces mice mammary carcinoma from the ductal elements of the mammary gland by increasing substantial oxidative stress. Tumor was induced (Barros et al., 2004) using DMBA as a carcinogen by a single dose of 20 mg/kg body weight, dissolved in olive oil (1 ml) given through an oral gavages. The test samples of the extracts were given daily through an oral gavage. During the experimental period, animals were weighed weekly. Palpation of mammary tumors began 4 week after animals received DMBA. Animals were observed daily to assess their general health. The volume of individual tumor was measured weekly. Tumor volume was calculated using the formula: Tumor volume (cc) = 4/3 πr^3. On 120th day, mice were sacrificed and tumors were removed from the animals and weighed. Each tumor was fixed in 10% buffered formal saline and processed for routine histological examination. Haematoxylin and eosin stained slides were studied.

FREE RADICAL SCAVENGING ACTIVITY

Different solvent extracts (Pt. ether, EtOAc, and MeOH) of the plant *T. occidentalis* (leaves) were tested for hydroxyl (Halliwell et al., 1992) and DPPH (Shimada et al., 1992) radical scavenging capacity using α-tocoferol as a positive control with ten increasing concentrations (10–100 µg/µl). Different test samples show percent inhibition of OH as follows: Pt. ether (6.42–63.04%), EtOAc (28.02–83.31%), MeOH (20.06–78.87%), and α-tocoferol (28.08–96.22%). The DPPH radical scavenging effect of different solvent extracts were as follows: Pt. ether (7.21–64.44%), EtOAc (28.06–82.31%), and MeOH (10.02–78.17%) with ten increasing concentrations (10–100 µg/µl). Standard antioxidant (α-tocoferol) inhibits DPPH radical formation (45.05–96.22%) at the same concentration range. A gradual increase in percent inhibition of DPPH with the increasing concentrations of test samples indicating its dose dependent nature. *In vitro* antioxidant assay revealed that among the various extracts studied, EtOAc extract was found to be the most potent antioxidant. The overall order of potency was: α-tocoferol (96%) > EtOAc (83%) > MeOH (79%) > Pt. ether (63%) at the concentration of 90 µg/µl (Table 1(a) and (b)).

Table 1. (a) Effect of various solvent extracts of the plant *Thuja occidentalis* on percent inhibition of hydroxyl radical against reference (α-tocoferol).

Concentration (µg/ml)	% Inhibition			
	Pt. ether	EtOAc	MeOH	Toco
10	6.42 ± 1.32	10.02 ± 1.31	20.21 ± 1.30	28.08 ± 1.28
20	16.11 ± 1.34	20.02 ± 1.36	29.92 ± 1.35	37.32 ± 1.30
30	20.05 ± 1.40	26.71 ± 1.39	43.32 ± 1.41	46.04 ± 1.33
40	28.64 ± 1.52	34.27 ± 1.48	51.01 ± 1.47	57.71 ± 1.39
50	37.91 ± 1.59	47.08 ± 1.51	56.46 ± 1.53	72.82 ± 1.42
60	44.02 ± 1.60	55.42 ± 1.58	67.09 ± 1.32	80.32 ± 1.46
70	52.08 ± 1.62	61.21 ± 1.60	78.82 ± 1.32	84.04 ± 1.51
80	58.26 ± 1.71	65.04 ± 1.67	86.72 ± 1.32	95.32 ± 1.59
90	62.55 ± 1.76	69.95 ± 1.72	78.75 ± 1.32	96.22 ± 1.64
100	63.04 ± 1.81	78.31 ± 1.75	80.87 ± 1.32	96.02 ± 1.69

Each value is mean ± SD (n = 3). $P < 0.05$ (petroleum ether extract) *vs.* α-tocoferol; $p > 0.05$ (ethyl acetate and methanol extract) *vs.* α-tocoferol (Khoobchandani et al., 2009a, 2009b).

Table 1. (b) Effect of various solvent extracts of the plant *Thuja occidentalis* on percent inhibition of DPPH radicals against reference (α-tocoferol).

Concentration (µg/ml)	% Inhibition			
	Pt. ether	EtOAc	MeOH	Toco
10	7.21 ± 1.24	10.02 ± 1.22	28.06 ± 1.24	45.05 ± 1.25
20	17.01 ± 1.28	15.52 ± 1.25	30.08 ± 1.25	48.09 ± 1.28
30	19.03 ± 1.31	20.41 ± 1.29	37.07 ± 1.29	52.09 ± 1.31
40	27.94 ± 1.35	32.26 ± 1.32	45.87 ± 1.31	58.43 ± 1.34
50	37.07 ± 1.38	47.08 ± 1.36	56.87 ± 1.37	65.52 ± 1.38
60	45.02 ± 1.42	50.04 ± 1.39	62.21 ± 1.40	72.65 ± 1.42
70	51.04 ± 1.44	61.21 ± 1.41	67.87 ± 1.44	88.05 ± 1.46
80	59.26 ± 1.47	64.48 ± 1.44	73.26 ± 1.47	94.42 ± 1.49
90	63.45 ± 1.50	69.95 ± 1.48	78.75 ± 1.50	96.22 ± 1.52
100	63.44 ± 1.54	72.31 ± 1.50	80.87 ± 1.52	96.02 ± 1.54

Each value is mean ± SD (n = 3). $P < 0.05$ (petroleum ether extract) *vs.* α-tocoferol; $p > 0.05$ ethyl acetate and methanol extract) *vs.* α-tocoferol (Khoobchandani et al., 2009a; 2009b).

In vivo antioxidative effect of solvent extracts (EtOAc and MeOH) of the plant leaves was estimated in terms of percentage of down regulation of reduced glutathione (GSH) in DMBA induced oxidative stress in female ICRC mice liver (Ojeswi et al., 2010). As Pt. ether extract did not show any marked antioxidative activity in earlier *in vitro* experiments, was not considered for *in vivo* studies. The EtOAc and MeOH extracts of the plant *T. occidentalis* (leaves) were considered in test concentration 5 and 10 mg/kg body weight of experimental mice separately and percentage of down regulation of reduced GSH was recorded as a function of days (20, 40, 60, and 120 days) against normal and cancerous control experimental mice. In normal, no DMBA and extracts were administered and in cancerous control, no extract was given while all other experimental conditions remained same as that of the treatments. An increased level of down regulation of reduced GSH in cancerous control animals was observed when compared with EtOAc extract (10 mg/kg body weight) treated animals. The percentage of down regulation of reduced GSH in doxorubicin drug treated group was near to EtOAc extract (10 mg/kg body weight) treated mice which indicate its protective role against DMBA induced oxidative stress (Figure 1).

The DMBA toxicity is associated with its oxidative metabolism leading to the formation of free radicals, which bind covalently to nucleophillic sites on cellular macromolecules eliciting cancerous responses. Free radicals and their biochemical reactions in each stage of the metabolic process are involved in cancer development (Kun-Young et al., 2003). Antioxidants act as the primary line of defense against reactive oxygen species and suggest their usefulness in estimating the risk of oxidative damage induced during carcinogenesis. The GSH is non-protein cellular thiol which in conjunction with GPx has a regulatory role in cell proliferation (Anbuselvam et al., 2007). The GSH and its dependent enzymes scavenge the electrophilic moieties involved in the cancer initiation (Sunde and Hoekstra, 1980) and serves as marker for the evaluation of oxidative stress (Comporti, 1989; Nam and Kang, 2008). We observed decreased down regulation of reduced GSH in EtOAc extract of the plant *T. occidentalis* treated animals which suggest the antioxidative properties of *T. occidentalis*.

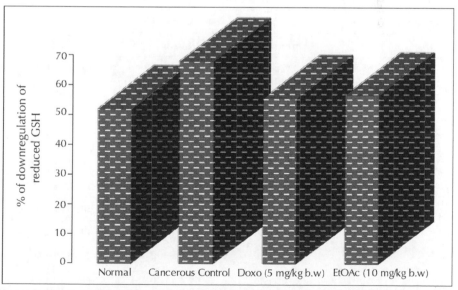

Figure 1. Effect of EtOAc extract of *Thuja occidentalis* (leaves) on reduced GSH in liver of experimental mice. Values are expressed as mean ± SD (n = 8); p < 0.05 *vs.* cancerous control (Ojeswi et al., 2010).

ANTIBREAST CANCER ACTIVITY

In vitro antibreast cancer activity of Pt. ether, EtOAc, and MeOH extracts of *T. occidentalis* (leaves) were screened against human breast cancer cell lines MCF-7 and MDA-MB-468 with ten increasing concentrations (10–100 µg/µl) for 24 hr by the TBE and MTT bioassays (Ojeswi et al., 2009). The Pt. ether extract did not show any marked cytotoxic activity. In case of EtOAc extract, maximum inhibition 51.42 and 51.21% of MDA-MB-468 cell lines was achieved at the concentration level of 90 µg/µl, by TBE and MTT assays respectively while in MeOH extract, the growth of MDA-MB-468 cells was inhibited up to 49.02 and 49.02% at the concentration level of 90 µg/µl by the above assays (Table 2(a) and (b)). The growth of MCF-7 cell line was inhibited by the EtOAc extract up to the maximum level of 91.42 and 94.06% at the concentration level of 90 µg/µl in TBE and MTT assays, respectively. In case of MeOH extract, maximum inhibition 88.02 and 92.04% of MCF-7 cell line was observed at the same concentration using respective assays (Table 3(a) and (b)). Percent inhibition resulting from *in vitro* bioassays demonstrated that both the extracts exhibit cytotoxicity (antibreast cancer activity) against the cell lines MDA-MB-468 and MCF-7. These extracts showed more pronounced efficacy on MCF-7 compared to MDA-MB-468 cell line (p < 0.05). It was also inferred that EtOAc extract is more significant antibreast cancer agent against cell line MCF-7 showing maximum inhibition 94.06% at the concentration 90 µg/µl at 24 hr. IC_{50} values calculated from MTT assay using probit analysis were as follows: Pt. ether (25.70), EtOAc (21.08), and MeOH (22.97).

Table 2(a). Percentage growth inhibitory activity of various solvent extracts of the plant. *Thuja occidentalis* on MDA-MB-468 Cell line by Trypan blue exclusion assay.

Concentration (µg/µl)	% Inhibition		
	Pt. ether	EtOAc	MeOH
10	7.52 ± 1.21	9.01 ± 1.23	11.01 ± 1.23
20	17.41 ± 1.24	19.02 ± 1.26	20.22 ± 1.27
30	22.07 ± 1.28	24.12 ± 1.29	31.06 ± 1.30
40	26.71 ± 1.31	31.88 ± 1.32	37.12 ± 1.33
50	30.09 ± 1.33	37.75 ± 1.35	40.44 ± 1.35
60	35.02 ± 1.35	42.16 ± 1.37	44.83 ± 1.38
70	37.24 ± 1.38	43.75 ± 1.39	46.43 ± 1.41
80	40.41 ± 1.39	48.02 ± 1.42	49.08 ± 1.44
90	42.5 ± 1.42	48.42 ± 1.45	49.42 ± 1.46
100	23.41 ± 1.45	49.2 ± 1.46	50.02 ± 1.48

Each value is mean ± SD (n = 3). P < 0.05 (Ojeswi et al., 2009)

Table 2. (b) Percentage growth inhibitory activity of various solvent extracts of the plant *Thuja occidentalis* on MDA-MB-468 Cell line by MTT assay.

Concentration (μg/μl)	% Inhibition		
	Pt. ether	EtOAc	MeOH
10	8.52 ± 1.12	10.11 ± 1.14	12.01 ± 1.42
20	18.41 ± 1.15	20.02 ± 1.21	22.22 ± 1.37
30	23.67 ± 1.18	27.12 ± 1.25	32.66 ± 1.31
40	28.37 ± 1.21	33.88 ± 1.32	39.11 ± 1.33
50	31.09 ± 1.23	38.75 ± 1.36	42.44 ± 1.37
60	36.02 ± 1.26	42.16 ± 1.38	45.83 ± 1.42
70	39.24 ± 1.29	44.75 ± 1.44	47.43 ± 1.44
80	42.41 ± 1.33	49.02 ± 1.48	50.08 ± 1.47
90	44.05 ± 1.35	49.01 ± 1.53	50.4 ± 1.49
100	45.08 ± 1.37	50.2 ± 1.61	51.02 ± 1.52

Each value is mean ± SD (n = 3), P < 0.05 (Ojeswi et al., 2009).

Table 3. (a) Percentage growth inhibitory activity of various solvent extracts of the plant. *Thuja occidentalis* on MCF-7 Cell line by Trypan blue exclusion assay

Concentration (μg/μl)	% Inhibition		
	Pt. ether	EtOAc	MeOH
10	15.02 ± 1.30	19.13 ± 1.27	20.42 ± 1.32
20	34.41 ± 1.33	38.24 ± 1.30	39.22 ± 1.34
30	46.12 ± 1.35	54.66 ± 1.33	59.66 ± 1.35
40	49.07 ± 1.39	70.08 ± 1.37	75.32 ± 1.39
50	60.01 ± 1.42	73.15 ±1.39	79.04 ±1.40
60	66.32 ± 1.44	70.06 ± 1.43	82.83 ± 1.44
70	73.21 ± 1.47	84.75 ± 1.45	86.43 ± 1.46
80	80.41 ± 1.49	86.02 ± 1.47	88.08 ± 1.50
90	84.05 ± 1.51	89.01 ± 1.49	88.9 ± 1.52
100	86.08 ± 1.58	88.42 ± 1.50	89.02 ± 1.54

Each value is mean ± SD (n = 3), P < 0.05 (Ojeswi et al., 2009).

Table 3. (b) Percentage growth inhibitory activity of various solvent extracts of the plant *Thuja occidentalis* on MCF-7 Cell line by MTT assay.

Concentration (µg/µl)	% Inhibition		
	Pt. ether	EtOAc	MeOH
10	18.52 ± 1.20	20.11 ± 1.22	21.01 ± 1.24
20	38.41 ± 1.23	40.02 ± 1.24	41.22 ± 1.26
30	46.67 ± 1.25	57.12 ± 1.27	61.66 ± 1.27
40	51.37 ± 1.28	73.88 ± 1.29	75.11 ± 1.29
50	61.09 ± 1.30	76.75 ± 1.31	82.44 ± 1.30
60	69.02 ± 1.33	82.16 ± 1.33	85.83 ± 1.32
70	76.24 ± 1.35	86.75 ± 1.35	87.43 ± 1.34
80	83.41 ± 1.37	89.02 ± 1.37	90.08 ± 1.38
90	85.05 ± 1.39	90.01 ± 1.39	94.06 ± 1.39
100	85.08 ± 1.40	92.42 ± 1.41	94.4 ± 1.41

Each value is mean ± SD (n = 3). P < 0.05 (Ojeswi et al., 2009).

In vivo experiment has been conducted to observe the preventive role of EtOAc and MeOH extracts of *T. occidentalis* (leaves) against DMBA induced mammary cancer (Ojeswi et al., 2010). As Pt. ether extract did not show any marked cytotoxic activity, therefore, was not considered for the present study. The EtOAc and MeOH extracts in two doses (5 and 10 mg/kg body weight) of the plant were tested for DMBA induced ICRC mice mammary carcinoma in terms of tumor weight, volume, increase in survival rate, body weight, histological variation, and mutagenicity against the standard drug doxorubicin. The effect of test samples on mean tumor volume was measured. It was found that tumor volume in the extracts treated was smaller than cancerous control group. The EtOAc extract (10 mg/kg body weight) showed significant reduction of tumor volume compared to cancerous control (p < 0.05). However, smallest tumor volume was observed in case of doxorubicin drug treated group. Thus, EtOAc extract (10 mg/kg body weight) administered in ICRC mice appeared to reduce tumor volume up to 50% compared to cancerous control group (Figure 2). The effect of doses (5 and 10 mg/kg body weight) of EtOAc and MeOH extracts of the plant *T. occidentalis* (leaves) on tumor weight was observed in cancerous control, EtOAc and MeOH extract treated, and doxorubicin drug treated groups. The EtOAc extract (10 mg/kg body weight) exhibited significant (p < 0.05) reduction in tumor weight (39%) compared to cancerous control group at 120th day. However, smallest tumor weight was observed in case of doxorubicin drug treated group. The tumor weight of mice in other groups was higher than EtOAc extract (10 mg/kg body weight) and lower than cancerous control groups (Table 4). A gradual increase in body weight was observed in all animals up to 48th day of experiment. The body weight of the mice in cancerous control group did not show any increase after 48th day and then started decreasing constantly. The body weight of the normal control group increased up to 120th day, demonstrating a normal growth pattern. There was a sharp and significant difference in body weight between the normal and cancerous control group and cancerous control and EtOAc extract (10 mg/kg body weight) group at the end of 120th day (p < 0.05). The body weight of doxorubicin drug treated group was near to cancerous control group. The body weight of mice in other groups was between cancerous control and EtOAc extract (10 mg/kg body weight) group. (Table 4)

The effect of test samples on percentage of survival was measured. It was concluded that in EtOAc extract (5 and 10 mg/kg body weight) and MeOH extract (10 mg/kg body weight) treated groups, 90% survival was observed at final day of experimentation. In case of MeOH extract (5 mg/kg body weight) treated, 80% survival while in doxorubicin drug treated group 66% survival were observed at the final 120th day. The lowest survival rate, 40% was observed in cancerous control group. Thus, EtOAc extract (10 mg/kg body weight) administered in ICRC mice appeared to increase life span of animals compared to cancerous control and doxorubicin drug treated groups (Figure 3).

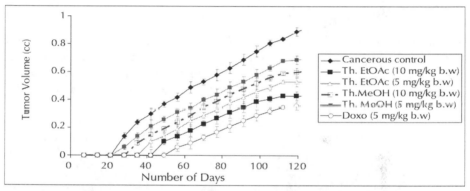

Figure 2. Effect of EtOAc and MeOH extracts of *Thuja occidentalis* (leaves) on palpable tumor volume. Each value is mean ± SD (n = 8). P > 0.05 *vs.* cancerous control. Th.: *Thuja occidentalis;* EtOAc: ethylacetate; MeOH: methanol; Doxo: doxorubicin. (Ojeswi et al., 2010).

Table 4. Effect of *Thuja occidentalis* extracts on body weight and tumor weight.

Animals	Parameters	
	Body weight (g)	Tumor weight (g)
Normal Control	62.25 ± 8.30	----
Cancerous Control	30.45 ± 6.90[2]	5.20 ± 0.29
EtOAc extract (5 mg/Kg body weight)	48.06 ± 3.71[2,3]	2.19 ± 0.12[5]
EtOAc extract (10 mg/Kg body weight)	51.24 ± 8.01[1,4]	2.01 ± 0.34[6]
MeOH extract (5 mg/Kg body weight)	40.02 ± 2.80[2,3]	4.02 ± 0.31[5]
MeOH extract (10 mg/Kg body weight)	42.31 ± 2.82[2,3]	3.76 ± 0.14[5]
Doxorubicin (5 mg/Kg body weight)	28.43 ± 2.21[2]	1.42 ± 0.02[6]

Values are expressed as mean ± SD (n = 8); 1p > 0.05 *vs.* normal control. 2p < 0.05 *vs.* normal control. 3p > 0.05 *vs.* cancerous control and doxorubicin. 4p < 0.05 *vs.* cancerous control and doxorubicin. 5p > 0.05 *vs.* cancerous control. 6p < 0.05 *vs.* cancerous control. (Ojeswi et al., 2010).

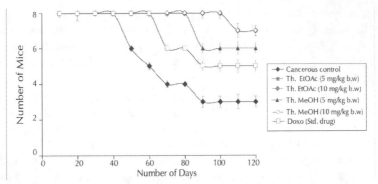

Figure 3. Effect of EtOAc and MeOH extracts of *Thuja occidentalis* (leaves) on percent survival. Each value is mean ± SD (n = 8). P < 0.05: EtOAc (5 and 10 mg/kg body weight) and MeOH (10 mg/kg body weight) extracts *vs.* cancerous control; p < 0.05: EtOAc (10 mg/kg body weight) *vs.* oxorubicin. Th: *Thuja occidentalis;* EtOAc: ethyl acetate; MeOH: methanol; Doxo: doxorubicin. (Ojeswi et al., 2010).

HISTOPATHOLOGICAL STUDY

Mammary tumors were excised from control and test samples treated animals for their histological evaluation at the 120th day. Histological evaluation revealed that all tumors from the cancerous control group were highly malignant cells and none of the tumors showed necrosis. In tumors excised from animals receiving EtOAc extract (10 mg/kg body weight), significant areas of necrosis were present compared to MeOH (10 mg/kg body weight) treated group while in case of doxorubicin treated tumors, large foci of necrosis areas were present which were distinctly appeared in Slide 1 (Ojeswi et al., 2010).

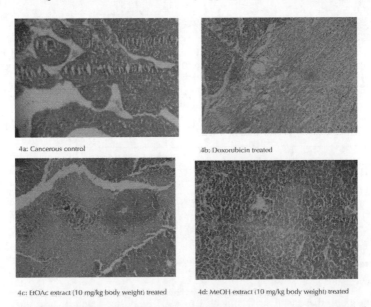

4a: Cancerous control

4b: Doxorubicin treated

4c: EtOAc extract (10 mg/kg body weight) treated

4d: MeOH extract (10 mg/kg body weight) treated

Slide 1. Microscopic view of Haematoxylin and eosin stained slides of cancerous control, doxorubicin treated, EtoAc extract (10 mg/kg body weight) and MeOH extract (10 mg/kg body weight) of *T. occidentalis*-treated tumors. Dark colored areas show well-developed tumor cells while light colored areas show necrosis. (Ojeswi et al., 2010).

ANTIMUTAGENIC ACTIVITY

Antimutagenic activity (Savage, 1993) of various solvent extracts of the plant *T. occidentalis* (leaves) was evaluated against DMBA induced cytogenetic damage in female ICRC mice bone marrow. The effect of test samples on percent of chromosomal aberration was measured in terms of chromatid breaks (CB), centric rings (CR), exchanges, acrocentric association (ACA), acentric fragments (FR), intracalary deletion (ICD), and total abnormal metaphases. Percent of aberrant metaphase in various groups were as follows: cancerous control–92.34%, doxorubicin treated (5 mg/kg body weight)–73.56%, EtOAc extract (5 mg/kg body weight)–53.34%, EtOAc extract (10 mg/kg body weight–45.25%, MeOH extract (5 mg/kg body weight)–51.90%, and MeOH extract (10 mg/kg body weight–57.74% (Table 5). The extracts under study reduce the chromosomal aberration like CB, CR, ACA, FR, ICD, and pulverization in bone marrow cells compared to cancerous control and standard drug doxorubicin treated groups. The EtOAc extract (10 mg/kg body weight) exhibited maximum reduction in chromosomal aberration in bone marrow of cancerous mice (p <0.05) while, doxorubicin was not found to exhibit the reduction in abnormal metaphases (Slide 2).

Table 5. Effect of various solvent extracts of the plant *Thuja occidentalis* on Percent aberrant metaphases in the bone marrow of experimental ICRC mice.

Group	CB	CR	FR	ACA	Pulvi	Abnormal metaphase
Normal Control	0.20 ± 0.40	0.0 ± 0	0.60 ± 0.54	0.0 ± 0	0.0 ± 0	0.8 ± 0.84
Cancerous Control	16.80 ± 1.28^2	6.70 ± 1.83^2	43.80 ± 3.49^2	57.20 ± 1.92^2	5.20 ± 1.45^2	92.34 ± 4.49^2
Doxorubicin (5mg/Kg body weight)	10.60 ± 3.36^2	5.60 ± 1.23^2	27.40 ± 2.30^2	46.60 ± 2.38^2	3.67 ± 2.96^2	73.56 ± 3.25^2
EtOAc extract (5 mg/Kg body weight)	8.20 ± 2.48^3	3.12 ± 2.18^3	11.25 ± 2.36^3	$22.4\,6\pm 3.46^3$	0.82 ± 0.45^3	53.34 ± 4.67^3
EtOAc extract (10 mg/Kg body weight)	6.34 ± 3.34^3	2.04 ± 2.18^3	10.36 ± 3.16^3	25.25 ± 2.41^3	0.0 ± 0^1	43.25 ± 6.56^3
MeOH extract (5 mg/Kg) body weight)	9.23 ± 2.09^3	4.03 ± 1.70^3	12.84 ± 2.93^3	38.84 ± 3.73^3	0.34 ± 0.28^3	57.74 ± 2.94^3
MeOH extract (10 mg/Kg body weight)	8.46 ± 1.59^3	3.23 ± 2.14^3	11.98 ± 2.51^3	34.92 ± 3.56^3	0.0 ± 0^1	51.90 ± 5.85^3

Mean ± SE (n = 8). Where; CB: Chromatid Break, CR: Centric Ring, DC: Dicentric, FR: Fragment, ACA: Acrocentric Association, Pulvi: Pulvirization, P value: [1]p > 0.05 *vs.* Normal Control; [2]p < 0.001 *vs.* Normal Control; [3]p < 0.01 *vs.* Normal control and Tumor Control.

The antibreast cancer bioassay of the extracts (EtOAc and MeOH) indicates that EtOAc extract of *T. occidentalis* (leaves) showed significant antibreast cancer activity against DMBA induced mammary carcinoma in ICRC mice. The EtOAc extract of the plant exhibit reduction of tumor volume (50%), tumor weight (39%) and chromosomal aberration (54%) compared to cancerous control group with the increase in body weight and life span in comparison with cancerous control and doxorubicin treated group. Therefore, EtOAc extract appears to be most effective for antibreast cancer activity. The observed results in all the bioassay parameters indicate the presence of some chemical moiety in the leaves of the plant *T. occidentalis*, responsible for its antibreast cancer activity. The EtOAc extract being potent antibreast cancer agent against DMBA induced mammary carcinoma in ICRC mice and is considered for characterization of bioactive principle.

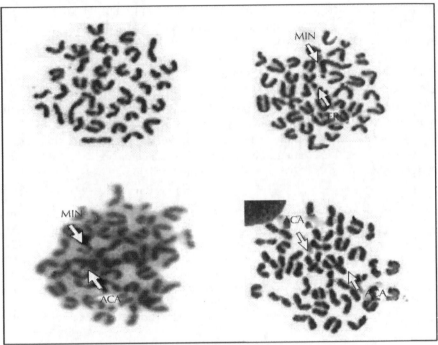

Slide 2. Chromosomal aberration in bone marrow of experimental mice (a) Normal Control, (b) Tumor Control, (c) Doxorubicin treated, (d) EtOAc extract (10 mg/kg body weight) treated.

ACTIVITY GUIDED CHROMATOGRAPHIC FRACTIONATION OF THE ETHYL ACETATE EXTRACT

The EtOAc extract was refluxed with Pt. ether for 20 hr to remove fat content. Defatted EtOAc soluble mass was subjected to chromatographic separation using a column (120 cm long and 4 cm diameter with stationary phase of 125 g of silica gel) eluted with CH_3OH: water (H_2O) (1:1). After the removal of solvent, a brown mass was obtained which was monitored by thin layer chromatography (TLC) using solvent system EtOAc ($CH_3COOC_2H_5$): formic acid (HCOOH): H_2O (8:1:1). The development of chromatogram in iodine chamber showed six spots. The brown mass was re-chromatographed using 150 cm long and 3 cm diameter column with stationary phase of 80 g silica gel and eluted with different composition of solvent mixture chloroform ($CHCl_3$): MeOH. Different fractions of 25 ml each were collected and subjected to TLC to ensure their purity using (EtOAc: $CHCl_3$: CH_3OH; 7:1:2) mobile phase. Fractions of same R_f values, fraction 13-24; $R_f = 0.44$ labeled as LEA[1] (first fraction of EtOAc extract; fraction 25-38; $R_f = 0.66$ labeled as LEA[2] (second fraction of EtOAc extract, fraction 39-53; $R_f = 0.81$ labeled as LEA[3] (third fraction of EtOAc extract, fraction 63-77; $R_f = 0.85$ labeled as LEA[4] (fourth fraction of EtOAc extract, fraction 78-99; $R_f = 0.94$ labeled as LEA[5] (fifth fraction of EtOAc extract and fraction 109-116; $R_f = 0.96$ labeled as LEA[6] (sixth fraction of EtOAc extract were mixed (Table 6). Removal of solvent furnished a white (LEA[2]), pale yellow (LEA[3]), and light yellow (LEA[5]) compounds. Compound LEA[1], LEA[4], and LEA[6] were found in trace amount.

Table 6. Details of chromatographic fractionation of ethyl acetate extract of *Thuja occidentalis* (leaves) (Ojeswi et al., 2010).

Fraction No.	Solvent System	TLC	R_f	Remarks
1–12	CHCl$_3$:MeOH (9:1)	Nil	-	-
13–24	CHCl$_3$:MeOH (9:1)	One Spot	0.04	LEA[1]
25–38	CHCl$_3$:MeOH (8:2)	One Spot	0.66	LEA[2]
39–53	CHCl$_3$:MeOH (7:3)	One Spot	0.81	LEA[3]
54–62	CHCl$_3$:MeOH (7:3)	Nil	-	-
63–77	CHCl$_3$:MeOH (6:4)	One Spot	0.85	LEA[4]
78–99	CHCl$_3$:MeOH (5:5)	One Spot	0.94	LEA[5]
100–108	CHCl$_3$:MeOH (4:6)	Nil	-	-
109–116	CHCl$_3$:MeOH (3:7)	One Spot	0.96	LEA[6]
117–124	CHCl$_3$:MeOH (2:8)	Nil	-	-
125–135	CHCl$_3$:MeOH (1:9)	Nil	-	-

ANTI BREAST CANCER BIOASSAY OF THE EtOAc FRACTIONS

The major compounds (LEA[2], LEA[3] and LEA[5]) recovered from EtOAc extract were screened for antibreast cancer activity in terms of cytotoxic activity against MCF-7 cell line. Compound LEA[2] and LEA[3] did not show noticeable cytotoxic activity, 30.04 and 32.86% inhibition of MCF-7 cell line at 24 hr. In case of LEA[5], maximum inhibition 93.88% of MCF-7 cells was observed at the concentration of 90 µg/µl. The compound LEA[5] was further assessed for antibreast cancer activity in terms of tumor weight and volume in ICRC mice. Improvement in the bioefficacy in terms of decrease in the treatment concentration from 10 mg/kg body weight to 4.5 mg/kg body weight has been observed in the compound (LEA[5]) exhibiting tumor weight: 1.99 ± 0.34 g; tumor volume: 0.40 ± 0.15 cc (Ojeswi et al., 2010). The compound (LEA[5]) also exhibited large necrosis area at the concentration of 4.5 mg/kg body weight in the histological slide of mammary tumor as equivalent to EtOAc extract (10 mg/kg body weight) treated tumors (Ojeswi et al., 2010). The compound LEA[5] was, therefore, considered for its chemical characterization which is in progress.

CONCLUSION

The present piece of work demonstrates that EtOAc extract of the plant *T. occidentalis* exhibited decreased tumor weight and volume compared to cancerous control with enhanced body weight and longevity compared to cancerous control and doxorubicin drug treated group. The chromatographic fractionation of the EtOAc extract to its derived compound LEA^{5}A (aglycone) has resulted into the lowering of effective test concentration from 10 mg/ml to 4.5 mg/ml and 5 mg/ml to 2.6 mg/ml with equivalent bioefficacy.

KEYWORDS

- **CHARGE syndrome**
- **Chromatin-remodeling enzyme KISMET (KIS)**
- **Circadian rhythmicity**
- **Constant darkness (DD)**
- **Cryptochrome (CRY)**
- **Day:night cycle**
- ***Drosophila***
- **Jetlag (JET)**
- **Light-dependent degradation**

ACKNOWLEDGMENT

The authors gratefully acknowledge Prof. V. G Dass, Director, Dayalbagh Educational Institute, Dayalbagh, Agra, for providing necessary research facilities. Authors acknowledge Board of Research in Nuclear Science, Mumbai for providing Financial Assistant.

Chapter 10

Antioxidants and Combinatorial Therapies in Cancer Treatment

Arpita Saxena

INTRODUCTION

Cancer has been posed as a major threat to humans not because there are no medications available, but because all available therapies have many side effects (Saxena et al., 2010). All the current chemotherapeutic agents cause a lot of damage to non-cancerous cells along with the cancerous cells. Plant derived anticancer drugs act through multi-targets simultaneously and/or synergistically. Many of these drugs are also chemo preventive, which prevent the both primary and secondary recurrence of the disease. Many cancer patients, who are undergoing the therapy, take antioxidant supplements in an effort to alleviate treatment toxicity and improve the long-term outcomes. The modulating effects of antioxidants in treatment depend on a wide range of factors, including the metabolic state of the patient, the stage and site of the disease, and the modality being used (Carmia, 2004). Agents used in chemotherapy damage a plethora of cellular molecules, increase lipid peroxidation of molecules, reduce antioxidant levels, and enhance oxidative stress (Sangeetha et al., 1990). Therefore, combination of antioxidants with conventional anticancer drug will be beneficial. Dietary and endogenous antioxidants prevent cellular damage by reacting with and eliminating oxidizing free radicals. Considerable laboratory evidence from chemical, cell culture, and animal studies indicate that antioxidants may slow or possibly prevent the development of cancer. Studies show that a high intake of antioxidant rich foods is inversely related to cancer risk. While clinical studies on the effect of antioxidants in modulating cancer treatment are limited in number and size. Experimental studies show that antioxidant vitamins and some phytochemicals selectively induce apoptosis in cancer cells but not in normal cells and prevent the angiogenesis and metastatic spread, suggesting a potential role for antioxidants as adjuvants in cancer therapy. Henceforth, this synergistic approach can lead to minimized side effects and effective dose of conventional chemotherapeutics.

Many studies target towards the lowering of the dose of known anticancer drugs or potent anti-neoplastic leads with higher efficacy (apoptotic potential) is using various antioxidants. Such studies assume that antioxidants may be helpful in the existing cancer therapies (Borek, 2004; Lee et al., 1999). The idea that drives them usually is that if a combination of antioxidants can reduce the dose, then the side-effects of conventional anticancer drugs like inflammation of adjoining tissues, interference with proper metabolism and hindering the normal activities can be avoided to a large extent. The consideration of whether to use antioxidants concomitantly with chemotherapy and radiation therapy has evolved into a heated debate. Great debates have sometimes spawned great breakthroughs in medical treatment, improving patient outcomes and saving lives. There are two groups of scientists who have asserted two different opinions about using antioxidants in the cancer therapy. One camp holds that taking antioxidants during cancer treatment could interfere with the way chemo and radiation work and diminish their benefits to the patient (Block, 2004). This is because radiation and some chemotherapy agents work by generating free radicals, which kill rapidly dividing cancer cells. Since, antioxidants scavenge free radicals, they might interfere with the therapeutic effects of these treatments. The opposing argument is that oxidation supports the proliferation of cancer cells and may itself interfere with treatment (Duthie et al., 1996). People who hold this view maintain that antioxidants may counter the harmful effects of oxidation in the malignant process and thereby increase the effects of drugs or radiation therapy in the benefit of the patient. Moreover, they note that some evidence suggests that antioxidant supplements to offer patient protection from the toxic effects of therapy and increase the efficacy (Lamson and Brignall, 1999, 2000; Prasad, 2004).

SYNERGISTIC ENHANCEMENT OF ANTICANCER POTENTIAL OF A LIGNIN COMPOSITION FROM *CEDRUS DEODARA* BY NATURAL ANTIOXIDANTS

In a recent chapter published by us, we tried to experiment with the synergy of two different antioxidant entities distinctly known for their anticancer properties. However, results showed the same extent of activities at one third the concentration of them by combining those (Saxena et al., 2010). The study involved AP9-cd, a standardized *lignan* from *Cedrus deodar,* which showed cytotoxicity and antitumor activity in various human cancer cell lines and different murine cancer models (Singh et al., 2007) and three different natural antioxidants namely Curcumin, Acteoside, and Silymarin. The AP9-cd has an optimum cytotoxic and growth inhibitory potential of 30 µg/ml in human leukaemia HL-60 and Molt-4 cells. This means that the apoptotic potential of AP9-cd was synergised by these antioxidants by three times and more.

The conclusion was that the cytotoxic and apoptotic potential of AP9-cd was significantly synergized by three natural antioxidants curcumin, acteoside, and silymarin in HL-60 cells. The mechanism of synergy involves the strong antioxidant effect of these antioxidants on HL-60 cells. All the three antioxidants reduce the reactive nitrogen oxygen species (RNOS) burst in HL-60 cells and inhibit the activation and translocation of NF-κB in the nucleus of HL-60 cells. Curcumin showed maximum synergy with AP9-cd in terms of cytotoxic and apoptotic potential than silymarin and acteoside in HL-60 cells. The combinations of antioxidants with AP9-cd provided an effective approach for cancer therapy that overcomes chemo-resistance and possible side effects.

SUPPLEMENTATION OF ANTIOXIDANT NUTRIENTS MAY PROTECT AGAINST CISPLATIN-INDUCED OXIDATIVE DAMAGE WHILE RETAINING THE ANTITUMOR EFFICACY

A study performed by Weij et al. (1998) states that cisplatin chemotherapy induces acute and more gradually occurring decreases in several major plasma antioxidants.

The observed fall in plasma antioxidant concentrations is probably determined by more than one mechanism, namely oxidative stress-induced consumption of antioxidants and renal loss of water-soluble low molecular weight antioxidants due to hyper filtration in combination with a specific cisplatin-related renal tubular defect. This is an undesirable situation as it may lead to diminished protection from chemotherapy induced oxidative stress and increased oxidative damage to normal tissues such as renal tubular cells. All in all, the results and findings of the authors suggested that supplementation of antioxidant nutrients may protect against cisplatin-induced oxidative damage while retaining the antitumor efficacy. It is the opinion of the authors of this chapter that the role of pro-oxidative metals, for example, copper and iron, and of antioxidants such as ceruloplasmin in the pathogenesis amelioration of chemotherapy-induced toxicity is further studied.

ENHANCEMENT OF CYTOTOXIC POTENTIAL OF CHEMOTHERAPEUTIC AGENTS IN COLORECTAL CANCER BY ANTIOXIDANTS

A study published by Chinery et al. (1997), showed that the antioxidants pyrrolidine dithiocarbamate (PDTC) and vitamin E induce apoptosis in CRC Cells. They further proved that this effect is mediated by induction of p21WAF1/CIP1, a powerful inhibitor of the cell cycle, through a mechanism involving C/EBP β (a member of the CCAAT/enhancer binding protein family of transcription factors), independent of p53. Despite a response rate of only 20%, five-fluorouracil (5FU) remains the single most effective treatment for advanced colorectal cancer (CRC), which is the second-leading cause of cancer deaths in the United States. Antioxidants significantly enhanced CRC tumor growth inhibition by cytotoxic chemotherapy *in vitro* (5FU and doxorubicin) and *in vivo* (5FU). Thus the authors insist that chemotherapeutic agents administered in the presence of antioxidants may provide a novel therapy for colorectal cancer.

ENHANCEMENT OF EFFECT OF DOXORUBICIN BY ANTIOXIDANTS

Another study by Liu and Tan published in 2002 states the fish oil and vitamin E appeared to enhance the antitumor effect of optimal doses of doxorubicin. In this study, four kinds of rodent diets, CO, FO, CVe, and FVe, were used by addition of canola oil, oil mixture (fish oil + canola oil), canola oil plus vitamin E, and oil mixture plus vitamin E, respectively, to a basic diet, AIN-93G, to investigate the influence of dietary fish oil and vitamin E on doxorubicin treatment in P388 ascitic mice. Animal life span (LS) and heart damage were recorded in mice fed the four different diets and treated with distinct doses of doxorubicin. The optimal doses of doxorubicin for antitumor effect as manifested by increased LS were 6.0 and 9.0 mg/kg. The work comprehensively investigated the influence of dietary fish oil and vitamin E, individually and in combination, on the therapeutic efficacy of doxorubicin and has shown their additively enhancing effects on optimal doses of doxorubicin in P388 ascitic mice. The authors, however, were honest to state that increasing doxorubicin dose led to severe heart damage, which was exacerbated by fish oil and vitamin E. Thus overall, it appeared to them that both fish oil and vitamin E modulate the effects of doxorubicin in the laboratory mouse like a double-edged sword, on the one hand, enhancing its antitumor effect and on the other, aggravating its cardiotoxicity.

CANCER PREVENTIVE AND CURATIVE ABILITY OF SILYMARIN

Silymarin is a naturally occurring polyphenolic antioxidantflavonoid extracted from the milk thistleplant [*Silybum marianum* (L.) Gaertneri]. Silymarin is the collective name for the active compounds derived from the plant, and silibinin is the most active and abundant constituent. Silymarin is one such agent, which has been extensively used since ages for the treatment of liver conditions, and thus has possibly the greatest patient acceptability. A study published in Hogan et al. (2007) opinions that silibinin significantly inhibits proliferation through cell-cycle arrest via inhibition of cyclin-CDK promoter activity. Despite its antioxidant profile, there is no effect on COX-2 expression. Apoptosis does not appear to be greatly increased in human colon cancer cell lines Fet, Geo, and HCT116. Rather, inhibition of cell cycle regulatory proteins play a fundamental role in silibinin's mechanism of action, and this may serve as a basis for combined use with conventional chemotherapeutics.

Another study published in the same year by Kaur and Agarwal (2007) reiterates that silymarin has cancer protective effects against skin, prostrate, breast, bladder, hepatocellular, lung, colon, and ovarian carcinomas. They have also performed clinical trials on cancer patients where patients were administered silymarin orally. Their observations have significant relevance for translating the basic research to clinical settings, as two major hurdles in this transition that is bioavailability and toxicity, have been somewhat defined for silymarin and silibinin. As they suggest, hepatoprotective effects of silymarin and silibinin confer added advantage of using them in adjuvant therapy, not limiting only to their cancer chemopreventive efficacy.

HEATED DEBATES OVER THE USE OF ANTIOXIDANTS IN COMBINATION WITH CANCER DRUGS

There is an Irish saying"Hope is the physician of each misery" and that "There is no hope unmingled with fear, and no fear unmingled with hope"Baruch Spinoza.

Numerous articles and several reviews have been published on the role of antioxidants, and diet and lifestyle modifications in cancer prevention. However, the potential role of these factors in the management of human cancer has been largely ignored (Kedar et al., 1999). Extensive *in vitro* studies and limited *in vivo* studies have revealed that individual antioxidants such as vitamin A (retinoids), vitamin E (primarily α-tocopheryl succinate), vitamin C (primarily sodium ascorbate), and carotenoids (primarily polar carotenoids) induce cell differentiation and growth inhibition to various degrees in rodent and human cancer cells by complex mechanisms. The proposed mechanisms for these effects include inhibition of protein kinase C activity, prostaglandin E_1-stimulated adenylate cyclase activity, expression of c-myc, H-ras, and a transcription factor (E_2F), and induction of transforming growth factor-β and p^{21}genes. Furthermore, antioxidant vitamins seperately or in combination enhance the growth-inhibitory effects of x-irradiation, chemotherapeutic agents, hyperthermia, and biological response modifiers on tumor cells, primarily *in vitro*. These vitamins, individually, also reduce the toxicity of several standard tumor therapeutic agents on normal cells. Low fat and high fiber diets can further enhance the efficacy of standard cancer therapeutic agents; the proposed mechanisms for these effects include the production of increased levels of butyric acid and binding of potential mutagens in the gastrointestinal tract by high fiber and reduced levels of growth promoting agents such as prostaglandins, certain fatty acids, and estrogen by low fat.

It was suggested in a recent publication that no supplementary antioxidants be given concurrently with chemotherapy agents who employ a free-radical mechanism (Labriola and Livingston, 1999). The present authors are by no means recommending any lack of caution about the use of antioxidants. On the contrary, published research indicates the cautious and judicious use of a number of antioxidants can be helpful in the treatment of cancer; as sole agents and as adjuncts to standard radiation and chemotherapy protocols (Lamson and Brignall, 1999). It is the opinion of the authors of this chapter that interactions between antioxidants and chemotherapeutics cannot be predicted solely based on the presumed mechanisms of action. The fact remains that physicians must be aware of the available research to help their patients take advantage of positive interactions existing between antioxidants and chemotherapy or radiation. Additionally, physicians need to remain aware of the large body of evidence showing a positive effect of antioxidants in the period following chemotherapy administration. The general protocol with standard oncologic therapies is to follow a watch-and-wait strategy after therapeutic administration is concluded. This is a period when supplemental therapies are highly indicated and have been demonstrated to result in a higher percentage of successful outcomes (Lamm et al., 1994; Whelan et al., 1999). In words of Derek (2009) reducing complicated interactions to a single sentence can be an oversimplification.

KEYWORDS

- **Antioxidants**
- **Colorectal cancer**
- **Cytotoxic**
- **Five-fluorouracil**
- **Life span**
- **Silymarin**

Chapter 11

Eruca sativa Inhibits Melanoma Growth: A Scientific Evidence

M. Khoobchandani, N. Ganesh, L. Valgimigli, and M. M. Srivastava

INTRODUCTION

Cancer is the abnormal growth of cells usually invades and destroys normal cells in our bodies. These cells are born due to imbalance in the body *viz.* metabolic disorder in cellular system and reactive oxygen species formation, triggering the morbidity, and mortality in living organisms. An overproduction of ROS from disrupted metabolism referred as oxidative stress may cause damage through mutations terminating into cancer (Nascimento et al., 2007; Shureiqi et al., 2000). Mutations are changes to the base pair sequence of genetic material and cause genetics and other degenerative disorders. The worldwide new incidence of cancer is about 6 million cases per year (Greenlee et al., 2001). Among various cancer forms, melanoma is a malignant neoplasm of melanocytes, most frequently arising from the skin. Melanoma is accounted for 2·6% of the global cancer incidence and 1·1% of cancer-related deaths (Hoey et al., 2007). Even if these data rank melanoma eighth or ninth in incidence, its doubling rate every 10–20 years is more worrying (Diepgen and Mahler, 2002). It is estimated that 68,130 men and women (38,870 men and 29,260 women) will be diagnosed with and 8,700 men and women will die of melanoma of the skin in 2010 (Altekruse et al., 2010). Multidisciplinary scientific investigations are making best efforts to combat this disease. The curative surgical treatment of melanoma remains a significant clinical challenge (Balch, 1992) and trials of post-surgical adjuvant therapy have proved largely unsuccessful with the majority inducing severe side effects at therapeutically effective doses (Balch et al., 2001).

An emphasis, recently, has been given towards the researches on complementary and alternative medicine that deals with cancer management. Epidemiological data indicates a beneficial effect of the "Mediterranean diet" on human health, on several degenerative diseases, including cancer (Cassileth, 2009). Encouraging intervention studies are now available (Tseng et al., 2008), however most investigations focus on main food products, such as olive oil (Pauwels and Covas, 2009), tomato (Tang et al., 2009), and red wine (Guerrero et al., 2009), while relatively little is known on food products consumed on less regular basis. Among the latter, *Eruca sativa* (rocket) certainly deserves attention. *E. sativa*, (Miller) Thell (Figure 1) belongs to the Cruciferous family and is originated in the Mediterranean region (Zeven and de Wet, 1982) but widely distributed all over the world (Warwick, 1994). The seeds are used for the production of spicy (taramira) oil while leaves are consumed as salads in India and European countries (Bianco, 1995). Investigations have been carried out to provide evidence that higher intakes of Cruciferous vegetables are associated with decreased cancer risk in humans (Higdon et al., 2007; Verhoeven et al., 1996). Glucosinolates and their derived products isothiocyanate found in Cruciferous vegetables have been reported to inhibit growth of melanoma cells (Melchini et al., 2009).

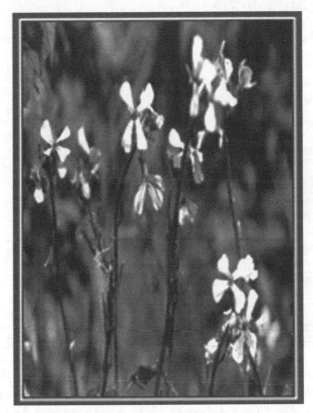

Figure 1. *Eruca sativa.*

The present chapter explains anti-melanoma activity of *E. sativa* plant (seed oil), demonstrating that the isothiocyanates found in seed oil play important role in inhibition of proliferation of cancerous cells. The intention behind this communication is to raise awareness and encourage implementation of herbalism for combating cancer.

FREE RADICAL SCAVENGING

Seed oil of plant *E. sativa* was tested for their free radical scavenging effect by using Fenton (Halliwell et al., 1992) and DPPH (Shimada et al., 1992) assays. Seed oil showed percent inhibition 95.55% against hydroxyl radicals at the concentration 100 µg/ml. Standard (α-tocoferol) antioxidant inhibited 99.46% of hydroxyl radicals for the same concentration. A gradual increase in percent inhibition of DPPH˙ with ten increasing concentrations of test samples was also found to be dose dependent (Figure 2).

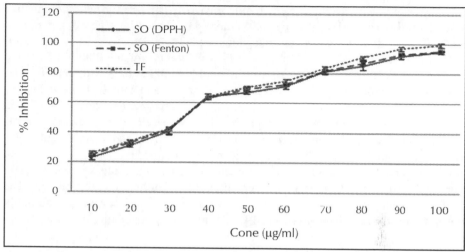

Figure 2. Percentage inhibition of hydroxyl and DPPH radicals, concentration dependency of seed oil against standard α-tocoferol. Each value is mean ± SD (n = 3). P > 0.05 (SO) vs. α-tocoferol.

Hydroxyl free radical is known to have damaging effect to almost every biological molecule found in living cells. *In vitro* Fenton assay involves hydroxyl radical generation through the incubation of Fe^{2+}-EDTA chelate at pH 7.4 which in turn degrade deoxyribose sugar (Khoobchandani et al., 2009; Ojeswi et al., 2009). The rate of degradation of deoxyribose sugar in test samples are compared with control in terms of appearance of pink chromogen with thiobarbituric acid. Seed oil exhibited maximum antioxidant activity as that of standard antioxidant α-tocoferol at the concentration of 90 µg/ml. A similar trend of free radical scavenging was found in DPPH assay.

Seed oil increased the level of down-regulation of reduced glutathione in *in vivo* study. Free radicals and their biochemical reactions in each stage of the metabolic process are involved in cancer development (Kun-Young et al., 2003). Antioxidants act as the primary line of defense against reactive oxygen species and suggest their usefulness in estimating the risk of oxidative damage induced during carcinogenesis. The GSH is non-protein cellular thiol which in conjunction with glutathione peroxydase has a regulatory role in cell proliferation. The GSH and its dependent enzymes scavenge the electrophilic moieties involved in the cancer initiation and serves as marker for the evaluation of oxidative stress (Comporti, 1989; Nam and Kang, 2008). Seed oil rendered significant protection against oxidative stress induced by melanoma in liver tissues in a dose dependent manner. Our observation supports the fact that melanoma cells induced oxidative stress is related to depletion of antioxidant system.

ANTITUMOR ACTIVITY

Seed oil inhibited the cell proliferation in a dose dependent manner. The inhibitions recorded with the two assays Trypan blue exclusion (Frieauff et al., 2001) and Methyl thiazole tetrazolium cell viability assay (Lee et al., 2002). Percent inhibition resulting from *in vitro* cell viability bioassays demonstrates that seed oil (IC50 24.78 µg/ml) is the most efficient candidate as cytotoxic bioagent. The percent inhibition against B16F10 cells was significantly ($p < 0.05$) more pronounced for seed oil, therefore it was further studied for *in vivo* anti-melanoma activity. Melanoma cells injected subcutaneously into mice grew to an average size of tumor volume 2,000 mm^3 in the control group. Seed oil produced significant inhibition of tumor growth in animals as compared to tumor control group. Seed oil at a dose of 1 and 2 mg/kg body weight inhibited 19.79 and 29.48% of melanoma growth respectively and doxorubicin reduced 37% of tumor growth at 21st day (Figure 3). The intraperitoneal route of seed oil was found to be effective in inhibiting melanoma growth. Both SO and reference doxorubicin reduced significantly ($p < 0.01$) tumor growth as compared to control tumor group. It is interesting to note that neither life threatening toxicity nor a loss of body weight during the seed oil treatment was observed as that of normal control animals. The finding is significant in comparison with side effects (loss of body weight) normally observed in adjuvant therapy (Balch, 1992), highlighting the ability of naturally occurring (seed oil) to inhibit melanoma growth with the view to develop new antitumor substances with low toxic potential.

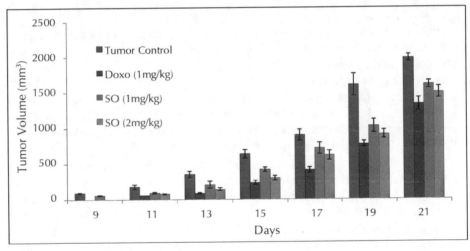

Figure 3. Effect of the *Eruca sativa* seed oil (every other day, from day 5th to 21st) on the melanoma growth. *Mean ± SE (n = 5). DOXO: Doxorubicin, SO: Seed Oil.*

ANTIMUTAGENIC ACTIVITY

Antimutagenic activity of seed oil was observed in terms of chromosomal aberration (Savage, 1993) and micronucleus assay (Schmid, 1975) by the induction of melanoma cells. The effect of the test samples on percent of chromosomal aberration was measured in terms of chromatid breaks, centric rings, acrocentric association, acentric fragments, intercalary deletion, and total abnormal metaphases (Slide 1). Percent of aberrant metaphase in various groups were found as: cancerous control (82.60%), doxorubicin treated (77.80%; 1 mg/kg) while for seed oil treated (51.20 and 47.50%) at two doses 1 and 2 mg/kg, respectively (Table 1). Seed oil exhibited significantly (p

< 0.01) reduction in chromosomal aberration like CB, CR, ACA, FR, ICD, and pulverization in bone marrow cells compared to tumor control and standard doxorubicin drug. The order of chromosomal aberration was found as: seed oil > doxorubicin drug > tumor control group.

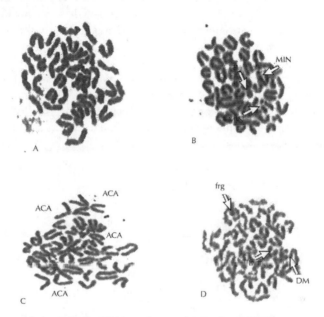

Slide 1. Chromosomal aberration in (A) Normal control animal and (B) Tumor control animal (C) *E. sativa* seed oil treated animal (D) Doxorubicin treated animal after induction of B16F10 melanoma cells.

Table 1. Effect of *Eruca sativa* seed oil on aberrant metaphases in the bone marrow of melanoma tumor induced mice.

Group	CB	CR	FR	ACA	Pulvi	ICD	Abnormal metaphase
Grp I	0.20 ± 0.40	0.0 ± 0	0.60 ± 0.54	0.0 ± 0	0.0 ± 0	0.0 ± 0	0.8 ± 0.84
Grp II	12.80 ± 2.28^b	6.20 ± 0.83^b	23.80 ± 2.49^b	34.20 ± 1.92^b	4.20 ± 1.09^b	4.40 ± 3.20^b	82.60 ± 2.49^a
Grp III	10.60 ± 3.36^b	5.60 ± 1.14^b	17.40 ± 2.30^b	33.60 ± 2.88^b	3.20 ± 1.92^b	5.40 ± 1.94^b	77.80 ± 3.76^a
Grp IV	8.60 ± 1.82^c	2.60 ± 1.14^c	11.24 ± 1.51^c	28.92 ± 3.12^c	0.0 ± 0^a	2.60 ± 1.14^c	51.20 ± 5.32^b
Grp V	8.20 ± 1.09^c	2.40 ± 0.70^c	10.30 ± 1.93^c	23.35 ± 3.42^c	0.0 ± 0^a	3.60 ± 1.14^c	47.50 ± 2.95^b

Mean ± SE (n = 5). [a]p > 0.05, [b]p < 0.001 vs. Normal Control; [c]p < 0.01 vs. Normal and Tumor Control.

Group I: Normal; Group II: Tumor control; Group III: Doxorubicin, Group IV: Seed oil (1 mg dose); Group V: Seed oil (2 mg dose). CB: Chromatid Break, CR: Centric Ring, FR: Fragment, ACA: Acrocentric Association, Pulvi: Pulvirization, ICD: Intracalary Deletion.

The effect of seed oil on melanoma induced mice was determined in terms of micronucleated polychromatic erythrocytes (MPCEs) and normochromatic erythrocytes

(MPCEs) per 1,000 cells. Percent of MPCE and MNCE in various groups were found as: cancerous control (100%), doxorubicin treated (84-89%; 1 mg/kg) while seed oil treated (14–15 and 6–10%) at two doses 1 and 2 mg/kg respectively (Figure 4). Seed oil treated mice were significantly (p <0.001) reduced the formation of micronuclei in PCEs and NCEs comparable with tumor control and doxorubicin treated group. The micronucleus assay has been used in cytogenetic studies to detect chromosomal changes such as acentric chromosome, chromatid fragments, and chromosome lagging at anaphase. Formation of MN in the interphase is dependent on factors such as cell cycle stage and types of mutagens. Micronuclei were considered an indication of a mutation effect (Auerbach, 1962). Results of this study indicate that the seed oil reduced the frequency of micronuclei per PCEs and NCEs. The decrease in PCEs and NCEs in tumor alone mice reflects the early effects on cell cycle leading to mitotic inhibition. The observed antimutagenic efficacy showed the similar trends of chromosomal aberration assay.

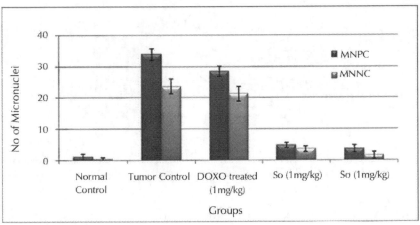

Figure 4. Effect of the *Eruca sativa* seed oil on frequency of micronuclei formation per PCEs and NCEs against standard doxorubicin.

HISTOPATHOLOGY STUDY

It is evidenced that tumor growth and lethality are dependent on angiogenesis. The decrease in tumor growth by test samples in mice may be attributed to decreased host angiogenesis. Representative photographs of melanoma after excision and photomicrographs of stained tumor micro sections are illustrated in Slide 2. A marked and dense microvasculature was observed in the control tumors. Tumors treated with SO (31.23 ± 6.3%) and doxorubicin (27.6 ± 6.7%) had significantly fewer micro-vessels compared with the control (62.6 ± 8.7%). The findings are in the harmony of earlier observation (Barnhill et al., 1998) that the suppression of melanoma is based on the triggering of apoptosis and angiogenesis. The improved angiogenesis inhibition observed with seed oil treatment is the indicative of high test sample accumulation in the tumor. The fact also finds support from the decreased tumor micro-vessel density resulting from seed oil treatment, suppressing the expression of angiogenic vascularization, tumor cell proliferation, and increased tumor cell apoptosis in melanoma.

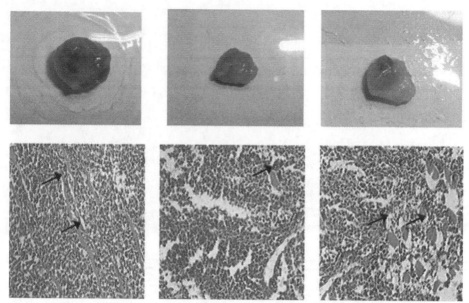

Slide 2. Histological observation of micro vessels among the tumor cells with solid tumor: (A) Control tumor (B) Doxorubicin treated (C) Seed oil treated are tissue sections stained by HE (200ꞁ). Arrows indicate micro vessels. Histological study demonstrated that numerous micro vessels with larger cavity and better integrity could be seen among the tumors of the mice injected with B16F10 cells. In contrast, micro vessels were few in the tumor of the mice treated with seed oil and doxorubicin.

CHEMISTRY PROFILE OF SEED OIL

Head Space/Solid Phase Micro Extraction analysis of the crude oil resulted in the identification of isothiocyanates by GC-MS. Identification of ITCs was accomplished by comparison with NIST 05 MS-library (f-fit > 700; r-fit > 650) and was confirmed using authentic standards in all cases (Figure 5). Seed oil revealed the presence of significant amount of allyl-ITC (40.30 µg/gm), 3-butenyl-ITC (259.60 µg/gm), 2-phenylethyl-ITC (158.50 µg/gm), 4-methyl sulfinyl butyl isothiocyanate (743.10 µg/gm) and bis(4-isothiocyanatobutyl)disulphide (~5000 µg/gm) and traces of erucin (Table 2) (Khoobchandani et al., 2010).

Table 2. Chemical structure of isothiocyanates identified in taramira seed oil.

Sulforaphane	Allyl isothiocyanate	2-phenylethylisothiocyanate
3-butenylisothiocyanate	Bis(4-isothiocyanatobytyl)disulfide	

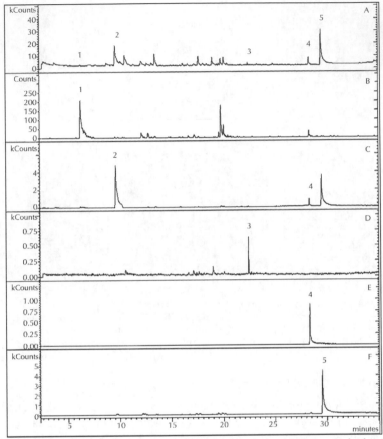

Figure 5. HS-SPME-GC-MS chromatograms obtained from analysis of *E. sativa* seed oil in Total ion Count (A) and in Selected Ion Monitoring of m/z 99 (B), m/z 72 (C), m/z91 (D), m/z 160 (E), m/z 86 (F).

Like other cruciferous vegetables, taramira plant is rich sources of sulfur-containing compounds known as glucosinolates, have recently garnered great interest for their potential role in the maintenance of human health. Chopping or chewing cruciferous vegetables results in the formation of bioactive glucosinolate hydrolysis products, such as isothiocyanates (Chen and Andreasson, 2001; Fahey et al., 1997; Zhang et al., 1992).

Formation of an isothiocyanate by hydrolysis of a glucosinolate
(Source: *Chen & Andreasson, 2001*)

Epidemiological studies suggest that high intake of cruciferous vegetables has been associated with lower risk of cancer (Jeffery and Jarrell, 2001; Poppel et al., 1999). Many organizations, including the National Cancer Institute, recommend the consumption of five to nine servings (2.5–4.5 cups) of fruits and vegetables daily. The isothiocyanates rich seed oil triggering of cell cycle arrest, enzymatic free radical scavenging, and blockage of DNA damage in the suppression of melanoma has been proposed in the schematic pattern (Figure 6).

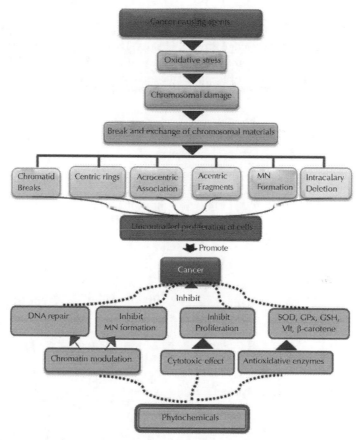

Figure 6. Tentative mechanism depicting isothiocyanates inhibition of cancer.

CONCLUSION

ITCs-rich seed oil was, notably, the only preparation of *E. sativa* capable of significant reduction of melanoma *in vivo* at 21st day, at doses only twice as large as those effective for the reference drug doxorubicin. Overall, the results nicely complement other investigations depicting the safe and health promoting value of dietary consumption of *E. sativa*, highlighting its potential for clinical applications and lend support to its use in traditional medicine without any toxicity and loss of body weight.

KEYWORDS

- **Cancer**
- ***Eruca sativa***
- **Melanoma**
- **Micronucleated polychromatic erythrocytes**
- **Mutations**

ACKNOWLEDGMENT

The authors gratefully acknowledge Prof. V. G Dass, Director, Dayalbagh Educational Institute, Dayalbagh, Agra, for providing necessary research facilities. M. Khoobchandani acknowledges Department of Science and Technology (New Delhi) for Financial Assistant.

Chapter 12

Optical and Mechanical Investigations of Nanostructures for Biomolecular Detection

G. Malegori, D. Nardi, F. Banfi, C. Giannetti, and G. Ferrini

INTRODUCTION

Since Luigi Galvani (1737–1798) began his studies, physics and biology have interacted and many tools from physics have been used in the biological sciences. Today the availability of new microscopic techniques has pushed the boundaries from the μm to the (sub-) nm level. These possibilities stimulate to find ever more creative ways of using physics, material science, and biology combined together.

In particular, the development of techniques capable of measuring the chemical and mechanical state of biological samples, *in vivo* and with attention to molecular dynamics localized at surfaces is of great interest. The way organic thin films properties are affected by molecular interactions at surfaces makes such films a model system for biological research and applications ranging from light-emitting diodes and solar cells to chemical sensors and nanomedicine. Moreover, the possibility of studying surface chemical reactions in biological samples without treatments and *in vivo* is an important issue for the understanding of the complex chemical machinery of living cells. Many cell functions depend on surface ligand-receptor complexes or surface chemical reactions and many kind of tumors start from the first cellular layer inside hollow organs. Therefore, non-invasive techniques that allow an *in vivo* study of chemical processes located at surfaces constitute important tools to develop and test biological models and target diseases.

An approach trying to combine these aspects will be reviewed here, based on the following techniques: (a) Optical detection based on evanescent wave spectroscopy, (b) femtosecond laser pulses used to excite thermal and mechanical transients in nanoengineered materials, (c) Non-Contact Atomic Force Microscopy (NC-AFM) and force spectroscopy.

The complementarity of these seemingly not related techniques aims to foster an approach beneficial for the problems at hand in nanomedicine and drug delivery. While chemical information is provided by optical spectroscopy, mechanical, and structural parameter could be retrieved by NC-AFM and optically induced mechanical transients. The measured parameters could in principle be related to a single theoretical model, thus characterizing the response of the system with a multimodal approach.

MOLECULAR DETECTION AT SURFACES USING EVANESCENT WAVE SPECTROSCOPY

One interesting possibility to develop surface sensitive spectroscopic techniques is the use of evanescent waves (Knoll, 1998). The term evanescent wave optics refers to a number of optical phenomena and techniques associated with the total internal reflection of light at the boundary between two media of different optical properties, usually described by their refraction indexes, as can be observed at the boundary between a glass prism and water (see Figure 1). In this case, glass is the incidence medium, with refraction index n_i, and water is the transmitting medium, with refraction index n_t.

A laser light beam (wavelength λ) impinging upon that interface from the glass side, that is from the side of the material with the higher refractive index, will be totally (internally) reflected if the angle of incidence exceeds a critical value $\theta_c = sin^{-1}(n_t/n_i)$. However in the transmitting medium the optical field does not fall abruptly to zero. The optical E-field in the rarer medium along the propagation direction, E_x, has the usual oscillatory character of an electromagnetic wave. Instead, the component perpendicular to the interface, E_z, is bounded and decays exponentially into the optically rarer medium with a decay length l which is a function of the angle of incidence,

$$l = \lambda/(2\pi ((nsin\theta)^2-1)^{1/2}), \text{ for } \theta > \theta_c.$$

Such inhomogeneous electromagnetic wave in the rarer medium is called an evanescent wave. The advantage using this kind of waves resides in the selective illumination of the near-interface range, resulting in a surface selectivity for optical experiments due to this surface-bounded light. Moreover, its intensity is enhanced compared to the incoming wave, which results in a sensitivity enhancement for optical experiments. When an absorbing layer of molecules is present at the interface, the evanescent field interacts with molecular resonances, giving an absorption spectrum comparable to that observed in a transmission experiment. When films are much thinner than the penetration depth and the electric field amplitude can be considered constant over the film thickness, it is possible to associate an "effective thickness" to the film equivalent to that of a transmission experiment (Harrick and and du Pré, 1966). It results that the electric field amplitude in the thin film is determined by the refractive indexes of the incidence and transmission media.

Using a broadband spectral source it is possible to retrieve absorbance spectra of the molecular species absorbed on the surface and thus obtain a selective spectral fingerprint of the molecules at the surface. A particularly promising broadband spectral source is constituted by the white light continuum produced in nonlinear fibers seeded by a femtosecond laser oscillator. In this way, broadband continuum, extending from 450 to 1,600 nm with a nearly flat spectral intensity, can be obtained from few nanojoule pulses produced by a standard 120 fs-800 nm Ti:sapphire oscillator (Cilento et al., 2010). The key elements in continuum generation by high repetition rate and low energy per pulse sources are the newly developed micro structured photonic-crystal fibers (PCF), engineered to be nearly dispersion-free at particular frequencies in the near-infrared/visible range (see Figure 1). Nonlinear interactions between an infrared laser pulse propagating into the fiber and the silica core generate a broadband pulse output.

To demonstrate that this kind of light source could be effectively used in evanescent wave spectroscopy of biomolecules, the formation of thin films of Methylene Blue (MB) in aqueous solution at a fused quartz surface was investigated with evanescent wave absorption spectroscopy (Ferrini et al., 2009). The MB has a variety of aggregation states (monomers, H-dimers, J-dimers, trimers) that depend on the concentration and surface proximity. The spectra of the various aggregates are known and can thus be used to test new optical techniques.

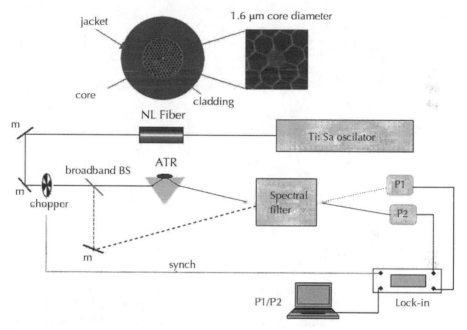

Figure 1. Evanescent wave optics.

The continuum spectrum is produced by delivering from 790 nm to 100 fs laser pulses with a maximum energy of 20 nJ from a Ti:Sapphire laser oscillator into a nonlinear fiber. The nonlinear fiber output is recollimated and split in two beams by a broadband beam splitter. One beam is sent into a fused quartz prism in a Kretchmann configuration, as shown schematically in Figure 1, the other is used as a reference. To directly probe MB in water solution, a drop of liquid is prepared on the surface of the prism. Both beams are collimated and successively spectrally filtered by the same monocromator, adjusting the angle with respect to the input slit to spatially separate the beams. The continuum is modulated by a chopper constituted by a photo elastic modulator at 50 kHz and the photodiode signal amplitude at the same frequency is detected by means of a lock-in amplifier. By taking the ratio between the probe beam and the reference beam, the attenuation produced by the MB solution can be measured at every wavelength.

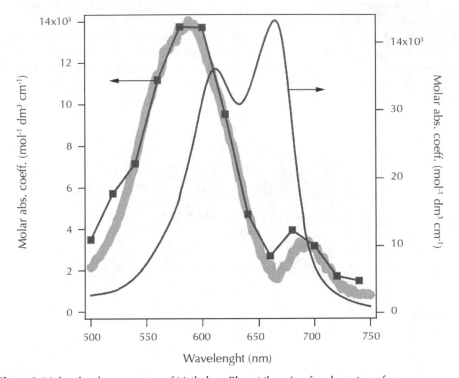

Figure 2. Molar absorbance spectra of Methylene Blue at the prism fused quartz surface.

The molar absorbance spectra of MB at the prism fused quartz surface are reported in Figure 2 (Ferrini et al., 2009). The thick gray line represent the retrieved spectrum for MB dimers at a fused silica surface after spin coating, complete solvent (ethanol) evaporation and reduction (Ohline et al., 2001). The square points represent the molar absorbance of the MB water solution retrieved from the evanescent white-light continuum absorption, with a surface molecular density of 10^{15} cm^{-2} (Ferrini et al., 2009) The continuous line is representative of the bulk molar absorption spectrum.

From the experimental data two main conclusions can be drawn. The first regards the aggregation state of MB near the fused silica surface. At the highest concentration available in this experiment, the MB at the surface is almost entirely organized in the form of dimers, as it is apparent from the prominence of the dimers peak in the absorbance data. The second regards the fact that the molar absorbance spectrum measured directly from a liquid water solution agree quantitatively with the dimer absorbance spectrum retrieved from an experiment using spin coating and complete solvent (ethanol) evaporation (Ohline et al., 2001), confirming that, at comparable concentrations, the dimers spectral features are the same in different experimental conditions.

From the spectra the aggregation state of MB near the fused silica surface was determined to be due almost entirely to dimers even if the molar concentration to obtain dimers aggregation in bulk water solution were much higher than that used in the experiment. This imply that MB dimer aggregation is favored by the vicinity of a quartz surface, a conclusion identical to those obtained by (Fujita, 2005) using optical waveguide spectroscopy with a broadband CW xenon lamp. While the combination of attenuated total internal reflection with a broadband light source allows to recover absorbance rapidly at all wavelengths, using short laser pulses opens the possibility to study the molecular dynamics at surfaces by means of pump and probe techniques. In fact, by adding a delayed pump pulse that excites the MB solution at the surface (either from the solution side or from the prism) it would be possible to study the temporal behavior of absorbance and/or orientation dynamics after an optical excitation, with a temporal resolution in the sub-ps time range. Moreover, the use of the asynchronous optical sampling technique (Bartels et al., 2007) to perform pump and probe experiments without mechanical delay line, with a time resolution below 100 fs in a 10 ns time measurement window and high speed scanning, opens the possibility to use evanescent wave absorption spectroscopy to follow in real time the modifications of the molecules electronic or vibrational dynamics in evolving chemical reactions.

Since, evanescent wave spectroscopy is a surface sensitive technique, its application in fluorescence resonance energy transfer (FRET) should give interesting insights, especially in situations where donor and acceptor chromophores labels molecules resident on surfaces and experiments in bulk solution are not possible.

MECHANICAL STUDY OF SURFACE NANOSTRUCTURES USING LASER GENERATED THERMAL TRANSIENTS

In recent years, the use of femtosecond laser pulses to excite thermal and mechanical transients in matter (Maris, 1998) led, in recent years, to the development of applied acoustics in the domains of material science and biology. Recently, this approach has been applied to nanoengineered materials to optically generate and detect acoustic waves in the gigahertz–terahertz frequency range. A review of the latest advances on ultrafast generation and detection of thermal gradients and pseudo-surface acoustic waves in lattices of metallic nanostructures, that is, elastic meta-materials, is of interest both to physicists and life scientists due to the development of new molecular sensors and manipulation techniques based on acoustic waves.

Nanostructured meta-materials emerged as model systems to investigate both the mechanical (Giannetti et al., 2009; Nardi et al., 2009) and thermal (Banfi et al., 2010) energy transfer at the nanoscale. The sensitivity of the all-optical time-resolved technique to deposited mass and thermal fluxes, coupled with the phononic crystal properties induced by the nanopatterned periodic lattices, opens the way to a variety of applications ranging from nanocalorimetry to mass sensors. The approach reported here is based on optical time-resolved experiments with femtosecond resolution over a 5 decades time window (100 fs to 10 ns) and does not require piezoelectric substrates. This approach extends the range of exploitable materials with respect to standard interdigital transducer-based mass sensor technology and paves the way to an increased miniaturization. The basic idea is to use a subpicosecond light pulse (pump pulse) focused to a small spot (the laser wavelength diffraction limit constituting the smaller achievable spot's diameter) to induce a nonequilibrium local heating of both electrons and lattice of the sample surface on the picosecond timescale. The local temperature increase triggers a sudden lattice expansion *via* the thermal expansion coefficient. The photoinduced thermoelastic stress launches strain pulses propagating away from the pump-excited spot, propagating at the sound velocity. Since the refractive index of the material depends on its local strain, through the photoelastic constant, it is possible to follow the propagation of the strain pulses monitoring the reflectivity variation of a second delayed pulse (probe pulse) focused at the same or different locations on the sample. An energy per pulse of the order of 1 nJ, which is easily available by means of Ti:sapphire oscillators producing 100 fs light pulses at 100 MHz repetition rate, can be exploited to impulsively heat semiconductor or metal samples, leading to temperature raises of the order of 0.1-10 K, implying thermoelastic stresses ranging from 0.1 to 1 Mbar.

Among the mechanical modes excited by short laser pulses, Surface Acoustic Waves (SAWs) have the greatest practical relevance. The SAWs are solutions of the elastic eigenvalue equation in which the displacement field is confined to the surface within a depth of the order of the wavelength (Landau and Lifschitz, 1986), very much like the evanescent electromagnetic waves addressed in the previous section. In particular, when the pump pulse is focused on a small area of $1-10$ μm^2 of a surface, the large Fourier spectrum of the excited acoustical waves allows launching of SAWs at different k-wave vectors. Time-resolved imaging techniques have been employed to follow the picosecond-timescale The SAW propagation on free surfaces (Sugawara et al., 2002), through grain boundaries (Hurley et al., 2006), in phononic crystals (Profunser et al., 2006), and in resonators (Maznev, 2009). In addition, SAWs in the hypersonic frequency range (> 1 GHz) are currently used to manipulate electrons in semiconductor devices (Cecchini et al., 2006) and photons in microcavities (de Lima et al., 2005).

Notably, the same pump-probe technique can be applied to study heat transport in matter (Stoner and Maris, 1993). The pump-induced temperature variation triggers a heat flow on the subnanosecond timescale from the heated volume to the rest of the sample. The dependence of the refractive index on the temperature enables following the propagation of heat pulses by means of the optical probe pulse. This technique, named time-domain thermo reflectance, has been employed to investigate the thermal conductance at metal–metal (Gundrum et al., 2005) and metal–dielectric (Lyeo and Cahill, 2006; Stoner and Maris, 1993) interfaces and to disentangle the energy transport related to electron diffusion (Gundrum et al., 2005), anharmonic phonon decay (Lyeo and Cahill, 2006), and ballistic phonon transport (Highland et al., 2007; Siemens et al., 2010). The signature of ballistic heat transport (von Gutfeld and Nethercot, 1966), has been recently reported at cryogenic temperatures in a GaAs crystal covered by a metallic thin film transducer (Perrin et al., 2006). The extension of this technique to the study of thermal transport between a single metallic nanoparticle and the environment is a more difficult task, due to the difficulties in controlling the properties of the nanoparticle-environment interface (Juvé et al., 2009; Voisin et al., 2000).

The frontier, in this intriguing research field, is the investigation of the thermo mechanical transients occurring between in lattices of metallic nanostructures and the underlying substrate (Giannetti et al., 2007; Hurley et al., 2006, 2008; Lin et al., 1993; Robillard et al., 2007; Siemens et al., 2009; Tobey et al., 2004). State-of-the-art nano-lithography and patterning techniques allow obtaining metallic nanostructures, whose shapes, dimensions, periodicities, and interface properties can be carefully tuned. The interest in these systems is inherent to the following features: (i) the periodicity, poten-tially scalable down to the 10 nm range (Chao et al., 2005), can be exploited to launch quasi-monochromatic SAWs in the substrate beyond the 10 GHz range (Siemens et al., 2009); (ii) the opening of a band gap in the acoustic modes (Nardi et al., 2009); and (iii) the fine control over the nanostructures/substrate interface, as required to investi-gate heat transport at the nanoscale.

The above-mentioned approach is here shown in a paradigmatic experiment. A scheme of the pump and probe experiment is shown in Figure 3.

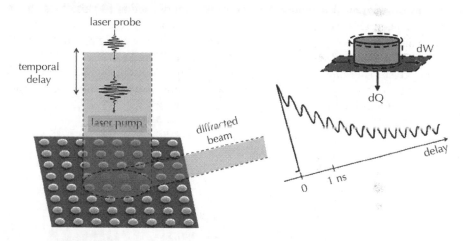

Figure 3. Schematic representation of the pump and probe experiment.

The pump beam selectively heats the permalloy (iron-nickel alloy, $Fe_{20}Ni_{80}$) nanodisks patterned in a square periodic array, leaving the temperature of the silicon substrate substantially unaltered. The sudden (ps time scale) thermal expansion of the nanodisk triggers two concurrent dynamics: (a) a SAW is launched in the substrate, finally transferring mechanical energy, dW, to the Si bulk (ns time scale), and (b) the disks thermalize with the silicon substrate transferring heat, dQ, on a ns timescale. The time-delayed probe pulse investigates these dynamics.

As the delay from the pump pulse increases, the disks temperature decreases and the transient average radius of the disks shrinks accordingly. The intensity of the dif-fracted probe pulse decreases because of a shrinking reflecting surface (nanosisks area). In the meanwhile the disks oscillate at the SAW frequency, inducing the oscilla-tions in the diffracted probe signal intensity. The oscillation is exponentially dumped due to mechanical energy radiation to the bulk (Giannetti et al., 2007; Nardi et al., 2009).

In Figure 4 (Giannetti et al., 2009), we report the time-resolved measurements on two-dimensional square lattices of permalloy nanodisks, with a thickness of 30-50 nm and a diameter of 400-600 nm. The laser source is a Ti:sapphire oscillator, delivering light pulses with 120 fs time duration, 30 nJ energy/pulse, and 790 nm wavelength, at a repetition rate of 76 MHz. The output is split into an intense component (pump, 10 nJ) and a weak component (probe, less than 1 nJ). The delay between the pump and probe pulses is changed by a mechanical delay-line. A feedback system that drives two piezo-nanomotors mounted on optical mirrors is used to keep the alignment between pump and probe. To optimize the optical signal-to-noise ratio, the pump and probe beams are focused on the same point of the sample with a diameter of 60 and 40 μm, respectively. This size allows exciting and probing a large number of nanostructures (about 3,000), while keeping the laser fluence high enough to significantly excite the system. A Peltier device is used to keep the sample back side temperature constant during the experiment. The pump beam intensity is modulated at 100 kHz by a photo-elastic modulator (PEM), placed between two crossed polarizers (chopper). In order to improve the signal to noise ratio the probe is detected recording the relative intensity variation of the first diffraction order spot, the nanostructured surface lattice (surface phononic crystal) serving as a diffraction grating. This technique avoids all nonperiodic contributions in the probe signal, such as Brillouin scattering from the acoustic pulses propagating into the substrate. The first-order diffracted beam is detected by a photodiode and filtered by a lock-in amplifier referenced at the PEM frequency (Giannetti et al., 2007). Relative intensity variations of the order of 10^{-6} can be measured with a time resolution of 120 fs in a time window of 3 ns.

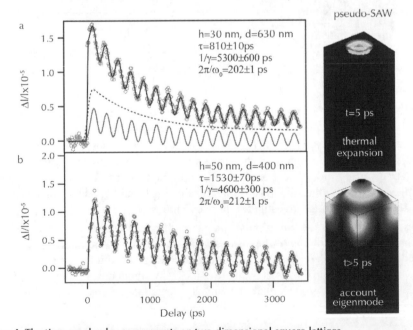

Figure 4. The time-resolved measurements on two-dimensional square lattices.

In the experimental trace (see Figure 4), at zero delay, it is possible to see a fast increase of the transient signal while a nanosecond decay superimposed to an oscillation with much shorter period is detected for positive delays. Considering the laser energy density absorbed by the nanostructures and by the silicon substrate, we can estimate that, within 5 ps, the temperature of the nanodisks is homogeneously increased by about 10 K. In contrast, the substrate temperature is essentially unvaried due to the different penetration depth of the 800 nm radiation (Giannetti et al., 2007, 2009).

The light penetration depth is comparable with the nanostructure height, hence a uniform heating of the nanodisks is obtained and the impulsive temperature mismatch triggers a nonequilibrium expansion of the nanostructures dimensions (of the order of 10^{-5} considering the effective thermal expansion coefficient of the Py/Si system). The expanded periodic nanostructures induce a spatially modulated stress on the silicon surface. Such stress launches a pseudo-SAW with a wavelength matching the nanodisks two-dimensional lattice periodicity. The variation of the diffracted light intensity as a function of the delay evidences that the nanostructures, due to the thermal expansion, oscillates around a larger diameter with respect to the unperturbed value, which is proportional to the average temperature. The transient average diameter decays following the disk cool down due to the energy exchange with the substrate. The oscillation dynamic is well represented by the fit function in Figure 4(a) (black line), obtained by the sum of a damped oscillating function (continuous gray line, representing the SAW) and a simple exponential decay (dashed gray line, due to disk cool down). The oscillating and the exponentially damped curves have been scaled for graphical reasons.

The period of the oscillations (T), superposed on the exponential decay, are related to the lattice spatial periodicity (λ), and are connected by the sound velocity (v): $\lambda/T = v$. The frequency $\upsilon = 1/T$ is the oscillation Eigen frequency of the surface waves associated to the 2D nanostructured lattice. Finally, the decaying amplitude of the oscillations is due to the elastic energy dissipation in the bulk, much like by a spring affected by viscous damping.

It is important to note that the disks thermalization with the silicon substrate on a nanosecond timescale can be followed by this technique, providing also important thermo dynamical information at the nanoscale. The reader is referred to (Banfi et al., 2010; Giannetti et al., 2007; Siemens et al., 2010) for a fuller account.

The possibility to optically control the excitation of SAW and thermal gradients in arrays of metallic nanostructures on substrates opens the way to fundamental applications in the field of hypersonic phononics, nanocalorimetry, and biology. The sensitivity of the time-resolved techniques can be exploited to develop mass sensors with picosecond time resolution. Considering that a difference of 10 ps in the oscillation period has been measured for the samples reported in Figure 4, we can easily estimate the sensitivity of these devices. The nanostructures volume difference in the two samples is $\Delta V = 5 \cdot 10^{-17}$ cm^3, corresponding to a mass difference/disk of $\Delta m = 5 \cdot 10^{-16}$ g/disk. In the probe area, the number of nanodisks is about 1,250, giving an absolute mass variation of $\Delta m = 625$ fg. Shorter SAW wavelengths imply higher surface confinement and, hence, higher surface sensitivity (Auld, 1990). The proposed device periodicity can be scaled to tens of nanometers, thus enhancing the sensitivity.

The experimental scheme reported in this work proves useful to access the specific heat, that is nanocalorimetry (Banfi et al., 2010), or thermal conductivity of mesoscale/ nanoscale samples (Wilson, 2007). Without entering in details, the quantities controlling the thermal dynamics can be extracted from the exponentially decaying contribution to the diffracted probe intensity, see Figure 4. Such informations could be of interest for the thermodynamics at the nanoscale of biomolecules or receptor aggregates.

A NEW APPROACH TO ATOMIC FORCE SPECTROSCOPY USING WAVELET TRANSFORMS

Atomic force microscopy (AFM) (Garcia and Perez, 2002; Giessibl, 2003; Morita et al., 2002) has developed into a powerful technique, delivering not only topographical images with sub-molecular resolution (Gross et al., 2009) but also providing sensitive force measurements on the atomic scale (Lantz et al., 2001; Sugimoto et al., 2007). Such force measurements are commonly referred to as force spectroscopy. The simplest technique used for quantitative force measurements exploit the static deflection of the cantilever, from which the force is determined using Hooke's law (Butt et al., 2005).

The investigation of mechanical properties of biological samples with AFM has received considerable attention in the past years (Cross et al., 2007; Radmacher et al., 1996; Rosenbluth et al., 2006). In addition to fundamental research interests, monitoring local mechanical properties of cells allows a better understanding of the mechanism of some diseases causing cell stiffness changes (Costa, 2003). The elastic properties of bacteria or cell walls can be determined by taking force curves using AFM. The stiffness of the exterior cell surfaces is measured by indenting them with a cantilever tip, achieving a lateral resolution of few tens of nm (Butt et al., 2005).

When the surface of a biological object is deformed by the pressure exerted by the tip of an AFM cantilever, the amount of displacement with respect to the under-formed surface (the indentation) carries information on its elastic properties. The deflection of the cantilever as its tip indents an object is usually described with models of linear elasticity theory (Landau et al., 1959).

In the literature there are examples of force spectroscopy applied to cell walls or soft samples in the absence of strong interaction between the tip and the surface. In this case, soft cantilevers can be used for indentation studies without taking into account instabilities caused by jump-to-contact or force modulations due to the interactions between tip and surface. However, in the natural environment, the presence of strong adhesion of the tip to the cell surfaces is often found. Moreover, there is frequently the need to immobilize mobile samples (cells, bacteria, spores). As an example, we mention that the Young modulus of the external surface of *Clostridium tyrobutyricum* spores, with an atomic force microscope and in air, can be reliably measured despite the strong tip-spore adhesion forces and the need to immobilize the spores due to their slipping on most substrates (Andreeva et al., 2009).

More refined techniques with respect to static force spectroscopy rely on measuring of the cantilever's dynamical parameters while it is excited at or near its resonant frequency and interacts with the force field provided by a sample surface (Albrecht et al., 1991). A recent development of this dynamic technique is known as three-dimensional (3D) force spectroscopy (Albers et al., 2009). It emerges that the so called "non-contact" atomic force microscopy (NC-AFM) is a powerful tool to study not only the surface topography, but also the mechanical and chemical characteristics of the sample at the nanoscale. The tip of an excited cantilever is sensitive to both forces and force gradients, when approaching the sample surface. The response of the interacting cantilever may show a modification of the oscillation amplitude, frequency, phase, or damping. The measurement of these cantilever parameters provides information on the physical properties of the sample with (sub) molecular resolution. In dynamical force spectroscopy, the influence of the local environment on the cantilever oscillations around the equilibrium position is usually detected by an optical beam deflection method, and the cantilever dynamics is analyzed by the Fourier transform (FT), that represents the temporal oscillations of the cantilever in the frequency domain. By doing so, the Eigen modes of the cantilever oscillations are displayed in the spectrum as resonance peaks. However, FT analysis is correctly interpreted only in the case of stationary systems that is, the frequency spectrum must be correlated with a temporally invariant physical system. In many cases, even if the interacting sample–cantilever system changes its spectral response during the acquisition, as in the tapping mode technique, the origin of the spectral features can be traced to the interaction dynamics from reasonable assumptions. However, in these cases, the FT of the signal only displays an average spectrum over the collection time and prevents a direct correlation of the frequency features with the signal modifications in time and their temporal evolution.

To go beyond these limitations, a mathematical tool that combines time domain and frequency domain analysis is useful for non-stationary signals. There are several mathematical approaches providing a time–frequency representation of a signal, using basis functions that do not extend indefinitely in time as the Fourier basis (e.g., windowed Fourier transform). One of the most refined approaches is the wavelet transform (WT) analysis (Mallat, 1999). The WTs are computed by correlating the signal $f(t)$ with families of time–frequency atoms, called wavelets. The wavelets are smooth functions $\Psi(t)$ with a limited support in time (unlike the Fourier basis) whose oscillation behavior sets the frequency resolution. Being limited in time, the wavelet functions are subjected to translation in time (d) and dilation by a positive scale factor (s). Time translation (d) is connected to time (t) and dilations (s) to frequency (f). By correlating the translated and dilated wavelets ($\Psi_{s,d}(t)$) with the signal for every delay (d) and every scale (s) in a range, a two dimensional map of "resemblance coefficients" $Wf(s,d)$ is obtained, giving at every delay (d) the resemblance of the signal with the wavelet scaled by the coefficients.

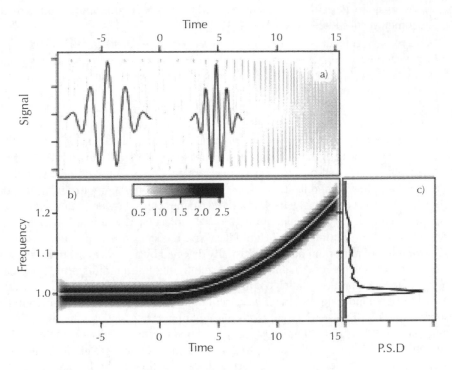

Figure 5. Comparision of Fourier transform (FT) and wavelet transform (WT). (a) Shows the time signal, a cosine function for negative times and a cosine with quadratic chirp. (b) WT of the signal, coded in gray scale describes the evolution of its spectral content.

In Figure 5 (Malegori and Ferrini, 2010(b)), the FT and the WT analysis are compared. Figure 5 (a) shows the time signal, a cosine function for negative times and a cosine with quadratic chirp (i.e., a frequency proportional to the square of time) for positive times. Two wavelet functions with different dilations and delays are superposed to the signal to show the local resemblance between signal and wavelet. The WT of the signal, coded in gray scale (see Figure 5(b)), correctly describes the evolution of its spectral content. The white line superposed on the WT is the calculated instantaneous frequency. In Figure 5(c) the FT (power spectral density) of the signal is displayed. Only an average of the signal instantaneous frequencies is observed.

From the previous example, it is clear that WT converts a one-dimensional time signal into a two-dimensional time–frequency image, which displays the time and frequency information of the signal in a time–frequency plane. The square modulus of the wavelet coefficients $|Wf(s,d)|^2$ is proportional to the local energy density of the signal at the given delay and scale. Thus, WT represents the temporal evolution of the spectral energy content of the signal (Malegori and Ferrini, 2010b, 2011a).

The dynamics of a free cantilever in air can be reasonably modeled as a harmonic oscillator with viscous dissipation. In NC-AFM, the frequency shift of the cantilever is proportional to the gradient of the interaction force for small frequency shifts (Morita et al., 2002). The frequency shift can be followed in real time by the WT, allowing to capture transient force interactions that could not be measured otherwise.

An example of this technique is presented in Figure 6 (Malegori and Ferrini, 2010b). In panel (a) is shown the power spectral density of the Brownian motion of the first flexural mode of the cantilever (Malegori and Ferrini, 2010a) while the tip is moved into interaction with a graphite surface.

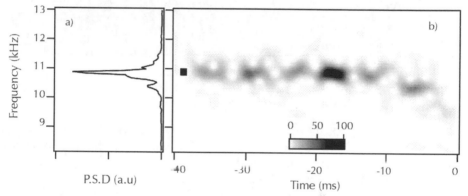

Figure 6. (a) Power spectral density of the Brownian motion of the first flexural mode of the cantilever. (b) WT of the same signal that is the cantilever thermal fluctuations around its instantaneous equilibrium position.

The Brownian motion is enhanced in correspondence of the first resonance frequency of the cantilever at about 11 kHz. However the power spectral density gives no information on the frequency shift due to the cantilever interaction. Figure 6(b) shows the WT of the same signal that is the cantilever thermal fluctuations around its instantaneous equilibrium position, as the tip approaches the surface at constant velocity of about 225 nm/s. The wavelet coefficients $|Wf(f,t)|$ are coded in grayscale. In this case, a clear frequency shift as a function of time is detected. The origin of the time axis corresponds to the jump-to-contact onset, a phenomenon due to strong surface forces that induce the cantilever tip to land on the surface almost at once. The wavelet frequency resolution $\Delta\Omega$ and time resolution Δt are limited by a time-frequency uncertainty principle, much like the Heisenberg principle in quantum mechanics, which states that $\Delta t \, \Delta\Omega \geq 1/2$. The black box at the left side of Figure 6(b) represents the so called Heisenberg box, the minimum uncertainty area for the analyzing wavelet. It is important to note that the entire measurement takes only a few tens of ms, a time compatible with force imaging acquisition rates.

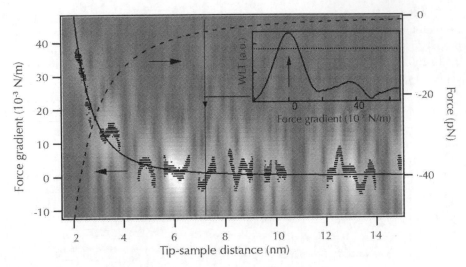

Figure 7. Quantitative analysis based on the WT of the Brownian motion.

Figure 7 (Malegori and Ferrini, 2010b) presented a quantitative analysis based on the WT of the Brownian motion shown in Figure 6. In this case the time axis of Figure 6 is converted into tip-sample distance taking into account tip velocity and cantilever static deflection. Then, the WT "ridges" are calculated to provide the instantaneous frequencies evolution within the limits of the wavelet resolution. The wavelet ridges are the crest of the wavelet coefficients, that is, the local maxima of the normalized WT above a specified threshold, as schematically shown in the inset. The threshold is represented by a horizontal line and the maximum point is indicated by an arrow for a vertical cut of the data at constant tip-sample distance. The frequency shift is converted into the interaction force gradient (Morita et al., 2002) allowing to map the force gradient versus tip-sample distance curve. The continuous black line is a Hamaker-like force-gradient function fitted to the wavelet ridges by considering a Van der Waals type interaction potential. The dashed line is the interaction force calculated by integration.

The technique used to retrieve the measurements contained in Figure 7 could be of interest not only to study the force fields near solid surfaces, but also to characterize force fields in the proximity of surfaces covered with receptors or other kinds of biomolecules, thus characterizing the chemical specificity *via* mechanical interactions. Moreover, the same analysis can be used to follow the frequency evolution of the cantilever torsional modes (Malegori and Ferrini, 2011b), which give important information on the friction between tip and sample and allow the nanotribology study of surfaces (Schirmeisen, 2010). Another important evolution of the wavelet analysis is towards force spectroscopy in liquid environments that are of great interest for biological studies (Fukuma et al., 2007).

CONCLUSIONS

Mechanical interactions and forces are fundamental to biology. Those of chemical origin govern transport on the molecular scale and determine motility and adhesion on the cellular scale. Measuring mechanical interactions at the nanoscale provides unique opportunities to measure forces, displacements, and mass changes from cellular and subcellular processes. Optical spectroscopy is a powerful technique that allows detecting and identifying various samples through the "fingerprint" of their specific molecular vibrations. The progress in the studies of biological sample has led to the possibility of realizing optical biodiagnostics. Femtosecond laser technology is mature enough to be part of complex optical systems to be used in potential applications not only in biochemistry but also as biodiagnostics of viruses, bacteria, or even cancer cells at the molecular level. The merging of mechanical interactions, probed with AFM force spectroscopy, with surface specific femtosecond optical spectroscopy techniques (evanescent wave optical spectroscopy) provides new opportunities to follow the dynamics of a single molecule in time. Moreover, the merging of femtosecond light excitation with mechanical surface waves prospects the possibility of manipulating the mechanical degrees of freedom of single molecules (e.g., vibrational modes) and having ultrasensitive and ultrafast mass diagnostics down to the femtogram level. The ultimate goal of these efforts is to create a multiprobe laboratory on a common platform to apply the techniques described in previous sections to the same (biological) system.

KEYWORDS

- **Atomic force microscopy**
- **Fluorescence resonance energy transfer**
- **Methylene Blue**
- **Photonic-crystal fibers**
- **Surface Acoustic Waves**

ACKNOWLEDGMENT

This work was partially supported by MIUR under contract PRIN 2008JWKYXB and by Università Cattolica through D.2.2 grants.

Chapter 13

Suffering and Comfort in Portuguese Cancer Patients

João Luís Alves Apystolo, Rita Susana Soares Capela,
and Inês Barata Sá Castro

INTRODUCTION

Someone who is diagnosed with a severe illness experiences feelings of threat, loss, uncertainty, finitude, anxiety, and of deprivation of basic needs, which cause discomfort and suffering. Suffering is part of the personal experience of cancer patients, particularly terminal patients who not only have to face physical symptoms, but are also confronted with the idea of death being near and, therefore, feel their integrity is threatened. In addition, cancer patients experience discomfort resulting from the treatment itself, which can add to this sense of threat to physical integrity.

Nevertheless, individuals may have health projects encompassing a vital capacity and resilience to fight for life, in order to overcome the ontological condition of suffering and try to achieve levels of comfort that are necessary for existence, for life to go on.

ANALYSING THE CONCEPT OF SUFFERING

Suffering is a fundamental and universal experience of the human condition. It has been described as an inevitable human experience (Frankl, 2004), as the state of severe distress associated with events that threaten the integrity or continued existence of the person as a whole (Cassell, 1991). Suffering involves the construction of personal meanings that carry a strong affective load. Therefore, the way in which people deal with suffering is highly subjective and individual, and in order to understand it, one must access the individual meanings attributed and ways of responding to suffering, that is the subjective experiences of suffering (Gameiro, 2000; Mcintyre, 2004).

Most people find it hard to distinguish pain from suffering; however, these are very different entities that can be inter-related. Suffering is not limited to physical pain. It is always experienced by the whole-person and not merely on the body level (Cassell, 1991; Cassel, 1999; Fleming, 2003; Neto, 2004).

OPERATIONALIZING THE CONCEPT OF SUFFERING

Suffering can be understood as a complex, personal, and multidimensional phenomenon comprising five dimensions: psychological, physical, existential, sociorelational, and positive experiences related to suffering (Gameiro, 2000).

Physical suffering covers pain, discomfort, and loss of physical strength. This type of suffering focuses on the dimensions of pain and management of symptoms resulting from the disease or treatments, and also on energy loss and functional limitations. To put it in a simple way, one can say that pain, physical symptoms, or other disabilities (such as loss of energy or strength) limit the patients' access to the world, thus causing suffering (Barbosa, 2006; Gameiro, 2000).

Psychological suffering covers cognitive (disturbing and pessimistic ideas, etc.) and emotional disorders (such as depressed mood, anxiety, irritability, and psychological tension). Mental suffering and emotional suffering are both dimensions of psychological suffering. Mental suffering is mainly due to memory loss and concentration problems, lack of cognitive control due to preoccupations and difficulty in solving problems. Emotional suffering includes mood disorders, insomnia, ideas of abandonment, and desire to die (suicidal ideation/intent) (Barbosa, 2006; Gameiro, 2000).

Existential suffering is related to changes in personal identity (low self-esteem; changes in body image; sense of loss of function etc.), changes in the sense of control (loss of self-control; loss of perceived control over the situation; fatalism; lack of confidence in one's own skills; perceived loss of freedom, of control over one's life etc.), existential limitations (loss of purpose in life; sense of futility and personal insignificance; disappointment etc.), limitations in life projects (perceived threat or inability to develop one's own project etc.), and lack of harmony with oneself. In other words, existential suffering expresses the loss of life's meaning and the sense of uselessness and despair that can be experienced (Barbosa, 2006; Gameiro, 2000).

Socio-relational suffering refers to affective relational changes (due to separation from loved ones, empathic suffering, inability to perform family role etc.) and socio-professional changes (due to changes in socio-professional status and roles, loss of income etc.). This type of suffering is divided into two main components: family and social. The social component includes problems with health professionals, economic and professional problems, and lack of social and community support. The family component is related to patient-family communication problems (conspiracy of silence), self-blame for being dependent, deep concerns about the future, and sexual problems (Barbosa, 2006; Gameiro, 2000).

The dimension of positive experiences of suffering during illness resulted from the validation of *"The Inventory of Subjective Suffering Experiences in Illness"*—ISSEI conducted on a sample of 125 hospitalized patients in central hospitals. This new dimension of suffering accounts for the possibility of there being positive aspects about suffering, such as optimism and hope, which result from the illness process (Gameiro, 2000). Whereas loss is inevitable in illness, its negative consequences, particularly in the psychosocial and existential domains, may not be inevitable (Mcintyre, 2004).

In fact, it is possible for someone to adjust to the situation of suffering. Even in face of the most adverse conditions, it is possible to cope with the existential crisis and find a purpose in life (Frankl, 2004). In order to do this, patients have to believe they are fulfilling a role and have a purpose that is unique, living life to its fullest in accordance with their human potential. In this way, they can achieve a sense of plenitude, inner peace, and even transcendence (Neto, 2004).

ANALYSING THE CONCEPT OF COMFORT

Comfort has come to acquire a significant role in health care philosophy and it is recognized as a holistic outcome related to the responses of the whole-person. The comfort theory has been used to explain and predict phenomena of human responses to the health-illness process, and has contributed to a proper evaluation of care and to the assessment of intervention outcomes (Kolcaba, 1991, 2003).

In this way, comfort as a process (of comforting) or as a product (of interventions) is a noble concept that underlies the interventions of health professionals in the health-illness continuum, as well as the human responses to this process (Kolcaba, 1991; Kolcaba, 2003).

The word comfort comes from the Latin word *confortare* which means "to give back strength, vigor, and energy; make strong, reinforce, invigorate" (Instituto de Lexicologia e Lexicografia da Academia das Ciências de Lisboa, 2001). In view of these meanings, the concept of comfort could be misunderstood and considered too vague to be studied and assessed as a health and well-being component. In addition, comfort has a much more complex and diverse meaning than the one inferred from its etymology. Comfort is a dimension composed of dynamic processes, experiences, and concepts, such as quality of life, hope, control, and decision-making. Thus, control and absence of pain are often considered a synonym for comfort, while the presence and feeling of pain very often describe the meaning of the word discomfort. At the same time, discomfort is usually referred to as unmet needs, and when needs are satisfied they result in the experience of comfort. However, the state of comfort does not pre-suppose complete absence of discomfort because sensitivity to discomfort is relative and individual (Kolcaba, 1991, 2003).

One can consider four different meanings of comfort. The first meaning has to do with comfort as a cause, either of the state of comfort itself or of relief from discomfort. The second meaning associates comfort with a state of ease and peaceful contentment. Thus, comfort as a cause (first meaning) is supposed to produce comfort as an effect (second meaning) (Kolcaba and Kolcaba, 1991).

Many of life's conditions, such as concerns, pain, or suffering, mean absence of the state of comfort. The existence of these conditions is designated as discomfort, whose outcome is contrary to the state of comfort. It should be stressed that the state of comfort can exist without a prior state of discomfort (ease). However, when discomfort cannot be avoided, it is often neutralized with additional comforts, relieving discomfort.

The third meaning of comfort is in the sense of relief from discomfort and it can be understood through the first two meanings. The cause of relief is specified by the first meaning, whereas the state of comfort is specified by the second meaning. *When relief itself is called comfort, it need not to be equivalent to the state of comfort as it may be* incomplete, partial, or temporary if, for example, it is relief from only one of many discomforts. It can be partial because only a degree of relief is attained and temporary as it may last only until discomfort arises again.

According to the fourth meaning, comfort is whatever makes life easy or pleasurable. This refers to the goal of maximizing pleasure and in this aspect it is not applicable to nursing care.

A fifth and a sixth meaning of comfort can also be considered: one that comes from the Latin word *confortare* meaning to "strengthen greatly" (expressing the actions of strengthening, encouragement, incitement, aid, succor, support, and countenance); and another one that indicates physical refreshment or sustenance. These meanings are related to causes of renewal, amplifications of power, positive mindsets, and readiness for action. Thus, comfort is based on things that strengthen and encourage, support and/or physically refresh or invigorate a person (Kolcaba and Kolcaba, 1991).

OPERATIONALIZING THE CONCEPT OF COMFORT

In order to operationalize the concept of comfort, Kolcaba described it as the immediate experience of feeling strengthened when the basic human needs of relief, ease, and transcendence are addressed in four contexts of experience (physical, psychospiritual, sociocultural, and environmental) (Kolcaba, 1991, 2003).

Relief is the state in which a need has been met, essential for the person to re-establish her/his normal functioning; ease is a state of calmness or contentment and it is necessary for an effective performance; transcendence is the state in which people feel they have skills or potential to plan, control their destiny, and resolve their problems.

These three states of comfort can be experienced in the following four contexts: physical, psychospiritual, sociocultural, and environmental. The physical context pertains to bodily sensations; the psychospiritual context pertains to the internal awareness of self (including self-concept, sexuality, and purpose in one's life) and can also encompass one's relationship to a higher order or being; the sociocultural context pertains to interpersonal, familiar, and societal relationships; the environmental context involves items such as light, noise, equipment (furniture), color, temperature, and natural versus synthetic elements.

These four contexts, when combined with the three senses of comfort form a taxonomic structure (TS) of 12 cells, which represents the total Gestalt of patient comfort from the perspective of patients' needs and their fulfillment (see Table 1).

Table 1. Kolcaba's conceptual framework of comfort (Kolcaba, 1991).

States Contexts	Relief	Ease	Transcendence
Physical	Physical Relief	Physical Ease	Physical Transcendence
Psychospiritual	Psychospiritual Relief	Psychospiritual Ease	Psychospiritual Transcendence
Sociocultural	Sociocultural Relief	Sociocultural Ease	Sociocultural Transcendence
Environmental	Environmental Relief	Environmental Ease	Environmental Transcendence

COMPARING THE FINDINGS OF STUDIES ON COMFORT AND SUFFERING OF PORTUGUESE CANCER PATIENTS AND RELATIVES

Instruments used in the different studies:

(1) Sociodemographic and clinical questions;

(2) Comfort Chemotherapy Scale (CCS) (Apóstolo et al., 2006): five point Likert-type scale with 33 items, based on the operational model of "comfort" to assess the three states of comfort (relief, ease, and transcendence) in the four contexts described;

(3) The Inventory of Subjective Suffering Experiences in Illness—ISSEI—(Gameiro, 2000): five point Likert-type scale with 44 items to assess the five dimensions of suffering (psychological, existential, sociorelational, and positive experiences of suffering).

Study 1

Descriptive-analytic study aiming to describe the characteristics of suffering and comfort experienced by female patients undergoing chemotherapy, to analyze the relationship between the comfort and suffering experienced by these patients and to determine whether these states would be related to the number of chemotherapy cycles and to the patients' age (Apóstolo et al., 2006).

The CCS and the ISSEI were administered to a consecutive sample of 50 female patients diagnosed with cancer (breast and gynecological) undergoing chemotherapy in outpatient care, in a hospital of the Centre Region of Portugal. Mean age 51.94; SD 12.41, ranging from 30 to 74 years. Regarding education (years), 46% 4, 26% between 5 and 9, 8% between 10 and 12, and 20% higher education. Data was collected between 16 August and 30 October, 2004.

Main results: Number of chemotherapy cycles: 64% less than 5; 14% between 6 and 10; 4% between 11 and 15; 6% between 16 and 20; 12% more than 20 cycles.

The analysis of the dimensions showed that female patients undergoing chemotherapy reported higher discomfort and suffering in the state of relief and in the physical context, as well as higher comfort in the sociocultural context.

The analysis of the scales' items that revealed higher levels of suffering (assessed by the ISSEI) showed that these were related to the sociorelational level, particularly to the items that addressed the concern with the fact that being ill would bring suffering to relatives, that is the aspects of empathic suffering[1] (see Figure 1). Nevertheless, the aspects that registered a higher level of perceived comfort (assessed by the CCS) were related to family support[2].

---

[1] "I wish my family would not suffer so much because I am ill; My disease makes me worry about the future of people close to me; The idea that I cannot help my family as I did before makes me worried; I dread the fact that I may have to leave the people I care about".

[2] "My family/friends help me face the disease; To know that I am loved gives me strength to go on; People's affection around me brings me comfort; Visits from friends make me happy; The state of mind of the people around me gives me strength; If I need help, I have people who take care of me".

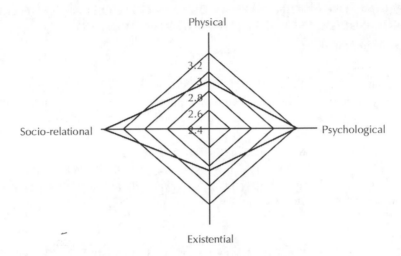

Figure 1. Profile of the suffering of patients undergoing chemotherapy.

These patients suffer because they understand how much suffering is brought to their loved ones due to the process of illness. On the other hand, being close to loved ones is understood as something that provides comfort, showing how important it is to have the presence and support of the family.

The high mean levels of suffering associated with inability to perform activities they used to assume before becoming ill and with the severity and worsening of health conditions are noteworthy. From a physical point of view, although there were few reports on high levels of pain, patients suffered with the anticipation of future pain and due to weariness and lack of physical vigor and energy.

Comfort and suffering were not correlated with the number of chemotherapy cycles or with the patients' age. Comfort correlated negatively with suffering and positively with the positive experiences of suffering. These two concepts are closely related and can be seen as part of a continuum in which one of the extremities--suffering/discomfort--corresponds to the existence of unmet human needs.

Study 2

Descriptive study aiming to characterize the patients' suffering in the context of oncology palliative care (Capela, 2010).

The ISSEI was administered to a consecutive sample of 50 inpatients or outpatients attending a palliative care unit in the North Region of Portugal. Mean age (years) 61,0; SD 14.0, ranging from 27-88 years; 48% male and 52% female; 66% married, 18 % widowed, 8% divorced, and 8% single. Regarding education (years), 58% 4, 20% 6, 2% 9, 4% 12, 6% undergraduate degree, 10% no education. Data was collected between 7 May and 15 October, 2009.

Main results: Patients showed high levels of sociorelational suffering, particularly affective-emotional suffering, that is they suffered from the negative impact of the disease on their closest relatives. The loss of physical vigor was also a great source of suffering because of its impact on the performance of activities of daily living, as well as psychological suffering, depressive mood, despair, existential limitations, loss of autonomy, and meaningfulness. The socio-professional changes are not a primary source of suffering. In addition, pain seems to be the symptom that brings less suffering to terminal patients.

Study 3
Descriptive-analytic study aiming to analyze the suffering of women undergoing chemotherapy after mastectomy and to identify the extent to which social support, physical and psychological morbidity, and some sociodemographic and clinical variables are related to such suffering (Ferreira, 2009).

The ISSEI was administered to a consecutive sample of 84 women undergoing chemotherapy after mastectomy in outpatient consultations in a day hospital. Mean age 52.99; SD 10.66, ranging from 35 to 76 years; 76.2% married, 11.8% widowed and 12% single, divorced or separated. Regarding education (years), 64.3% between 4 and 9, 25.0% between 13 and 19, 10.7% between 10 and 12. Data was collected between 24 July and 5 September, 2003.

Main results: number of chemotherapy cycles: 54.8% less than 8, 34.5% between 8 and 15, 10.7% between 16 and 25.

These findings revealed that patients experienced high psychological and sociorelational suffering and few positive experiences of suffering.

The patients who received more social support experienced less suffering, whereas those with more physical and psychological morbidity showed higher levels of suffering, namely older and single patients.

Patients with higher academic qualifications experienced less suffering and, as the number of chemotherapy cycles increased, patients experienced more and more suffering in all dimensions (except in the sociorelational dimension in the case of number of chemotherapy cycles).

Patients who were given information about breast reconstruction and those who planned to take this step showed less suffering when compared to those who were not informed and those who did not consider having a reconstruction.

Suffering was positively correlated with age.

Study 4
Qualitative phenomenological study aiming to describe the experience lived by relatives of inpatients with oncological illness in terminal condition, in a palliative care unit, with a sample of five close relatives (three male and two female participants) (Apóstolo et al., 2004).

Results revealed that families of cancer patients experienced a process that was focused on the patient and on themselves and that was surrounded by circumstantial elements typical of hospital environments.

The feelings and emotions shared by these relatives were essentially related to pain (because of the anticipation of an inevitable loss), impairment, sadness, anguish, anger, emptiness, and uncertainty. They suffered from witnessing the suffering of their ill relatives, their physical and psychological deterioration, and subsequent loss of role in the family system.

Daily life experienced a deep change when family members decided to be close to their ill relatives, that is, in the hospital setting where everything could be done to provide the best possible quality of life. Family needs became secondary in face of the patient's needs and they felt that they were losing their social identity.

However, there were some experiences that can be considered as positive, such as a feeling of personal growth since this experience can make the family reflect on the purpose of life and the importance of the patient in their lives.

CONCLUSION

The relation between suffering, number of chemotherapy cycles and patients' age is not unanimous in all studies. Results from study 3, unlike the ones from study 1, showed that suffering is positively correlated with the number of chemotherapy cycles and with age. Both studies included women undergoing chemotherapy after mastectomy with similar mean ages. However, study 1 comprised a smaller sample that included also women with gynecological cancer hampering the possibility of comparing both samples. In addition, 64% of patients in study 1 had undergone less than 5 cycles, whereas in study 3 45.2% of patients had undergone between 8 and 25 cycles.

Nevertheless, the main results from all studies point to the great importance of the family in the comfort and suffering of cancer patients. Family members are a source of comfort, making these patients feel loved. They help them cope with the disease and provide support, encouragement and comfort in the most difficult times, easing their sense of loss, and of impending threat to their integrity. However, family is also a source of concern and suffering for patients because of their fear of becoming a burden. Because the patients' close relatives are seen both as a source of comfort and as a potential focus of suffering, health care interventions should encompass not only physical relief, but also an understanding of the patients' sociorelational contexts, in order to help them finding a purpose in their life, suffering and existence.

Therefore, it seems that in order for interventions intending to relief suffering to be effective, they will have to include some support of family relationships because of the major importance assigned by these patients to the negative impact of the disease on their families. Health professionals can intervene to alleviate patients' suffering, particularly by establishing an open patient-family communication and adopting attitudes of sincerity, respect and trust that facilitate the sharing of vulnerabilities, experiences, thoughts, emotions, and feelings. In this way, a conspiracy of silence can be avoided while mutual personal development and relief from suffering are promoted.

KEYWORDS

- **Comfort**
- **Comfort Chemotherapy Scale**
- **Existential suffering**
- **Psychological suffering**
- **Relief**
- **Taxonomic structure**

References

1

Abdollahi, A., Hahnfeldt, P., Maercker, C., Grone, H. J., Debus, J., Ansorge, W., Folkman, J., Hlatky, L., and Huber, P. E. (2004). Endostatin's anti-angiogenic signaling network. *Mol. Cell.* **13**, 649–663.

Akao, Y., Nakagawa, Y., and Naoe, T. (2006). Let-7 microRNA functions as a potential growth suppressor in human colon cancer cells. *Biological and Pharmaceutical Bulletin* **29**, 903–906.

Ambros, V. (2001). microRNAs: Tiny regulators with great potential. *Cell* **107**, 823–826.

Ambros, V. (2004). The functions of animal microRNAs. *Nature* **431**, 350–355.

Antonelli-Orlidge, A., Saunders, K. B., Smith, S. R., and D'Amore, P. A. (1989). An activated form of transforming growth factor beta is produced by cocultures of endothelial cells and pericytes. *Proc. Natl. Acad. Sci. USA* **86**, 4544–4548.

Aznavoorian, S., Murphy, A. N., Stetler-Stevenson, W. G., and Liotta, L. A. (1993). Molecular aspects of tumor cell invasion and metastasis. *Cancer* **71**, 1368-1383.

Baratchi, S., Kanwar, R. K., and Kanwar, J. R. (2010). Survivin: A target from brain cancer to neurodegenerative disease. *Critical Reviews in Biochemistry and Molecular Biology* **45**, 535–554.

Baratchi, S., Kanwar, R. K., Khoshmanesh, K., Vasu, P., Ashok, C., Hittu, M., Parratt, A., Krishnakumar, S., Sun, X., Sahoo, S. K., and Kanwar, J. R. (2009). Promises of nanotechnology for drug delivery to brain in neurodegenerative diseases. *Current Nanoscience* **5**, 15–25.

Bartlett, D. W. and Davis, M. E. (2006). Insights into the kinetics of siRNA-mediated gene silencing from live-cell and live-animal bioluminescent imaging. *Nucleic Acids Res.* **34**, 322–333.

Bawa, R. (2009). NanoBiotech 2008: Exploring global advances in nanomedicine. *Nanomedicine* **5**, 5–7.

Benny, O., Fainaru, O., Adini, A., Cassiola, F., Bazinet, L., Adini, I., Pravda, E., Nahmias, Y.,

Koirala, S., Corfas, G., D'Amato, R. J., and Folkman, J. (2008). An orally delivered small-molecule formulation with anti-angiogenic and anticancer activity. *Nat. Biotechnol.* **26**, 799–807.

Blind, M., Kolanus, W., and Famulok, M. (1999). Cytoplasmic RNA modulators of an inside-out signal-transduction cascade. *Proc. Natl. Acad. Sci. USA* **96**, 3606–3610.

Brooks, P. C. (1996). Role of integrins in angiogenesis. *Eur. J. Cancer* **32A**, 2423–2429.

Calin, G. A., Dumitru, C. D., Shimizu, M., Bichi, R., Zupo, S., Noch, E., Aldler, H., Rattan, S., Keating, M., Rai, K., Rassenti, L., Kipps, T., Negrini, M., Bullrich, F., and Croce, C. M. (2002). Frequent deletions and down-regulation of micro- RNA genes miR-15 and miR-16 at 13q14 in chronic lymphocytic leukemia. *Proceedings of the National Academy of Sciences of the United States of America* **99**, 15524–15529.

Caplen, N. J., Parrish, S., Imani, F., Fire, A., and Morgan, R. A. (2001). Specific inhibition of gene expression by small double-stranded RNAs in invertebrate and vertebrate systems. *Proc. Natl. Acad. Sci. USA* **98**, 9742–9747.

Cavallaro, U. and Christofori, G. (2000). Molecular Mechanisms of Tumor Angiogenesis and Tumor Progression. *Journal of Neuro-Oncology* **50**, 63–70.

Cevc, G. (2004). Lipid vesicles and other colloids as drug carriers on the skin. *Adv. Drug. Deliv. Rev.* **56**, 675–711.

Chan, J. A., Krichevsky, A. M., and Kosik, K. S. (2005). MicroRNA-21 is an antiapoptotic factor in human glioblastoma cells. *Cancer Research* **65**, 6029–6033.

Chen, Y. and Gorski, D. H. (2008). Regulation of angiogenesis through a microRNA (miR-130a) that down-regulates anti-angiogenic homeobox genes GAX and HOXA5. *Blood* **111**, 1217–1226.

Cherian, A. K., Rana A. C., and Jain, S. K. (2000). Self-assembled carbohydrate-stabilized ceramic nanoparticles for the parenteral delivery of insulin. *Drug Dev. Ind. Pharm.* **26**, 459–463.

Cheung, C. G. A., Kanwar, J. R., and Krissansen, G. W. (2006). A cell-permeable dominant-negative survivin protein as a tool to understand how Survivin maintains tumour cell survival. *European Journal of Cancer* **4**, 149.

Clark, R. A., Tonnesen, M. G., Gailit, J., and Cheresh, D. A. (1996). Transient functional expression of alphaVbeta 3 on vascular cells during wound repair. *Am. J. Pathol.* **148**, 1407–1421.

Cleland, J. L. (1997). Protein delivery from biodegradable microspheres. *Pharm. Biotechnol.* **10**, 1–43.

Conradi, R. A., Hilgers, A. R., Ho, N. F., and Burton, P. S. (1992). The influence of peptide structure on transport across Caco-2 cells. II. Peptide bond modification which results in improved permeability. *Pharm. Res.* **9**, 435–439.

Das, M. and Sahoo, S. K. (2010). Epithelial cell adhesion molecule targeted nutlin-3a loaded immunonanoparticles for cancer therapy. *Acta Biomater* **7**, 355–369.

Devalapally, H., Duan, Z., Seiden, M. V., and Amiji, M. M. (2008). Modulation of drug resistance in ovarian adenocarcinoma by enhancing intracellular ceramide using tamoxifen-loaded biodegradable polymeric nanoparticles. *Clin. Cancer Res.* **14**, 3193–3203.

Devi, G. R. (2006). SiRNA-based approaches in cancer therapy. *Cancer Gene Ther.* **13**, 819–829.

Dews, M., Homayouni, A., Yu, D., Murphy, D., Sevignani, C., Wentzel, E., Furth, E. E., Lee, W. M., Enders, G. H., Mendell, J. T., and Thomas-Tikhonenko, A. (2006). Augmentation of tumor angiogenesis by a Myc-activated microRNA cluster. *Nat. Genet.* **38**, 1060–1065.

Duncan, R. (2006). Polymer conjugates as anticancer nanomedicines. *Nat. Rev. Cancer* **6**, 688–701.

Elbashir, S. M., Harborth, J., Lendeckel, W., Yalcin, A., Weber, K., and Tuschl, T. (2001). Duplexes of 21-nucleotide RNAs mediate RNA interference in cultured mammalian cells. *Nature* **411**, 494–498.

Fasanaro, P., D'Alessandra, Y., Di Stefano, V., Melchionna, R., Romani, S., Pompilio, G., Capogrossi, M. C., and Martelli, F. (2008). MicroRNA-210 modulates endothelial cell response to hypoxia and inhibits the receptor tyrosine kinase

ligand ephrin-A3. *Journal of Biological Chemistry* **283**, 15878–15883.

Ferrara, N., Gerber, H. P., and LeCouter, J. (2003). The biology of VEGF and its receptors. *Nat. Med.* **9**, 669–676.

Fire, A., Xu, S., Montgomery, M. K., Kostas, S. A., Driver, S. E., and Mello, C. C. (1998). Potent and specific genetic interference by double-stranded RNA in *Caenorhabditis elegans*. *Nature* **391**, 806–811.

Fish, J. E., Santoro, M. M., Morton, S. U., Yu, S., Yeh, R. F., Wythe, J. D., Ivey, K. N., Bruneau, B. G., Stainier, D. Y. R., and Srivastava, D. (2008). miR-126 Regulates Angiogenic Signaling and Vascular Integrity. *Developmental Cell* **15**, 272–284.

Foley, S., Crowley, C., Smaihi, M., Bonfils, C., Erlanger, B. F., Seta, P., and Larroque, C. (2002). Cellular localisation of a water-soluble fullerene derivative. *Biochem. Biophys. Res. Commun.* **294**, 116–119.

Folkman, J. (1990). How the field of controlled-release technology began, and its central role in the development of angiogenesis research. *Biomaterials* **11**, 615–618.

Folkman, J. (1995). Angiogenesis in cancer, vascular, rheumatoid and other disease. *Nat. Med.* **1**, 27–31.

Folkman, J. (1996). New perspectives in clinical oncology from angiogenesis research. *Eur. J. Cancer* **32A**, 2534–2539.

Folkman, J. and Kalluri, R. (2004). Cancer without disease. *Nature* **427**, 787.

de Fougerolles, A., Vornlocher, H. P., Maragan-ore, J., and Lieberman, J. (2007). Interfering with disease: A a progress report on siRNA-based therapeutics. *Nat. Rev. Drug Discov.* **6**, 443–453.

Gregory, R. I. and Shiekhattar, R. (2005). MicroRNA biogenesis and cancer. *Cancer Res.* **65**, 3509–3512.

Griffin, L. C., Tidmarsh, G. F., Bock, L. C., Toole, J. J., and Leung, L. L. (1993). *In vivo* anticoagulant properties of a novel nucleotide-based thrombin inhibitor and demonstration of regional anticoagulation in extracorporeal circuits. *Blood* **81**, 3271–3276.

Haas, T. L., Milkiewicz, M., Davis, S. J., Zhou, A. L., Egginton, S., Brown, M. D., Madri, J. A., and Hudlicka, O. (2000). Matrix metalloproteinase activity is required for activity-induced angiogenesis in rat skeletal muscle. *Am. J. Physiol. Heart Circ. Physiol.* **279**, H1540–1547.

Harris, S. L. and Levine, A. J. (2005). The p53 pathway: Positive and negative feedback loops. *Oncogene* **24**, 2899–2908.

Hockenbery, D., Nunez, G., Milliman, C., Schreiber, R. D., and Korsmeyer, S. J. (1990). Bcl-2 is an inner mitochondrial membrane protein that blocks programmed cell death. *Nature* **348**, 334–336.

Isik, F. F., Rand, R. P., Gruss, J. S., Benjamin, D., and Alpers, C. E. (1996). Monocyte chemoattractant protein-1 mRNA expression in hemangiomas and vascular malformations. *J. Surg. Res.* **61**, 71–76.

Jiang, G., Li, J., Zeng, Z., and Xian, L. (2006). Lentivirus-mediated gene therapy by suppressing survivin in BALB/c nude mice bearing oral squamous cell carcinoma. *Cancer Biology and Therapy* **5**, 435–440.

Johnson, S. M., Grosshans, H., Shingara, J., Byrom, M., Jarvis, R., Cheng, A., Labourier, E., Reinert, K. L., Brown, D., and Slack, F. J. (2005). RAS is regulated by the Let-7 microRNA family. *Cell* **120**, 635–647.

Josephson, L., Tung, C. H., Moore, A., and Weissleder R. (1999). High-efficiency intracellular magnetic labeling with novel superparamagnetic Tat-peptide conjugates. *Bioconjug. Chem.* **10**, 186–191.

Kanwar, J., Berg, R., Lehnert, K., and Krissansen, G. (1999). Taking lessons from dendritic cells: Mmultiple xenogeneic ligands for leukocyte integrins have the potential to stimulate anti-tumor immunity. *Gene Ther.* 6, 1835–1844.

Kanwar, J. R., Berg, R. W., Yang, Y., Kanwar, R. K., Ching, L. M., Sun, X., and Krissansen, G. W. (2003). Requirements for ICAM-1 immunogene therapy of lymphoma. *Cancer Gene Ther.* **10**, 468–476.

Kanwar, J. R., Kanwar, R. K., Pandey, S., Ching, L. M., and Krissansen, G. W. (2001b). Vascular attack by 5, 6-dimethylxanthenone-4-acetic acid combined with B7.1 (CD80)-mediated immunotherapy overcomes immune resistance and leads to the eradication of large tumors and multiple tumor foci. *Cancer Res.* **61**, 1948–1956.

Kanwar, J. R., Mahidhara, G., and Kanwar, R. K. (2009). Recent advances in nanoneurology for drug delivery to the brain. *Current Nanoscience* **5**, 441–448.

Kanwar, J. R., Mahidhara, G., and Kanwar, R. K. (2010). MicroRNA in human cancer and chronic inflammatory diseases. *Front. Biosci. (Schol Ed.)* **2**, 1113–1326.

Kanwar, J. R., Mohan, R. M., Kanwar, R. K., Roy, K., and Bawa, R. (2010). Application of aptamers in nano-delivery systems in cancer, eye and inflammatory diseases. *Nanomedicine* **5**, 1435–1445.

Kanwar, J. R., Palmano, K. P., Sun, X., Kanwar, R. K., Gupta, R., Haggarty, N., Rowan, A., Ram, S., and Krissansen, G. W. (2008). "Iron-saturated" lactoferrin is a potent natural adjuvant for augmenting cancer chemotherapy. *Immunol. Cell Biol.* **86**, 277–288.

Kanwar, J. R., Shen, W. P., Kanwar, R. K., Berg, R. W., and Krissansen, G. W. (2001a). Effects of survivin antagonists on growth of established tumors and B7-1 immunogene therapy. *J. Natl Cancer Inst.* **93**, 1541–1552.

Kerr, J. F., Wyllie, A. H., and Currie, A. R. (1972). Apoptosis: A basic biological phenomenon with wide-ranging implications in tissue kinetics. *British Journal of Cancer* **26**, 239–257.

Khalil, I. A., Kogure, K., Futaki, S., and Harashima, H. (2006). High density of octa arginine stimulates macropinocytosis leading to efficient intracellular trafficking for gene expression. *J. Biol. Chem.* **281**, 3544–3551.

Knudson, A. G., Jr. (1971). Mutation and cancer: Statistical study of retinoblastoma. *Proc. Natl. Acad. Sci. USA* **68**, 820–823.

Kobayashi, N., Matsui, Y., Kawase, A., Hirata, K., Miyagishi, M., Taira, K., Nishikawa, M., and Takakura, Y. (2004). Vector-based *in vivo* RNA interference: dose- and time-dependent suppression of transgene expression. *J. Pharmacol. Exp. Ther.* **308**, 688–693.

Kondo, K. and Kaelin, W. G., Jr. (2001). The von Hippel-Lindau tumor suppressor gene. *Exp. Cell Res.* **264**, 117–125.

Krammer, P. H. (2000). CD95's deadly mission in the immune system. *Nature* **407**, 789–95.

Krissansen, G. W., Singh, J., Kanwar, R. K., Chan, Y. C., Leung, E., Lehnert, K. B., Kanwar,

J. R., and Yang, Y. (2006). A pseudosymmetric cell adhesion regulatory domain in the beta7 tail of the integrin alpha4beta7 that interacts with focal adhesion kinase and src. *Eur. J. Immunol.* **36**, 2203–2214.

Kuehbacher, A., Urbich, C., Zeiher, A. M., and Dimmeler, S. (2007). Role of Dicer and Drosha for endothelial microRNA expression and angiogenesis. *Circulation Research* **101**, 59–68.

Kulshreshtha, R., Ferracin, M., Wojcik, S. E., Garzon, R., Alder, H., Agosto-Perez, F. J., Davuluri, R., Liu, C. G., Croce, C. M., Negrini, M., Calin, G. A., and Ivan, M. (2007). A microRNA signature of hypoxia. *Molecular and Cellular Biology* **27**, 1859–1867.

Kuwabara, K., Ogawa, S., Matsumoto, M., Koga, S., Clauss, M., Pinsky, D. J., Lyn, P., Leavy, J., Witte, L., Joseph-Silverstein, J. et al. (1995). Hypoxia-mediated induction of acidic/basic fibroblast growth factor and platelet-derived growth factor in mononuclear phagocytes stimulates growth of hypoxic endothelial cells. *Proc. Natl. Acad. Sci. USA* **92**, 4606–4610.

Lameiro, M. H., Lopes, A., Martins, L. O., Alves, P. M., and Melo, E. (2006). Incorporation of a model protein into chitosan-bile salt microparticles. *Int. J. Pharm.* **312**, 119–130.

Lee, D. Y., Deng, Z., Wang, C. H., and Yang, B. B. (2007). MicroRNA-378 promotes cell survival, tumor growth, and angiogenesis by targeting SuFu and Fus-1 expression. *Proceedings of the National Academy of Sciences of the United States of America* **104**, 20350–20355.

Lee, R. C., Feinbaum, R. L., and Ambros, V. (1993). The *C. elegans* heterochronic gene lin-4 encodes small RNAs with antisense complementarity to lin-14. *Cell* **75**, 843–854.

Lee, Y., Ahn, C., Han, J., Choi, H., Kim, J., Yim, J., Lee, J., Provost, P., Radmark, O., Kim, S., and Kim, V. N. (2003). The nuclear RNase III Drosha initiates microRNA processing. *Nature* **425**, 415–419.

Lee, Y., Jeon, K., Lee, J. T., Kim, S., and Kim, V. N. (2002). MicroRNA maturation: Stepwise processing and subcellular localization. *EMBO J.* **21**, 4663–4670.

Lewin, M., Carlesso, N., Tung, C. H., Tang, X. W., Cory, D., Scadden, D. T., and Weissleder, R. (2000). Tat-peptide-derivatized magnetic nanoparticles allow *in vivo* tracking and recovery of progenitor cells. *Nat. Biotechnol.* **18**, 410–414.

Li, F. (2003). Survivin study: What is the next wave? *J. Cell Physiol.* **197**, 8–29.

Li, F. and Ling, X. (2006). Survivin study: An update of "what is the next wave"? *J. Cell Physiol.* **208**, 476–486.

Liang, J. F. and Yang, V. C. (2005). Synthesis of doxorubicin-peptide conjugate with multidrug resistant tumor cell killing activity. *Bioorg. Med. Chem. Lett.* **15**, 5071–5075.

Luo, L., Qiao, H., Meng, F., Dong, X., Zhou, B., Jiang, H., Kanwar, J. R., Krissansen, G. W., and Sun, X. (2006). Arsenic trioxide synergizes with B7H3-mediated immunotherapy to eradicate hepatocellular carcinomas. *Int. J. Cancer* **118**, 1823–1830.

Mahidhara, G., Kanwar, R. K., and Kanwar, J. R. (2011). A novel nanoplatform for oral delivery of anti-cancer biomacromolecules. *International Journal of Nanotechnology* (Accepted).

Maisonpierre, P. C., Suri, C., Jones, P. F., Bartunkova, S., Wiegand, S. J., Radziejewski, C., Compton, D., McClain, J., Aldrich, T. H., Papadopoulos, N., Daly, T. J., Davis, S., Sato, T. N., and Yancopoulos, G. D. (1997). Angiopoietin-2, a natural antagonist for Tie2 that disrupts *in vivo* angiogenesis. *Science* **277**, 55–60.

Maliyekkel, A., Davis, B. M., and Roninson, I. B. (2006). Cell cycle arrest drastically extends the duration of gene silencing after transient expression of short hairpin RNA. *Cell Cycle* **5**, 2390–2395.

Martin, C. R. and Kohli, P. (2003). The emerging field of nanotube biotechnology. *Nat. Rev. Drug Discov.* **2**, 29–37.

Matsumura, Y. and Maeda, H. (1986). A new concept for macromolecular therapeutics in cancer chemotherapy: Mechanism of tumor itropic accumulation of proteins and the antitumor agent smancs. *Cancer Res.* **46**, 6387–6392.

Maxwell, P. H., Dachs, G. U., Gleadle, J. M., Nicholls, L. G., Harris, A. L., Stratford, I. J., Hankinson, O., Pugh, C. W., and Ratcliffe, P. J. (1997). Hypoxia-inducible factor-1 modulates gene expression in solid tumors and influences both angiogenesis and tumor growth. *Proceed-*

ings of the National Academy of Sciences of the United States of America 94, 8104–8109.

Meade, B. R. and Dowdy, S. F. (2008). Enhancing the cellular uptake of siRNA duplexes following noncovalent packaging with protein transduction domain peptides. Adv. Drug Deliv. Rev. 60, 530–536.

Mi, J., Zhang, X., Rabbani, Z. N., Liu, Y., Reddy, S. K., Su, Z., Salahuddin, F. K., Viles, K., Giangrande, P. H., Dewhirst, M. W., Sullenger, B. A., Kontos, C. D., and Clary, B. M. (2008). RNA aptamer-targeted inhibition of NF-kappa B suppresses non-small cell lung cancer resistance to doxorubicin. Mol. Ther. 16, 66–73.

Michael, M. Z., O'Connor, S. M., Van Holst Pellekaan, N. G., Young, G. P., and James, R. J. (2003). Reduced Accumulation of Specific MicroRNAs in Colorectal Neoplasia. Molecular Cancer Research 1, 882–891.

Morimoto, K., Yamaguchi, H., Iwakura, Y., Miyazaki, M., Nakatani, E., Iwamoto, T., Ohashi, Y., and Nakai, Y. (1991). Effects of proteolytic enzyme inhibitors on the nasal absorption of vasopressin and an analogue. Pharm. Res. 8, 1175–1179.

Naumov, G. N., Akslen, L. A., and Folkman, J. (2006). Role of angiogenesis in human tumor dormancy: Animal models of the angiogenic switch. Cell Cycle 5, 1779–1787.

O'Rourke, G. E. and Ellem, A. O. (2000). John Kerr and apoptosis. Medical Journal of Australia 173, 616–617.

Ota, A., Tagawa, H., Karnan, S., Tsuzuki, S., Karpas, A., Kira, S., Yoshida, Y., and Seto, M. (2004). Identification and Characterization of a Novel Gene, C13orf25, as a Target for 13q31-q32 Amplification in Malignant Lymphoma. Cancer Research 64, 3087–3095.

Paddison, P. J., Caudy, A. A., Bernstein, E., Hannon, G. J., and Conklin, D. S. (2002). Short hairpin RNAs (shRNAs) induce sequence-specific silencing in mammalian cells. Genes Dev. 16, 948–958.

Paduano, F., Villa, R., Pennati, M., Folini, M., Binda, M., Grazia, M., and Zaffaroni, N. (2006). Silencing of suvivin gene by small interfering RNAs produces supra-additive growth suppression in combination with 17-allylamino-17-demethoxygeldanamycin in human prostate

cancer cells. Molecular Cancer Therapeutics 5, 179–186.

Pasquinelli, A. E., Reinhart, B. J., Slack, F., Martindale, M. Q., Kuroda, M. I., Maller, B., Hayward, D. C., Ball, E. E., Degnan, B., Muller, P., Spring, J., Srinivasan, A., Fishman, M., Finnerty, J., Corbo, J., Levine, M., Leahy, P., Davidson, E., and Ruvkun, G. (2000). Conservation of the sequence and temporal expression of Let-7 heterochronic regulatory RNA. Nature 408, 86–99.

Peer, D., Karp, J. M., Hong, S., Farokhzad, O. C., Margalit, R., and Langer, R. (2007). Nanocarriers as an emerging platform for cancer therapy. Nat. Nanotechnol. 2, 751–760.

Plank, M. J., Sleeman, B. D., and Jones, P. F. (2004). The role of the angiopoietins in tumour angiogenesis. Growth Factors 22, 1–11.

Plate, K. H., Breier, G., Weich, H. A., and Risau, W. (1992). Vascular endothelial growth factor is a potential tumour angiogenesis factor in human gliomas in vivo. Nature 359, 845–848.

Poliseno, L., Tuccoli, A., Mariani, L., Evangelista, M., Citti, L., Woods, K., Mercatanti, A., Hammond, S., and Rainaldi, G. (2006). MicroRNAs modulate the angiogenic properties of HUVECs. Blood 108, 3068–3071.

Prokop, A., Kozlov, E., Newman, G. W., and Newman, M. J. (2002). Water-based nanoparticulate polymeric system for protein delivery: Permeability control and vaccine application. Biotechnol. Bioeng. 78, 459–466.

Rawat, M., Singh, D., and Saraf, S. (2006). Nanocarriers: Promising vehicle for bioactive drugs. Biol. Pharm. Bull. 29, 1790–1798.

Rawat, M., Singh, D., and Saraf, S. (2008). Development and in vitro evaluation of alginate gel-encapsulated, chitosan-coated ceramic nanocores for oral delivery of enzyme. Drug Dev. Ind. Pharm. 34, 181–188.

Reinhart, B. J., Slack, F. J., Basson, M., Pasquinelli, A. E., Bettinger, J. C., Rougvie, A. E., Horvitz, H. R., and Ruvkun, G. (2000). The 21-nucleotide let-7 RNA regulates developmental timing in Caenorhabditis elegans. Nature 403, 901–906.

Rothbard, J. B., Garlington, S., Lin, Q., Kirschberg, T., Kreider, E., McGrane, P. L., Wender, P. A., and Khavari, P. A. (2000). Conjugation of arginine oligomers to cyclosporin A facilitates topical delivery and inhibition of inflammation. *Nat. Med.* **6**, 1253–1257.

Salcedo, R., Ponce, M. L., Young, H. A., Wasserman, K., Ward, J. M., Kleinman, H. K., Oppenheim, J. J., and Murphy, W. J. (2000). Human endothelial cells express CCR2 and respond to MCP-1: Direct role of MCP-1 in angiogenesis and tumor progression. *Blood* **96**, 34–40.

Sargiannidou, I., Zhou, J., and Tuszynski, G. P. (2001). The role of thrombospondin-1 in tumor progression. *Exp. Biol. Med. (Maywood)* **226**, 726–733.

Sarraf-Yazdi, S., Mi, J., Moeller, B. J., Niu, X., White, R. R., Kontos, C. D., Sullenger, B. A., Dewhirst, M. W., and Clary, B. M. (2008). Inhibition of *in vivo* tumor angiogenesis and growth via systemic delivery of an angiopoietin 2-specific RNA aptamer. *J. Surg. Res.* **146**, 16–23.

Scaffidi, C., Fulda, S., Srinivasan, A., Friesen, C., Li, F., Tomaselli, K. J., Debatin, K. M., Krammer, P. H., and Peter, M. E. (1998). Two CD95 (APO-1/Fas) signaling pathways. *EMBO J.* **17**, 1675–1687.

Schaffert, D. and Wagner, E. (2008). Gene therapy progress and prospects: Synthetic polymer-based systems. *Gene Ther.* **15**, 1131–1138.

Semenza, G. L. (1996). Transcriptional Regulation by Hypoxia-Inducible Factor 1 Molecular Mechanisms of Oxygen Homeostasis. *Trends in Cardiovascular Medicine* **6**, 151–157.

Sengupta, S., Eavarone, D., Capila, I., Zhao, G., Watson, N., Kiziltepe, T., and Sasisekharan, R. (2005). Temporal targeting of tumor cells and neovasculature with a nanoscale delivery system. *Nature* **436**, 568–572.

Shah, M. H. and Paradkar, A. (2005). Cubic liquid crystalline glyceryl monooleate matrices for oral delivery of enzyme. *Int. J. Pharm.* **294**, 161–171.

Shichiri, M. and Hirata, Y. (2001). Antiangiogenesis signals by endostatin. *FASEB J.* **15**, 1044–1053.

Shweiki, D., Itin, A., Soffer, D., and Keshet, E. (1992). Vascular endothelial growth factor induced by hypoxia may mediate hypoxia-initiated angiogenesis. *Nature* **359**, 843–845.

Smyth, S. S. and Patterson, C. (2002). Tiny dancers: The integrin-growth factor nexus in angiogenic signaling. *J. Cell Biol.* **158**, 17–21.

Stamatovic, S. M., Keep, R. F., Mostarica-Stojkovic, M., and Andjelkovic, A. V. (2006). CCL2 regulates angiogenesis via activation of Ets-1 transcription factor. *J. Immunol.* **177**, 2651–2661.

Suárez, Y., Fernández-Hernando, C., Pober, J. S., and Sessa, W. C. (2007). Dicer dependent microRNAs regulate gene expression and functions in human endothelial cells. *Circulation Research* **100**, 1164–1173.

Sudhakar, A., Sugimoto, H., Yang, C., Lively, J., Zeisberg, M., and Kalluri, R. (2003). Human tumstatin and human endostatin exhibit distinct anti-angiogenic activities mediated by alpha v beta 3 and alpha 5 beta 1 integrins. *Proc. Natl. Acad. Sci. USA* **100**, 4766–4771.

Sun, X., Kanwar, J. R., Leung, E., Lehnert, K., Wang, D., and Krissansen, G. W. (2001). Angiostatin enhances B7.1-mediated cancer immunotherapy independently of effects on vascular endothelial growth factor expression. *Cancer Gene Ther.* **8**, 719–727.

Sun, X., Kanwar, J. R., Leung, E., Vale, M., and Krissansen, G. W. (2003a). Regression of solid tumors by engineered overexpression of von Hippel-Lindau tumor suppressor protein and antisense hypoxia-inducible factor-1alpha. *Gene Ther.* **10**, 2081–2089.

Sun, X., Vale, M., Leung, E., Kanwar, J. R., Gupta, R., and Krissansen G., W. (2003b). Mouse B7-H3 induces antitumor immunity. *Gene Ther.* **10**, 1728–1734.

Sun, X., Qiao, H., Jiang, H., Zhi, X., Liu, F., Wang, J., Liu, M., Dong, D., Kanwar, J. R., Xu, R., and Krissansen, G. W. (2005). Intramuscular delivery of anti-angiogenic genes suppresses secondary metastases after removal of primary tumors. *Cancer Gene Ther.* **12**, 35–45.

Szebenyi, G. and Fallon, J. F. (1999). Fibroblast growth factors as multifunctional signaling factors. *Int, Rev, Cytol.* **185**, 45–106.

Tam, W., Hughes, S. H., Hayward, W. S., and Besmer, P. (2002). Avian bic, a gene isolated from a common retroviral site in avian leukosis virus-induced lymphomas that encodes a noncoding RNA, cooperates with c-myc in lymphomagenesis and erythroleukemogenesis. *Journal of Virology* **76**, 4275–4286.

Thai, T. H., Calado, D. P., Casola, S., Ansel, K. M., Xiao, C., Xue, Y., Murphy, A., Frendewey, D., Valenzuela, D., Kutok, J. L., Schmidt-Supprian, M., Rajewsky, N., Yancopoulos, G., Rao, A., and Rajewsky, K. (2007). Regulation of the germinal center response by microRNA-155. *Science* **316**, 604–608.

Thompson, C. B. (1995). Apoptosis in the pathogenesis and treatment of disease. *Science* **267**, 1456–1462.

Tili, E., Michaille, J.-J., Cimino, A., Costinean, S., Dumitru, C. D., Adair, B., Fabbri, M., Alder, H., Liu, C. G., Calin, G. A., and Croce, C. M. (2007). Modulation of miR-155 and miR-125b Levels following Lipopolysaccharide/TNF-{alpha} Stimulation and Their Possible Roles in Regulating the Response to Endotoxin Shock. *J. Immunol.* **179**, 5082–5089.

Tonini, T., Rossi, F., and Claudio, P. P. (2003). Molecular basis of angiogenesis and cancer. *Oncogene* **22**, 6549–6556.

Torchilin, V. P., Rammohan, R., Weissig, V., and Levchenko, T. S. (2001). TAT peptide on the surface of liposomes affords their efficient intracellular delivery even at low temperature and in the presence of metabolic inhibitors. *Proc. Natl. Acad. Sci. USA* **98**, 8786–8791.

Torchilin, V. P., Tischenko, E. G., Smirnov, V. N., and Chazov, E. I. (1977). Immobilization of enzymes on slowly soluble carriers. *J. Biomed. Mater. Res.* **11**, 223–235.

Tuerk, C. and Gold, L. (1990). Systematic evolution of ligands by exponential enrichment: RNA ligands to bacteriophage T4 DNA polymerase. *Science* **249**, 505–510.

Volinia, S., Calin, G. A., Liu, C. G., Ambs, S., Cimmino, A., Petrocca, F., Visone, R., Iorio, M., Roldo, C., Ferracin, M., Prueitt, R. L., Yanaihara, N., Lanza, G., Scarpa, A., Vecchione, A., Negrini, M., Harris, C. C., and Croce, C. M. (2006). A microRNA expression signature of human solid tumors defines cancer gene targets. *Proceedings of the National Academy of Sciences of the United States of America* **103**, 2257–2261.

Voorhoeve, P. M., le Sage, C., Schrier, M., Gillis, A. J. M., Stoop, H., Nagel, R., Liu, Y. P., van Duijse, J., Drost, J., Griekspoor, A., Zlotorynski, E., Yabuta, N., De Vita, G., Nojima, H., Looijenga, L. H. J., and Agami, R. (2006). A Genetic Screen Implicates miRNA-372 and miRNA-373

As Oncogenes in Testicular Germ Cell Tumors. *Cell* **124**, 1169–1181.

Wajant, H. (2002). The Fas signaling pathway: More than a paradigm. *Science* **296**, 1635–1636.

Wang, S., Aurora, A. B., Johnson, B. A., Qi, X., McAnally, J., Hill, J. A., Richardson, J. A., Bassel-Duby, R., and Olson, E. N. (2008). The Endothelial-Specific MicroRNA miR-126 Governs Vascular Integrity and Angiogenesis. *Developmental Cell* **15**, 261–271.

Weber, K. S., Nelson, P. J., Grone, H. J., and Weber C. (1999). Expression of CCR2 by endothelial cells: Implications for MCP-1 mediated wound injury repair and *in vivo* inflammatory activation of endothelium. *Arterioscler Thromb. Vasc. Biol.* **19**, 2085–2093.

Wooddell, C. I., Van Hout, C. V., Reppen, T., Lewis, D. L., and Herweijer, H. (2005). Long-term RNA interference from optimized siRNA expression constructs in adult mice. *Biochem. Biophys. Res. Commun.* **334**, 117–127.

Xin Hua, Z. (1994). Overcoming enzymatic and absorption barriers to non-parenterally administered protein and peptide drugs. *Journal of Controlled Release* **29**, 239–252.

Yagihashi, A., Ohmura, T., Asanuma, K., Kobayashi, D., Tsuji, N., Torigoe, T., Sato, N., Hirata, K., and Watanabe, N. (2005). Detection of autoantibodies to survivin and livin in sera from patients with breast cancer. *Clin. Chim. Acta.* **362**, 125–130.

Yang, W. J., Yang, D. D., Na, S., Sandusky, G. E., Zhang, Q., and Zhao, G. (2005). Dicer is required for embryonic angiogenesis during mouse development. *Journal of Biological Chemistry* **280**, 9330–9335.

Yi, R., Qin, Y., Macara, I. G., and Cullen, B. R. (2003). Exportin-5 mediates the nuclear export of pre-microRNAs and short hairpin RNAs. *Genes Dev.* **17**, 3011–3016.

Zapata, J. M., Pawlowski, K., Haas, E., Ware, C. F., Godzik, A., and Reed, J. C. (2001). A diverse family of proteins containing tumor necrosis factor receptor-associated factor domains. *J. Biol. Chem.* **276**, 24242–24252.

Zhang, L., Gao, L., Li, Y., Lin, G., Shao, Y., Ji, K., Yu, H., Hu, J., Kalvakolanu, D. V., Kopecko, D. J., Zhao, X., and Xu, D. Q. (2008). Effects of plasmid-based Stat3-specific short hairpin RNA and GRIM-19 on PC-3M tumor cell growth. *Clin. Cancer Res.* **14**, 559–568.

Zhang, S., Zhao, B., Jiang, H., Wang, B., and Ma, B. (2007). Cationic lipids and polymers mediated vectors for delivery of siRNA. *J. Control Release* **123**, 1–10.

Zhang, Y., Boado, R. J., and Pardridge, W. M. (2003). *In vivo* knockdown of gene expression in brain cancer with intravenous RNAi in adult rats. *J. Gene Med.* **5**, 1039–1045.

Zhou, X. H. and Li Wan, Po A. (1991). Comparison of enzyme activities of tissues lining portals of absorption of drugs: Species differences. *International Journal of Pharmaceutics* **70**, 271–283.

Zuhorn, I. S., Engberts, J. B., and Hoekstra, D. (2007). Gene delivery by cationic lipid vectors: Overcoming cellular barriers. *Eur. Biophys. J.* **36**, 349–362.

2

Ball, G. F. M. (1998). Bioavilability and Analysis of Vitamins in Food. In *Methods of Biochemical Analysis*. Chapman and Hall, London, vol. 10, pp. 293-313.

Burger, P. C. and Green, S. B. (1987). Patient age, histologic features, and length of survival in patients with glioblastoma multiforme. *Cancer* **59**(9), 1617-1625.

Butte, P. V., Pikul, B. K., Hever, A., Young, W. H., Black, K. L., and Marcu, L. (2005). Diagnosis of meningioma by time resolved fluorescence spectroscopy. *J. Biomed. Opt.* **10**(6), 064026.

Chung, Y. G., Schwartz, J. A., Gardner, C. M., Sawaya, R. E., and Jacques, S. L. (1997). Diagnostic Potential of Laser-Induced Autofluorescence Emission in Brain Tissue. *J. Korean Med. Sci.* **12**(2), 135-142.

Croce, A. C., Fiorani, S., Locatelli, D., Nano, R., Ceroni, M., Tancioni, F., Giombelli, E., Benericetti, E., and Bottiroli, G. (2003). Diagnostic Potential of Autofluorescence for an Assisted Intraoperative Delineation of Gioblastoma Resection Margins. *Photochem. Photobiol.* **77**(3), 309-318.

DaCosta, R. S., Andersson, H., and Wilson, B. C. (2003). Molecular Fluorescence Excitation Emission Matrices Relevant to Tissue Spectroscopy. *Photochem. Photobiol.* **78**(4), 384-392.

Frappaz, D., Chinot, O., Bataillard, A., Ben Hassel, M., Capelle, L., Chanalet, S., Chatel, M., Figarella-Branger, D., Guegan, Y., Guyotat, J., Hoang-Xuan, K., Jouanneau, E., Keime-Guibert, F., Laforet, C., Linassier, C., Loiseau, H., Maire, J. P., Menei, P., Rousmans, S., Sanson, M., and Sunyach, M. P. (2003). Summary version of the Standards, Options and Recommendations for the management of adult patients with intracranial glioma (2002). *Br. J. Cancer* **89**(S1), S73-83.

Haberland, C. (2007). *Clinical Neuropathology. Text and color atlas.* Demos Medical Publishing, LLC, New York.

Hochberg, F. H. and Pruitt, A. (1980). Assumptions in the radiotherapy of glioblastoma. *Neurology* **30**, 907–911.

International Agency for Research on Cancer (2008). World Cancer Report. http://www.iarc.fr/en/publications/pdfs-online/wcr/2008/index.php (accessed 17/08/10).

Katz, A. and Alfano, R. R. (1996). Optical Biopsy: Detecting Cancer with Light. In *Biomedical Optical Spectroscopy and Diagnostics*. E. Sevick-Muraca and D. Benaron (Eds.). OSA Trends in Optics and Photonics Series (Optical Society of America), 3, paper FT1.

Kuri Morales, P., Vargas Cortés, M., López Sibaja, Z., and Rizo Ríos, P. (2010). Registro Histopatológico de Neoplasias Malignas (Histopathological Register of Malignant Neoplasia). http://www.dgepi.salud.gob.mx/diveent/RHNM.htm (accessed 17/08/10).

Lin, W. C., Toms, S. A., Johnson, M., Jansen, E. D., and Mahadevan-Jansen, A. (2001). *In vivo* Brain Tumor Demarcation Using Optical Spectroscopy. *Photochem. Photobiol.* **73**(4), 396-402.

López, T., Figueras, F., Manjarrez, J., Bustos, J., Alvarez, M., Silvestre-Albero, J., Rodríguez-Reinoso, F., Martínez-Ferre, A., and Martínez, E. (2010). Catalytic nanomedicine: A new field in antitumor treatment using supported platinum nanoparticles. *In vitro* DNA degradation and *in vivo* tests with C6 animal model on Wistar rats. *Eur. J. Med. Chem.* **45**(5), 1982-1990.

López, T., Recillas, S., Guevara, P., Sotelo, J., Alvarez, M., and Odriozola, J. A. (2008). Pt/TiO₂ brain biocompatible nanoparticles: GBM treatment using C6 model in Wistar rats. *Acta Biomaterialia* **4**(6), 2037-2044.

Marcu, L., Jo, J. A., Butte, P. V., Yong, W. H., Pikul, B. K., Black, K. L., and Thompson, R. C. (2004). Fluorescence Lifetime Spectroscopy of Gioblastoma Multiforme. *Photochem. Photobiol.* **80**, 98-103.

Policard, A. (1924). Etude sur les aspects offerts par des tumeurs experimentales examinees a la lumiitre de Wood. *CR. Soc. Biol. Paris* **91**, 1423-1424.

Ricchelli, F., Gobbo, S., Jori, G., Salet, C., and Moreno, G. (1995). Temoperature-induced changes in fluorescence properties as a probe of porphyrin microenviroment in lipid membranes. 2. The partition of hematoporphyrin and protoporphyrin in mitochondria. *Eur. J. Biochem.* **233**(1), 165-170.

Rimington, C. (1960). Spectral-absorption Coefficients of some Porphyrins in the Soret-Band Region. *Biochem. J.* **75**(3), 620-623.

Roggan, A., Albrecht, H. J., Doerschel, K., Minet, O., and Mueller, G. J. (1995). Experimental set-up and Monte-Carlo model for the determination of optical tissue properties in the wavelength range 330-1100 nm. *Proc. SPIE.* **2323**, 21-36.

Saraswathy, A., Jayasree, R. S., Baiju, K. V., Gupta, A. K., and Pillai, V. P. (2009). Optimum wavelenght for the differentiation of brain tumor tissue using autofluorescence spectroscopy. *Photomed. Laser Surg.* **27**(3), 425-433.

Scott, T. G., Spencer, R. D., Leonard, N. G., and Weber, G. (1970). Emission properties of NADH: Studies of fluorescence lifetimes and quantum efficiencies of NADH, AcPyADH, and simplified synthetic models. *J. Am. Chem. Soc.* **92**, 687-695.

Stupp, R., Mason, W. P., Van den Beuf, M. J., Weller, M., Fisher, B., Taphoorn, M. J., Belanger, K., Brandes, A. A., Marosi, C., Bogdahn, U., Curschmann, J., Janzer, R. C., Ludwin, S. K., Gorlia, T., Allgeier, A., Lacombe, D., Cairncross, J. G., Eisenhauer, E., and Mirimanoff, R.O. (2005). Radiotherapy plus concomitant and adjuvant temozolomide for newly diagnosed glioblastoma. *N. Engl. J. Med.* **352**(10), 987–996.

Terasaki, M., Ogo, E., Fukushima, S., Sakata, K., Miyagi, N., Abe, T., and Shigemori, M. (2007). Impact of combination therapy with repeat surgery and temozolomide for recurrent or progressive glioblastoma multiforme: A prospective trial. *Surg. Neurol.* **68**(3), 250-254.

Wagnieres, G., MacWilliams, A., and Lam, S. (2003). Lung Cancer Imaging with Fluorescence Endoscopy. In *Handbook of Biomedical Fluorescence*. M. A. Mycek and B. W.Pogue (Eds.). Marcel Dekker, Inc., New York, p. 365.

Wallner, K. E., Galicich, J. H., Krol, G., Arbit E., and Malkin, M.G. (1989). Patterns of failure following treatment for glioblastoma multiforme and anaplastic astrocytoma. *Int. J. Radiat. Oncol. Biol. Phys* **16**(6), 1405–1409.

3

Allan, I., Newman, H., and Wilson, M. (2001). Antibacterial activity of particulate bioglass against supra- and subgingival bacteria. *Biomaterials* **22**, 1683-1687.

Allen, M., Bulte, J. W., Liepold, L., Basu, G., Zywicke, H. A., Frank, J. A., Young, M., and Douglas, T. (2005). Paramagnetic viral nanoparticles as potential high-relaxivity magnetic resonance contrast agents. *Magn. Reson. Med.* **54**, 807-812.

Balakrishnan, B., Mohanty, **M.**, Umashankar, **P. R., and** Jayakrishnan, **A.** (2005). Evaluation of an in situ forming hydrogel wound dressing based on oxidized alginate and gelatin. *Biomaterials* **26**, 6335-6342.

Batrakova, E. V. and Kabanov, A. V. (2008). Pluronic block copolymers: Evoltion of drug delivery concept from inert nanocarriers to biological response modifiers. *Journal of controlled release* **130**, 98-106.

Brand, G. D., Leite, J. R., de Sá Mandel, S. M., Mesquita, D. A., Silva, L. P., Prates, M. V., Barbosa, E. A., Vinecky, F., Martins, G. R., Galasso, J. H., Kuckelhaus, S. A., Sampaio, R. N., Furtado, J. R. Jr., Andrade, A. C., and Bloch, C. Jr. (2006). Novel dermaseptins from *Phyllomedusa hypochondrialis* (Amphibia). *Biochem. Biophys. Res. Commun.* **347**, 739-746.

Bruno, J. G. and Kiel, J. L. (1999). *In vitro* selection of DNA aptamers to anthrax spores with electrochemiluminescence detection. *Biosensors and Bioelectronics* **14**(5), 457-464.

Costerton, J. W., Stewart, P. S., and Greenberg, E. P. (1999). Bacterial biofilms: A common cause of persistent infections. *Science* **284**, 1318-1322.

Croy, S. R. and Kwon, G. S. (2004). The effects of Pluronic block copolymers on the aggregation state of nystatin. *J. Control. Release* **95**, 161-171.

Croy, S. R. and Kwon, G. S. (2005). Polysorbate 80 and Cremophor EL micelles deaggregate and solubilize nystatin at the core-corona interface. *J. Pharm. Sci.* **94**, 2345-2354.

Dong, H., Huang, J., Koepsel, R. R., Ye, P., Russell, A. J., and Matyjaszewski, K. (2011). Recyclable antibacterial magnetic nanoparticles grafted with quaternized poly (2-(dimethyl amino) ethyl methacrylate) brushes. *Biomacromolecules* **12**(4), 1305-1311.

Edgar, R., McKinstry, M., Hwang, J., Oppenheim, A. B., Fekete, R. A., Giulian, G., Merril, C., Nagashima, K., and Adhya, S. (2006). High-sensitivity bacterial detection using biotintagged phage and quantum-dot nanocomplexes. *Proc. Natl. Acad. Sci. USA* **103**(13), 4841-4845.

Faulk, W. P. and Taylor, G. M. (1971). An immunocolloid method for the electron microscope. *Immunochemistry* **8**(11), 1081-1083.

Flenniken, M. L., Liepold, L. O., Crowley, B. E., Willits, D. A., Young, M. J., and Douglas, T. (2005). Selective attachment and release of a chemotherapeutic agent from the interior of a protein cage architecture. *Chem. Commun.* 447–449.

Flenniken, M. L., Willits, D. A., Harmsen, A. L., Liepold, L. O., Harmsen A. G., Young, M. J., and Douglas, T. (2006). Melanoma and lymphocyte cell-specific targeting incorporated into a heat shock protein cage architecture. *Chem. Biol.* **13**, 161-170.

Hermerén, G., Marczewski, K., and Nielsen, L. (2007). Ethicasl aspects of nanomedicine: A condensed version of the EGE opinion 21.

Huang, L., Li, D. Q., Lin, Y. J., Wei, M., Evans, D. G., and Duan, X. (2005). Controllable preparation of Nano-MgO and investigation of its bactericidal properties. *J. Inorg. Biochem.* **99**(5), 986-993.

Ignatova, M., Starbova, K., Markova, N., Manolova, N. and, Rashkov, I. (2006a). Electrospun nanofibre mats with antibacterial properties from quaternised chitosan and poly(vinyl alcohol). *Carbohydr. Res.* **341**, 2098-2107.

Ignatova, M., Starbova, K., Markova, N., Manolova, N., and Rashkova, I. (2006b). Electrospun nanofibre mats with antibacterial properties from quaternised chitosan and poly(vinyl alcohol). *Carbohydr. Res.* **341**(12), 2098-2107.

Jia, H., Hou, **W.**, Wei, L., Xu, **B., and** Liu, **X.** (2008). The structures and antibacterial properties of nano-SiO$_2$ supported silver/zinc silver materials. *Dent. Mater.* **24**(2), 244-249.

Jones, N., Ray, B., Ranjit, K. T., and Manna, A. C. (2008). Antibacterial activity of ZnO nanoparticle suspensions on a broad spectrum of microorganisms FEMS. *Microbiol. Lett.* **279**(1), 71-76.

Kabanov, A., Nazarova, I. R., Astafieva, I. V., Batrakova, E. V., Alakhov, V. Y., Yaroslavov, A. A., and Kabanov, V. A. (1995). Micelle formation and solubilization of fluorescent probes in poly(oxyethylene-boxypropilene-b-oxyethylene) solutions. *Macromolecules* **28**, 2303-2314.

Kang, S., Pinault, M., Pfefferle, L. D., and Elimelech, M. (2007) Single-walled carbon nanotubes exhibit strong antimicrobial activity. *Langmuir* **23**, 8670-8673.

Kanwar, J. R., Mohan, R. R., Kanwar, R. K., Roy, K., and Bawa, R. (2010). Applications of aptamers in nanodelivery systems in cancer, eye, and inflammatory diseases. *Nanomedicine* **5**(9), 1435-1445.

Kostarelos, K. (2006). The emergence of nanomedicine: A field in the making. *Nanomedicine* **1**(1), 1-3.

Matthews, L. Kanwar, R. K., Zhou, S., Punj, V., and Kanwar, J. R. (2010). Application of nanomedicine in antibacterial medicine therapeutics and diagnostics. *Open Tropical Medicine Journal* **3**(1), 1-9.

Merli, D., Ugonino, M., Profumo, A., Fagnoni, M., Quartarone, E., Mustarelli, P., Visai, L., Grandi, M. S., Galinetto, P., and Canton, P. (2011). Increasing the antibacterial effect of lysozyme by immobilization on multi-walled carbon nanotubes. *Journal of Nanoscience and Nanotechnology* **11**(4), 3100-3106(7).

Muzzarelli, R. A., Guerrieri, M., Goteri, G., Muzzarelli, C., Anneni, T., Ghiselli, R., and Cornelissen, M. (2005). The biocompatibility of dibutyryl chitin in the context of wound dressings. *Biomaterials* **26**, 5844-5854.

Leite, J. R., Brand, G. D., Silva, L. P., Kückelhaus, S. A., Bento, W. R., Araújo, A. L., Martins,

G. R., Lazzari, A. M., and Bloch, C., Jr. (2008). Dermaseptins from *Phyllomedusa oreades* and *Phyllomedusa distincta*: Secondary structure, antimicrobial activity, and mammalian cell toxicity. *Comp. Biochem. Physiol. A Mol. Integr. Physiol.* **151**, 336-343.

LiPuma, J. J., Rathinavelu, S., Foster, B. K., Keoleian, J. C., Makidon, P. E., Kalikin, L. M., and Baker, J. R., Jr. (2009). *In vitro* activites of a novel nanoemulsion against burkholderia and other multi-drug-resistant cystic fibrosis-associated bacterial species. *Antimicob. Agents Chemother.* **53**, 249-255.

Lyon, D. Y., Fortner, J. D., Sayes, C. M., Colvin, V. L., and Hughes, J. B. (2005). Bacterial cell association and antimicrobial activity of a C60 water suspension. *Environ. Toxicol. Chem.* **24**, 2757-2762.

Pini, A., Giuliani, A., Falciani, C., Runci, Y., Ricci, C., Lelli, B., Malossi, M., Neri, P., Rossolini, G. M., and Bracci, L. (2005). Antimicrobial activity of novel dendrimeric peptides obtained by phage display selection and rational modification. *Antimicrob. Agens Chemother.* **49**, 2665-2672.

Salmaso, S., Elvassore, N., Bertucco, A., Lante, A., and Caliceti, P. (2004). Nisin-loaded poly-l-lactide nano-particles produced by CO_2 antisolvent precipitation for sustained antimicrobial activity. *Int. J. Pharma.* **287**(1/2), 163-173.

Saski, W. and Shah, S. G. (1965a). Availability of drugs in the presence of surface-active agents II. Effects of some oxyethylene oxypropylene polymers on the biological activity of hexetidine. *J. Pharm. Sci.* **54**, 277-280.

Saski, W. and Shah, S. G. (1965b). Availability of drugs in the presence of surface-active agents I. Critical micelle concentrations of some oxyethylene polymers. *J. Pharm. Sci.* **54**, 71-74.

Sepulveda, P., Jones, J. R., and Hench, L. L. (2002). *In vitro* dissolution of melt-derived 45S5 and sol-gel derived 58S bioactive glasses. *J. Biomed. Mater. Res.* **61**, 301-311.

Sondi, I. and Salopek-Sondi, B. (2004). Silver nanoparticles as antimicrobial agent: A case study on *E coli* as a model for Gram-negative bacteria. *J. Coll. Inter. Sci.*, **275**(1), 177-182.

Suci, P. A., Berglund, D. L., Liepold, L., Brumfield, S., Pitts, B., Davisonn, W., Oltrogge, L.,

Hoyt, K. O., Codd, S., Stewart, P. S., Young, M., and Douglas, T. (2007). High-density targeting of a viral multifunctional nanoplatform to a pathogenic, biofilm-forming bacterium. *Chemistry & Biology* **14**, 387-398.

Tam, P. J., Lu, Y. A., and Yang, J. L. (2002). Antimicrobial dendrimeric peptides. *Eur. J. Biochem.* **269**, 923-932.

Waltimo, T., Brunner, T. J., Vollenweider, M., Stark, W. J., and Zehnder, M. (2007). Antimicrobial effect of nanometric bioactive glass 45S5. *J. Dent. Res.* **86**, 754-757.

Wang, Y., Zhang, C. L., Zhang, Q., and Li, P. (2011). Composite electrospun nanomembranes of fish scale collagen peptides/chito-oligosaccharide antibacterial properties and potential for wound dressing. *International Journal of Nanomedicine*, **6**, 667-676.

Yacoby, I. (2006). Targeting antibacterial agents by using drug-carrying filamentous bacteriophages. *Antimicrob. Agents Chemother.* **50**, 2087-2097.

Yacoby, I., Bar, H., and Benhar, I. (2007). Targeted drug-carrying bacteriophages as anti bacterial nanomedicines. *Antimicrob. Agents Chemother.* **51**(6), 2156-2163.

Yacoby, I. and Benhar, I. (2008). Antibacterial nanomedicine. *Nanomedicine* **3**(3), 329-341.

Zampa, M. F., Araújo, I. M., Costa, V., Nery Costa, C. H., Santos, J. R. Jr., Zucolotto, V., Eiras, C., and Leite, J. R. (2009). Leishmanicidal activity and immobilization of dermaseptin 01 antimicrobial peptides in ultrathin films for nanomedicine applications. *Nanomedicine: Nanotechnology, biology, and medicine* **5**(3), 352-358.

Zhang, L. and Falla, T. J. (2006). Antimicrobial peptides: Therapeutic potential. *Exp. Opin. Pharmacother.* **7**, 653-663.

4

Agnihotri, S. A., Mallikarjuna, N. N., and Aminabhavi, T. M. (2004). Recent advances on chitosan-based micro- and nanoparticles in drug delivery. *Journal of Controlled Release* **100**, 5–28.

Agrawal, P., Strijkers, G. J., and Nicolay, K. (2010). Chitosan-based systems for molecular imaging. *Advanced Drug Delivery Reviews*, **62** 42–58.

Arhewoh, I. M., Ahonkhai, E. I., and Okhamafe, A. O. (2005). Optimising oral systems for the delivery of therapeutic proteins and peptides. *African Journal of Biotechnology* **4**(13), 1591-1597.

Badawi, A. A., Laithy, H. M. E., Qidra, R. K. E., Mofty, H. E., and Dally, M. E. (2008). Chitosan Based Nanocarriers for Indomethacin Ocular Delivery. *Arch. Pharm. Res.* **31**(8), 1040-1049.

Bae, K. H., Moon, C. W., Lee, Y., and Park, T. G. (2009). Intracellular Delivery of Heparin Complexed with Chitosan-g-Poly(Ethylene Glycol) for Inducing Apoptosis. *Pharmaceutical Research* **26**(1), 93-100.

Banerjee, T., Mitra, S., Singh, A. K., Sharma, R. K., and Maitra, A. (2002). Preparation, characterization and biodistribution of ultrafine chitosan nanoparticles. *International Journal of Pharmaceutics* **243**, 93–105.

Bao, H., Li, L., and Zhang, H. (2008). Influence of cetyltrimethylammonium bromide on physicochemical properties and microstructures of chitosan–TPP nanoparticles in aqueous solutions. *Journal of Colloid and Interface Science* **328**, 270–277.

Bhumkar, D. R. and Pokharkar, V. B. (2006). Studies on Effect of pH on Cross-linking of Chitosan with Sodium Tripolyphosphate: A Technical Note. *AAPS PharmSciTech.* 7(2) Article 50 (http://www.aapspharmscitech.org)

Borges, O., Silva, A. C. da., Romeijn, S. G., Amidi, M., Sousa, A. de, Borchard, G., and Junginger, H. E. (2006). Uptake studies in rat Peyer's patches, cytotoxicity and release studies of alginate coated chitosan nanoparticles for mucosal vaccination. *Journal of Controlled Release* **114**, 348–358.

Calvo, P., Lopez, C. R., Jato, J. L. V., and Alonso, M. (1997). Chitosan and chitosan/ethylene oxide- propylene oxide block copolymer nanoparticles as Novel carriers for proteins and vaccines. *Pharmaceutical research* **14**(10), 1431-1436

De Campos, A. M., Diebold, Y., Carvalho, E. L. S., Sanchez, A., and Alonso, M. J. (2004). Chitosan Nanoparticles as New Ocular Drug Delivery Systems: *In Vitro* Stability, *In Vivo* Fate, and Cellular Toxicity. *Pharmaceutical Research* **21**(5), 803-810.

De Campos, A. M., Sanchez, A., and Alonso, M. J. (2001). Chitosan nanoparticles: a new vehicle for the improvement of the delivery of drugs to the ocular surface-Application to cyclosporin A. *International Journal of Pharmaceutics* **224**, 159–168.

Chakravarthi, S. S, Robinson, D. H., and De, S. (2007). Nanoparticles prepared using natural and synthetic polymers. In *Nanoparticulate Drug Delivery Systems*. D. Thassu,, M. Deleers, and Y. Pathak (Eds.). Informa Healthcare, New York, USA, pp. 51-60.

Chang, Y. C., Shieh, D. B., Chang, C. H. and Chen, D. H. (2005). Conjugation of Monodisperse Chitosan-bound Magnetic Nanocarrier with Epirubicin for Targeted Cancer Therapy. *Journal of Biomedical Nanotechnology* **1**, 196–201.

Chen, F., Zhang, Z. R., Yuan, F., Qin, X., Wang, M., and Huang, Y. (2008). *In vitro* and *in vivo* study of N-trimethyl chitosan nanoparticles for oral protein delivery. *International Journal of Pharmaceutics* **349**, 226–233.

Chen, Y., Mohanraj, V. J., and Parkin, J. E. (2003). Chitosan-dextran sulfate nanoparticles for delivery of an anti-angiogenesis Peptide. *Letters in Peptide Science* **10**, 621–629.

Chen, Y., Mohanraj, V. J., Wang, F., and Benson, H. A. E. (2007). Designing Chitosan–Dextran Sulfate Nanoparticles Using Charge Ratios. *AAPS PharmSciTech.* **8**(4), Article 98 (http://www.aapspharmscitech.org).

Chun, W., Xiong, F., and Sheng, Y. L. (2007). Water-soluble chitosan nanoparticles as a novel carrier system for protein delivery. *Chinese Science Bulletin* **52**(7), 883-889.

Coppi, G. and Iannuccelli, V. (2009). Alginate/chitosan microparticles for tamoxifen delivery to the lymphatic system. *International Journal of Pharmaceutics* **367**, 127–132.

Coppi, G., Sala, N., Bondi, M., Sergi, S., and Iannuccelli, V. (2006). *Ex-vivo* evaluation of alginate microparticles for Polymyxin B oral Administration. *Journal of Drug Targeting* **14**(9), 599–606.

Csaba, N., Fuentes, M. G., and Alonso, M. J. (2008). *Nanoparticles for nasal vaccination*. Advance drug delivery reviews. Doi: 10.1016/j.addr.2008.09.005.

Dudhani, A. R. and Kosaraju, S. L. (2008). Bio-adhesive Chitosan Nanoparticles: Preparation and Characterisation. *Carbohydrate Polymers*, doi:10.1016/j.carbpol.2010.02.026.

Hamidi, M., Azadi, A., and Rafiei, P. (2008). Hydrogel nanoparticles in drug delivery. *Advanced Drug Delivery Reviews* **60**, 1638–1649.

Huang, H. N., Li, T. L., Chan, Y. L, Chen, C. L., and Wu, C. J. (2009). Transdermal immunization with low-pressure-gene-gun mediated chitosan-based DNA vaccines against Japanese encephalitis virus. *Biomaterials* **30**, 6017–6025.

Illum, L., Gill, I. J., Hinchcliffe, M., Fisher, A. N., and Davis, S. S. (2001). Chitosan as a novel nasal delivery system for vaccines. *Advanced Drug Delivery Reviews* **51**, 81–96.

Issa, M. M., Hoggard, M. K., and Artursson, P. (2005). Chitosan and the mucosal delivery of biotechnology drugs. *Drug Discovery Today: Technologies* **2**(1), 1-6.

Janes, K. A., Calvo, P., and Alonso, M. J. (2001). Polysaccharide colloidal particles as delivery systems for Macromolecules. *Advanced Drug Delivery Reviews* **47**, 83–97.

Janes, K. A., Fresneau, M. P., Marazuela, A., Fabra, A., and Alonso, M. J. (2001). Chitosan nanoparticles as delivery systems for doxorubicin. *Journal of Controlled Release* **73**, 255–267.

Kadiyala, I., Loo, Y., Roy, K., Rice, J., and Leong, K. W. (2010). Transport of chitosan–DNA nanoparticles in human intestinal M-cell model versus normal intestinal enterocytes. *European Journal of Pharmaceutical Sciences* **39**, 103–109.

Kao, H. J., Lin, H. R., Lo, Y. L., and Yu, S. P. (2006). Characterization of pilocarpine-loaded chitosan/Carbopol nanoparticles. *Journal of pharmacy and pharmacology* **58**, 179-186.

Kumar, M. N. V. R. (2000). Nano and Microparticles as Controlled Drug Delivery Devices. *J. Pharm. Pharmaceut. Sci.* **3**(2), 234-258.

Li, G., Liu, Z., Liao, B., and Zhong, N. (2009). Induction of Th1-Type Immune Response by Chitosan Nanoparticles Containing Plasmid DNA Encoding House Dust Mite Allergen Der p 2 for Oral Vaccination in Mice. *Cellular & Molecular Immunology* **6**(1), 45-50.

Ma, Z., Yoeh, H. H., and Lim, L. Y. (2002). Formulation pH Modulates the Interaction of Insulin with Chitosan Nanoparticles. *Journal of pharmaceutical Sciences* **91**(6), 1396-1404.

Mao, S., Sun, W., and Kissel, T. (2010). Chitosan-based formulations for delivery of DNA and siRNA. *Advanced Drug Delivery Reviews* **62**, 12–27.

Mladenovska, K., Raicki, R. S., Janevik, E. I., Ristoski, T., Pavlova, M. J., Kavrakovski, Z., Dodov, M. G., and Goracinova, K. (2007). Colon-specific delivery of 5-aminosalicylic acid from chitosan-Ca-alginate microparticles. *International Journal of Pharmaceutics* **342**, 124–136.

Motwani, S. K., Chopra, S., Talegaonkar, S., Kohli, K., Ahmad, F. J., and Khar, R. K. (2008). Chitosan–sodium alginate nanoparticles as submicroscopic reservoirs for ocular delivery: Formulation, optimization and *in vitro* characterization. *European Journal of Pharmaceutics and Biopharmaceutics* **68**, 513–525.

Nagamoto, T., Hattori, Y., Takayama, K., and Maitani, Y. (2004). Novel Chitosan Particles and Chitosan-Coated Emulsions Inducing Immune Response via Intranasal Vaccine Delivery. *Pharmaceutical Research* **21**(4), 671-674.

Patel, J. K. and Jivani, N. P. (2009). Chitosan Based Nanoparticles in Drug Delivery. *International Journal of Pharmaceutical Sciences and Nanotechnology* **2**(2), 517-522.

Prego, C., Paolicelli, P., Diaz, B., Vicente, S., Sanchez, A., Fernandezb, A. G., and Alonso, M. J. (2010). Chitosan-based nanoparticles for improving immunization against hepatitis B infection. *Vaccine* **28**, 2607–2614.

Qi, L., Xu, Z., Jiang, X., Hu, C., and Zou, X. (2004). Preparation and antibacterial activity of chitosan nanoparticles. *Carbohydrate Research* **339**, 2693–2700.

Rieux, A. des., Fievez, V., Garinot, M., Schneider, Y. J., and Preat, V. (2006). Nanoparticles as potential oral delivery systems of proteins and vaccines: A mechanistic approach. *Journal of Controlled Release* **116**, 1–27.

Sandri, G., Poggi, P., Bonferoni, M. C., Rossi, S., Ferrari, F., and Caramella, C. (2006). Histological evaluation of buccal penetration enhancement properties of chitosan and trimethyl chitosan. *Journal of pharmacy and pharmacology* **58**, 1327-1336.

Sarmento, B., Ribeiro, A., Veiga, F., Sampaio, P., Neufeld, R., and Ferreira, D. (2007). Alginate/Chitosan Nanoparticles are Effective for Oral Insulin Delivery. *Pharmaceutical Research* **24**(12), 2198-2206.

Schmidt, C. and Lamprecht, A. (2009). Nanocarriers in drug delivery-design, manufacture and physicochemical properties. In *Nanotherapeutics- drug delivery concepts in nanoscience.* A. Lamprecht (Ed.). Pan Standford Publishing Pte Ltd, Mainland Press Pvt Ltd, Singapore, pp. 1-38.

Schmitt, F. et al. (2010). Chitosan-based nanogels for selective delivery of photosensitizers to macrophages and improved retention in and therapy of articular joints. *Journal of Control Release,* doi:10.1016/j.jconrel.2010.02.008.

Singh, D. (2010). Development and characterization of chitosan nanoparticles loaded with amoxicillin. [Online] available from Pharmainfo.net (accessed 5th May, 2010)

Slutter, B., Plapied, L., Fievez, V., Sande, M. A., Rieux, A. des., Schneider, Y. J., Riet, E. V., Jiskoot, W., and Preat, V. (2009). Mechanistic study of the adjuvant effect of biodegradable nanoparticles in mucosal vaccination. *Journal of Controlled Release* **38**, 113–121.

Soppimath, K. S., Aminabhavi, T. M., Kulkarni, A. R., and Rudzinski, W. E. (2001). Biodegradable polymeric nanoparticles as drug delivery devices. *Journal of Controlled Release* **70**, 1–20.

Tiyaboonchai, W. and Limpeanchob, N. (2007). Formulation and characterization of amphotericin B–chitosan–dextran sulfate nanoparticles. *International Journal of Pharmaceutics* **329**, 142–149.

Tokumitsu, H., Ichikawa, H., and Fukumori, Y. (1999). Chitosan-Gadopentetic acid complex nanoparticles for gadolinium neutron capture therapy of cancer: Preperation by novel emulsion droplet coalescence technique and characterization. *Pharmaceutical research* **16**(12), 1830-1835.

Urrusuno, R. F., Calvo, P., Lopez, C. R., Jato, J. L. V., and Alonso, M. J. (1999). Enhancement of nasal absorption of insulin using chitosan nanoparticles. *Pharmaceutical research* **16**(10), 1576-1581.

Weecharangsan, W., Opanasopit, P., Ngawhirunpat, T., Rojanarata, T., and Apirakaramwong, A. (2006). Chitosan Lactate as a Nonviral Gene Delivery Vector in COS-1 Cells. AAPS *PharmSciTech.* **7**(3), Article 66 (http://www.aapspharmscitech.org)

Wilson, B., Samanta, M. K., Santhi, K., Kumar, K. P. S., Ramasamy, M., and Suresh, B. (2010). Chitosan nanoparticles as a new delivery system for the anti-Alzheimer drug tacrine. *Nanomedicine: Nanotechnology, Biology, and Medicine* **6**, 144–152.

Wu, Y., Yang, W., Wang, C., Hu, J., and Fu, S. (2005). Chitosan nanoparticles as a novel delivery system for ammonium glycyrrhizinate. *International Journal of Pharmaceutics* **295**, 235–245.

Yan, C., Chen, D., Gu, J., and Qin, J. (2006). Nanoparticles of 5-fluorouracil (5-FU) loaded N-succinyl-chitosan (Suc-Chi) for cancer chemotherapy: Preparation, characterization-*in-vitro* drug release and anti-tumour activity. *Journal of pharmacy and pharmacology* **58**, 1177–1181.

Yang, S. J., Shieh, M. J., Lin, F. H., Lou, P. J., Peng, C. L., Wei, M. F., Yao, C. J., Lai, P. S., and Young, T. H. (2009a). Colorectal cancer cell detection by 5-aminolaevulinic acid-loaded chitosan nano-particles. *Cancer Letters* **273**, 210–220.

Yang, S. J., Shieh, M. J., Lin, F. H., Lou, P. J., Peng, C. L., Wei, M. F. et al. (2009b). Colorectal cancer cell detection by 5-aminolaevulinic acid-loaded chitosan nano-particles. *Cancer Letters* **273**, 210–220.

Yu, S., Zhao, Y., Wu, F., Zhang, X., Lu, W., Zhang, H., and Zhang, Q. (2004). Nasal insulin delivery in the chitosan solution: *In vitro* and *in vivo* studies. *International Journal of Pharmaceutics* **281**, 11–23.

5

Abid, J. P., Wark, A. W., Brevet, P. F., and Girault, H. H. (2002). Preparation of silver nanoparticles in solution from a silver salt by laser irradiation. *Chemical communications* (Cambridge, England) **7**, 792-793.

Ahmad A., Mukherjee P., Senapati S., Mandal D., Khan M. I., Kumar R. and M. (2003). Extracellular biosynthesis of silver nanoparticles using the fungus *Fusarium oxysporum*. *Colloids Surf. B. Biointerf.* **28**, 313–318.

Ahmad, A., Senapati, S., Khan, M. I., Kumar, R., and Sastry, M. (2003). Extracellular biosynthesis of monodisperse gold nanoparticles by a novel extremophilic actinomycete *Thermomonospora* sp. *Langmuir* **19**, 3550.

Ahmad, N., Sharma, S., Singh, V. N., Shamsi, S. F., Anjum F., and Mehta, B. R. (2011) Biosynthesis of Silver Nanoparticles from *Desmodium triflorum*: A Novel Approach towards Weed Utilization. *Biotechnology Research International* **2011**, 8.

Ahmad, R. S., Ali, F., Hamid, R. S., and Sara, M. (2007). Synthesis and effect of silver nanoparticles on the antibacterial activity of different antibiotics against *Staphylococcus aureus* and *Escherichia coli*. *Nanomedicine: Nanotechnology, Biology and Medicine* **3**(2), 168-171.

Alfredo, R., Vilchis-Nestor, Victor Sánchez-Mendieta, Marco Camacho-López, A., Rosa, M.,Gómez-Espinosa, Miguel, A., Camacho-López, and Jesús Arenas-Alatorre, A. (2008), Solventless synthesis and optical properties of Au and Ag nanoparticles using *Camellia sinensis* extract. *Materials Letters* **62**, 3103-3105.

Amanulla, M. F., Balaji, K., Girilal, M., Yadav, R., Pudupalayam Thangavelu Kalaichelvan, and Ramasamy Venketesan. (2010). Biogenic synthesis of silver nanoparticles and their synergistic effect with antibiotics: A study against gram-positive and gram-negative bacteria. *Nanomedicine: Nanotechnology, Biology and Medicine* **6**, 103-109.

Ankamwar, B, Damle, C, Ahmad, A, and Sastry M. (2005a). Biosynthesis of gold and silver nanoparticles using *Emblica officinalis* fruit extract, their phase transfer and transmetallation in an organic solution. *Journal of Nanoscience and Nanotechnology* **5**, 1665-1671.

Ankamwar, B., Chaudhary, M., and Mural, S. (2005b). Gold nanotriangles biologically synthesized using Tamarind leaf extract and potential application in vapor sensing. *Synthesis and Reactivity in Inorganic and Metal-Organic Chemistry* **35**, 19.

Atiyeh, B. S., Costagliola, M., Hayek, S. N., and Dibo, S. A. (2007). Effect of silver on burn wound infection control and healing: Review of the literature. *Burn* **33**(2), 139-148.

Bae, C. H., Nam, S. H., and Park, S. M. (2002). Formation of silver nanoparticles by laser ablation of a silver target in NaCl solution. *Applied Surface Science* **197**, 628–634.

Baker, R. A. and Tatum, J. H. (1998). Novel anthraquinones from stationary cultures of *Fusarium oxysporum*. *Journal of Fermentation and Bioengineering* **85**, 359-361.

Balaji, D. S., Basavaraja, S., Deshpande, R., Bedre Mahesh, D., Prabhakar, B. K., and Venkataraman, A. (2009) Extracellular biosynthesis of functionalized silver nanoparticles by strains of *Cladosporium cladosporioides* fungus. *Colloids Surf. B Biointerfaces* **68**, 88-92.

Basavaraja, S., Balaji, S. D., Arun kumar, L., Rajasab, S., and Venkataraman, A. (2007). Extracellular biosynthesis of silver nanoparticles using the fungus *Fusarium semitectum*. *Materials Research Bulletin* **43**, 1164-1170.

Bell, A. A., Wheeler, M. H., Liu, J., Stipanovic, R. D., Puckhaber, L. S., and Orta, H. (2003). United States Department of Agriculture--Agricultural Research Service studies on polyketide toxins of *Fusarium oxysporum* f sp vasinfectum: Potential targets for disease control. *Pest Management Science* **59**, 736–747.

Beveridge, T. J., Hughes, M. N., Lee, H., Leung, K. T., Poole, R. K., Savvaidis, I., Silver, S., and Trevors, J. T. (1997). Metal–microbe interactions: Contemporary approaches. *Advances in Microbial Physiology* **38**, 177-243.

Beveridge, T. Y. and Murray, R. G. E (1980). Sites of metal deposition in the cell wall of *Bacillus subtilis*. *Journal of Bacteriology* **141**, 876-887.

Bhainsa, K. C. and D'Souza, S. F. (2006). Extracellular Biosynthesis of Silver Nanoparticles using the Fungus *Aspergillus fumigatus*. *Colloids Surf. B Biointerfaces* **47**(2) 160-164.

Birla, S. S., Tiwari, V. V., Gade, A. K., Ingle, A. P., Yadav, A. P., and Rai, M. K. (2009). Fabrication of silver nanoparticles by *Phoma glomerata* and its combined effect against *Escherichia coli*, *Pseudomonas aeruginosa* and *Staphylococcus aureus*. *Letters in Applied Microbiology* **48**, 173-179.

Blakemore, R. P. (1982). Magnetotactic bacteria. *Annual Review of Microbiology* **36**, 217–238.

Bonneman, H., Brijoux, W., Brinkmann, R., Tilling, A. S., Schilling, T., Tesche, B., Seevogel, K., Franke, R., Hormes, J. G., Pollmann, J. R., and Jvogel, W. (1998). Selective oxidation of glucose on bismuth-promoted Pd-Pt/C catalysts prepared from NOct$_4$Cl-stabilized Pd-Pt colloids. *Inorganica. Chimica. Acta* **270**, 95–110.

Brierley, J. A. (1990). Production and application of a Bacillus–based product for use in metals biosorption. In *Biosorption of heavy metals*. B. Volesky (Ed.) Boca Raton, FL CRC Press, pp. 305-312.

Brown, T. and Smith, D. (1976). The effects of silver nitrate on the growth and the ultrastructure of the yeast *Cryptococuss albidus*. *Microbios letters* **3**, 155-162.

Bruins, R. M., Kapil, S., and Oehme, S. W. (2000). Microbial resistance to metal in the environment. *Ecotoxicology and Environmental Safety* **45**, 198–207.

Brust, M. and Kiely, C. J. (2002). Some recent advances in nanostructure preparation from gold and silver particles: A short topical review. *Colloids and Surfaces A: Physicochem. Eng. Aspects* **202**, 175–186.

Burda, C. X., Chen, R., Narayanan, M. A., and El-Sayed (2005). Chemistry and properties of nanocrystals of different shapes. *Chem. Rev.* **105**, 1025-1102.

Callegari, A., Tonti, D., and Chergui, M. (2003). Photo chemically grown silver nanoparticles with wave length–controlled size and shape. *Nano Letters* **3**, 1565-1568.

Canizal, G., Ascencio, J. A., Gardea-Torresday, J., and Jose-Yacaman, M. (2001). *J. Nanopart. Res.* **3**, 475–481.

Cao, G. (Ed.). (2004). *Nanostructures and Nanomaterials: Synthesis, properties and applications*. Imperial college press, London.

Cao, Y. C., Jin, R., and Mirkin, C. A. (2002). Nanoparticles with Raman Spectroscopic Fingerprints for DNA and RNA Detection. *Science* **297**, 1536-1540.

Castro-Longoria, E., Vilchis-Nestor, A. R., and Avalos-Borja, M. (2011). Biosynthesis of silver, gold, and bimetallic nanoparticles using the filamentous fungus *Neurospora crassa*. *Colloids and Surfaces B: Biointerfaces* **83**(1), 42-48.

Chaki, N. K., Sudrik, S. G., Sonawane, H. R., and Vijayamohanan, K. (2002). Single phase preparation of monodispersed silver nanoclusters using a unique electron transfer and cluster stabilising agent. *Triethylamine, Chemical Communications* **8**(1), 76-77.

Chan, W. C. W. and Nie, S. M. (1998). Quantum dot bioconjugates for ultrasensitive nonisotopic detection. *Science* **281**, 2016–2018.

Chandran, S. P., Chaudhary, M., Pasricha, R., Ahmad, A., and Sastry, M. (2006). Synthesis of gold nanotriangles and silver nanoparticles using *Aloe vera* plant extract. *Biotechnology Progress* **22**, 577–583.

Chen, D., Qiao, X., Qui, X., and Chen, J. (2009). Synthesis and electrical properties of uniform silver nanoparticles for electronic applications. *Journal of Materials Science* **44**, 1076-1081.

Chen, J, Wang, K, Xin, J., and Jin, Y. (2008). *Mater. Chem. Phys.* **108**, 421.

Chen, J. C., Lin, Z. H., and Ma, X. X. (2003). Evidence of the production of silver nanoparticles via pretreatment of *Phoma* sp 32883 with silver nitrate. *Letters in Applied Microbiology* **37**, 105-108.

Chen, X. and Schluesener, H. J. (2008). Nanosilver: A nanoproduct in medical application. *Toxicology Letters* **176**(1), 1-12.

Chen, Y. Y., Wang, C., Liu, L. H., Qiu, J. S., and Bao, X. H. (2005). *Chemical Communications, Cambridge* **42**, 5298.

Cho, K. H., Park, J. E., Osaka, T., and Park, S. G. (2005).The study of antimicrobial activity and preservative effects of nanosilver ingredient, *Electrochimica Acta* **51**(5), 956-960.

Chu, C. S., McManus, A. T., Pruitt, B. A., and Mason, A. D. (1988). Therapeutic effects of silver nylon with weak direct current *Pseudomonas aeruginosa* infected burn wounds. *The Journal of Trauma* **28**(10), 1488-1492.

Corinne, P., Dewilde, A., Pierlot, C., and Aubry, J. M. (2000). Bactericidal and virucidal activities of singlet oxygen generated by thermolysis of naphthalene endoperoxides. *Methods in Enzymology* **319**, 197-207.

Cushing, B. L., Kolesnichenko, V. L., and Connor, C. J. O. (2004). Recent Advances in the Liquid-Phase Syntheses of Inorganic Nanoparticles. *Chemical Reviews* **104**, 3893–3946.

Daizy, P. (2009). Spectrochim. Biosynthesis of Au, Ag and Au-Ag nanoparticles using edible mushroom extract. *Acta A* **73**, 374-381.

Darnall, D. W., Greene, B., Henzl, M. J., Hosea, M., Mc Pherson, R. A., Sneddon, J., and Alexander, M. D. (1986). Selective recovery of gold and other metal ions from an algal biomass. *Environment and Science and Technology* **20**, 206-208.

Darroudi, M., Ahmad, M. B., Shameli, K., Abdullah, A. H., and Ibrahim, N. A. (2009). Synthesis and characterization of UV-irradiated silver/montmorillonite nanocomposites. *Solid State Sciences* **11**, 1621–1624.

Darroudi, M., Ahmad, M. B., Zamiri, R., Zak, A. K., Abdullah, A. H., and Ibrahim, N. A. (2011). Time dependent effect in green synthesis of silver nanoparticles. *International journal of nanomedicine* **6**, 677–681.

David S. G. (2004). *Bionanotechnology: Lessons from Nature.* John Wiley and sons, Inc., Publication.

Deendayal, M., Bolander, E. M., Mukhopadhyay, D., Sarkar, G., and Mukherjee, P. (2006). The use of microorganisms for the formation of metal nanoparticles and their application. *Applied Microbiology and Biotechnology* **69**, 485-492.

Deitch, E. A., Marino, A. A., Malaleonok, V., and Albricht, J. A. (1987). Silver nylon cloth: *In vitro* and *in vivo* evaluation of antimicrobial activity. *The Journal of Trauma* **27**, 301.

Devendra, J., Hemant, K. D., Sumita, K., and Kotharia, S. L. (2009). *Digest Journal of Nanomaterials and Biostructures* **4**(4), 723.

Dunn, K. and Edwards-Jones, V. (2004). The role of Acticoat with nanocrystalline silver in the management of burns. *Burns* **30**(1), S1-9.

Duran, N., Teixeria, M. P. S., De Conti, R., and Esposito (2002). Ecological-friendly pigments from fungi. *Critical Reviews in Food Science and Nutrition* **42**, 53-66.

Duran, N., Marcato, P. L., Alves, O. L., and De Souza, G. I. (2005). Mechanistic aspects of biosynthesis of silver nanoparticles by several *Fusarium oxysporum* strains. *Journal of Nanobiotechnology* **3**(8), 1-7.

Egorova, E. M. and Revina, A. A. (2000). Synthesis of metallic nanoparticles in reverse micelles in the presence of quercetin. *Colloids and Surfaces, ser.A* **168**, 87.

Elechiguerra, J. L., Justin L Burt, Jose R. Morones, Alejandra Camacho-Bragado, Xiaoxia Gao, Humberto H Lara, and Miguel Jose Yacaman (2005). Interaction of silver nanoparticles with HIV-1. *Journal of Nanobiotechnology* **3**, 6.

Elumalai, E. K., Prasad, T. N. V. K. V., Venkata Kambala, Nagajyothi, P. C., and David, E. (2010). Green synthesis of silver nanoparticle using *Euphorbia hirta* L and their anti fungal activities. *Archives of Applied Science Research* **2**(6), 76-81.

Ershov, B. G., Janata, E., Henglein, A., and Fojtlk A. (2007) unplublished report.

Esau, S. R., Roberto, S. B., Ocotlan-Flores, J., and Saniger, J. M. (2010). Synthesis of AgNPs by sonochemical induced reduction applications in SERS. *Journal of Nanoparticle Research* **9**, 77.

Eutis, S., Krylova, G., Eremenko, A., Smirnova, N., Schill, A. W., and El-Sayed, M. (2005). Growth and fragmentation of silver nanoparticles in their synthesis with a fs laser and CW light by photo-sensitization with benzophenone. *Photochemical and Photobiological Sciences* **4**, 154-159.

Falletta, E., Massimo Bonini, Emiliano Fratini, Antonella Lo Nostro, Giovanna Pesavento, Alessio Becheri, Pierandrea Lo Nostro, Patrizia Canton., and Piero Baglioni. (2008). Clusters of Poly(acrylates) and Silver Nanoparticles: Structure and Applications for Antimicrobial Fabrics. *The Journal of Physical Chemistry C* **112**(31), 11758–11766.

Fortin, D. and Beveridge, T. J. (2000). In *Biomineralisation.* E. Baeuerlein (Ed.). Wiley-VCH, Verlag, Germany,p.294.

Frilis, N. and Myers-Keith, P. (1986). Biosorptionof uranium and lead by *Streptomyces longwoodensis*. *Biotechnology and Bioengineering* **28**, 21-28.

Furno, F., Morley, K. S., Wong, B., Sharp, B. L., Arnold, P. L., Howdle, S. M., Bayston, R., Brown, P. D.,Winship, P. D., and Reid, H. J.(2004). *Journal of Antimicrobial Chemotherapy* **54**(6), 1019-1024.

Furr, J. R. and Russell, A. D. (1994). Antibacterial activity of Actisorb Plus, Actisorb and silver nitrate. *Journal of Hospital Infection* **27**, 201-208.

Gad, F., Zahra, T., Francis, K. P., Hasan, T., and Hamblin, M. R. (2004). Targeted photodynamic therapy of established soft-tissue infections in mice. *Photochemical and Photobiological Sciences* **3**, 451-458.

Gao, F., Lu, Q.,and Komarneni, S. (2005). Interface reaction for the self-assembly of silver nanocrystals under microwave-assisted solvothermal conditions. *Chemistry of Materials* **17**, 856-860.

Gardea-Torresdey, J. L., Parsons, J. G., Gomez, E., Peralta-Videa, J., Troiani, H., Santiago, P., and Jose-Yacaman, M. (2002). Formation and Growth of Au Nanoparticles Inside Live Alfalfa Plants. *Nano letters* **2**, 397-401.

Gericke, M and Pinches, A. (2006). Biological synthesis of metal nano particles. *Hydrometallurgy* **83**, 132–140.

Ghosh, S. K., Kundu, S., Mandal, M., Nath, S., and Pal, T. (2003). Studies on the evolution of silver nanoparticles in micelle by UV-photoactivation. *Journal of Nanoparticle Research* **5**, 577-587.

Gogoi, S. K., Chattopadhyay, A., and Ghosh, S. S. (2006). Activities of silver nanoparticles. *Langmuir*, **22**(22), 9322-9328.

Goia, E. and Matijevic, N. (1998). Preparation of monodispersed metal particles. *Journal of Chemical Education* **22**, 1203-1215.

Golab, Z. (1981). Bioaccumulation of heavy metals by the bacterium *Bacillus mycoides*. *Probl. Mineralurgii* **13**, 217-224.

Gopidas K. R., Whitesell, J. K., and Fox, M. A. (2003). Synthesis, Characterization, and Catalytic Applications of a Palladium-Nanoparticle-Cored Dendrimer. *Nano Letters* **3**, 1757-1760.

Govindaraju, K., Tamilselvan, S., Kiruthiga, V., and Singaravelu, G. (2010). Biogenic Silver anopartilces by *Solanum torvum* and their promising antimicrobial activity. *Journal of Biopesticides* **3**(1), 394–399.

Gulbranson, S. H., Hud, J. A., and Hansen, R. C. (2000). Argyria following the use of dietary supplements containing colloidal silver protein. *Cutis* **66**, 373–374.

Gurunathan, S., Kalishwaralal, K., Vaidyanathan, R., Venkataraman, D., Pandian, S. R. K., Muniyandi, J., Hariharan, N., and Eom, S. H. (2009). Biosynthesis, purification and character-

ization of silver nanoparticles using *Escherichia coli*. *Colloids and Surfaces B: Biointerfaces* **74**, 328-335.

Haes, A. J. and Van Duyne, R. P. (2002). A Nanoscale Optical Biosensor: Sensitivity and Selectivity of an Approach Based on the Localized Surface Plasmon Resonance Spectroscopy of Triangular Silver Nanoparticles. *Journal of the American Chemical Society* **124**(35), 10596-10604.

Haoran, Z., Qingbiao, L., Huixuan, W., and Daohua, S. (2005). *Journal of Chemical Technology & Biotechnology* **80**, 285-290.

Harekrishna, B., Bhui, D. K., Gobinda, P. S., Priyanka, S., Sankar, P. De., and Ajay Misra. (2009a). Green synthesis of silver nanoparticles using latex of *Jatropha curcas*. *Colloids and Surfaces A-physicochemical and Engineering Aspects* **339**, 134-139.

Harekrishna, B., Bhui, D. K., Gobinda, P. S., Priyanka, S., Santanu Pyne, and Misra, A. (2009b). Green synthesis of silver nanoparticles using seed extract of *Jatropha curcas*. *Colloids and Surfaces A: Physicochemical and Engineering Aspects* **348**, 212-216.

Harfenist, St A., Wang, Z. L., Alvarez, M. M., Vezmar, I., and Whetten, R. L. (1996). Highly Oriented Molecular Ag Nanocrystal Arrays. *The Journal of Physical Chemistry* **100**, 13904.

Hayat, M. A. (1989). *Colloidal Gold: Principles, methods and applications*. Acdemic Press, California.

He, S. T., Yao, J. N., Jiang, P., Shi, D. X., Zhang, H. X., Xie, S. S., Pang, S. J., and Gao, H. J. (2001). Formation of Silver Nanoparticles and Self-Assembled Two-Dimensional Ordered Superlattice. *Langmuir* **17**, 1571-1575.

He, Y., Wu, Y., Lu, G., and Shi, G. (2006). A facile route to silver nanosheet. *Materials Chemistry and Physics* **98**(1),178-182.

Henglein, A. (2001), Article ChemPort. *Langmuir* **17**, 2329–2333.

Henglein, A. and Giersig, M. (1999). Formation of Colloidal Silver Nanoparticles: Capping Action of Citrate. *The Journal of Physical Chemistry* **103**(44), 9533-9539.

Huang, C. P., Juang, C. P., Morehart, K., and Allen, L. (1990). The removal of copper (II) from dilute aqueous solutions by *Saccharomyces cerevisiae*. *Water Research* **24**, 433-439.

Huang, H. H., Ni, X. P., Loy, G. H., Chew, C. H., Tan, K. L., Loh, F. C., Deng, J. F., and Xu, G. Q. (1996). Photo chemaical formation of silver nanoparticles in poly(N–vinyl pyrrolidone). *Langmuir* **12**, 909-912.

Huang, J., Li Q., Sun, D., Lu, Y., Su, Y., Yang, X., Wang, H., Wang, Y., Shao, W., He, N., Hong, J., and Chen C. (2007). Biosynthesis of silver and gold nanoparticles by novel sundried *Cinnamomum camphora* leaf. *Nanotechnology* **18**, 105104-105114.

Huang, J., Lin, L., Li, Q., Sun, D., Wang, Y., Lu, Y., He, N., Yang, K., Yang, X., Wang, H., Wang, W., and Lin, W. (2008). Continuous-Flow Biosynthesis of Silver Nanoparticles by Lixivium of Sundried *Cinnamomum camphora* Leaf in Tubular Microreactors. *Industrial & Engineering Chemistry Research* **47**, 6081-6090.

Hussain, Brust, M., Papworth, A. J., and Cooper, A. I. (2003). Preparation of acrylate-stabilized gold and silver hydrosols and gold-polymer composite films. *Langmuir* **19**, 4831–4835.

Ingle, A. P., Gade, A. K., Pierrat, S., Sonnichsen, C., and Rai, M. K. (2008a). Mycosynthesis of silver nanoparticles using the fungus *Fusarium acuminatum* and its activity against some human pathogenic bacteria. *Current Nanoscience* **4**, 141-144.

Ingle, A., Rai, M., Gade, A. and Bawaskar, M. (2008b). *Fusarium solani*: A novel biological agent for the extracellular synthesis of silver nanoparticles. *Journal of nanoparticle research* **11**(8), 2079-2085.

Jae, Y. S. and Beom, S. K. (2009). Rapid Biological Synthesis of Silver Nanoparticles Using Plant Leaf Extracts. *Bioprocess and Biosystems Engineering* **32**, 79-84.

Jain, D., Daima, H. K., Kachhwaha, S., and Kothari, S. L. (2009). Synthesis of plant mediated silver nanoparticles using papaya fruit extract and evaluation of of their anti microbial activities. *Digest Journal of Nanomaterials and Biostructures* **4**(3), 557.

Jana, N. R., Gearheart, L., and Murphy, C. (2001a). Wet Chemical Synthesis of Silver Nanorods and Nanowires of Controllable Aspect Ratio. *The Journal of Chemical Communications* **7**, 617-618.

Jana, N. R., Gearheart, L., and Murphy, C. J. (2001b). Seeding Growth for Size Control of 5–40 nm Diameter Gold Nanoparticles. *Langmuir* **17**, 6782.

Joerger, R., Klaus, T., and Granqvist, C. G. (2000). Biologically Produced Silver–Carbon Composite Materials for Optically Functional Thin-Film Coatings. *Advanced Materials* **12**, 407-409.

Jortner, J. and Rao, C. N. R. (2002). Nanostructured Advanced Materials: Perspectives and Directions. *Pure and Applied Chemistry* **74**, 1491.

Kalimuthu, K., Suresh Babu, R., Venkataraman, D., Bilal, M., and Gurunathan, S. (2008). Biosynthesis of silver nanocrystals by Bacillus licheniformis. *Colloids Surf. B Biointerfaces* **65**(1)150-153.

Kalishwaralal, K., Deepak, V., and Gurunathan, S. (2010). Biosynthesis of silver and gold nanoparticles using *Brevibacterium casei*. *Colloids and Surfaces B. Biointerfaces* **77**, 257–262.

Kamala Nalini, S. P. (2008). *Synthesis of silver nanoparticles using flower extract of Hibiscus sabdariffa*. Nati. level symposium biotech vel Tech, India, 34-38.

Kamat, P. V. (2002). Photochemical and photocatalytic aspects of metal nanoparticles. *The Journal of Physical Chemistry B* **106**, 7729–7744.

Karbasian, M., Atyabi, S. M., Siadat, S. D., Momen, S. B., and Norouzian, D. (2008). Optimizing Nano-silver Formation by *Fusarium oxysporum* PTCC 5115 Employing Response Surface Methodology. *American Journal of Agricultural and Biological Sciences* **3**(1), 433-437.

Kauffman, C. A. and Carver, P. L. (1997). Antifungal agents in the 1990s: Current status and future developments. *Drugs* **53**, 539-549.

Kearns, G. J., Foster, E. W., and Hutchison, J. E. (2006). Substrates for direct imaging of chemical functionalized SiO_2 surfaces by transmission electron microscopy. *Analytical Chemistry* **78**, 298-303.

Khomutov, G. B. and Gubin, S. P (2002). Interfacial synthesis of noble metal nanoparticles. *Materials Science and Engineering: C* **22**, 141–146.

Kim, J. S., Kuk, E., Yu, K. N., Kim, J. H., Park, S. J., and Lee, H. J. (2007). Antimicrobial effects of silvernanoparticles. *Nanomedicine: Nanotechnology, Biology and Medicine* **3**, 95-101.

Kim, K. J., Sung, W. S., Moon, S. K., Choi, J. S., Kim, J. G., and Lee, D. G. (2008). Antifungal effect of silver nanoparticles on dermatophytes. *Journal of Microbiology and Biotechnology* **18**(8), 1482-1484.

Kim, Y. H., Lee, D. K., and Kang, Y. S. (2005). *Colloids Surf. A, Physio. Chemical and Engineering Aspects* **273**, 257-258.

Kishimoto, N., Takeda, Y., and Okubo, S. (2004). *Jap. Patent* JP2004091817.

Klaus, T., Jeorger, R., Olsson, E., and Granqvist, C., (2004). Bacteria as workers in the living factory: Metal accumulating bacteria and their potential for material science. *Trends in Biotechnology* **19**, 15-20.

Klaus, T., Joerger, R., Olsson, E., and Granqvist, C. G. (1999). Silver-based crystalline nanoparticles, microbially fabricated. *Proceedings of the National Academy of Sciences* **96**(24), 13611-13614.

Kloepfer, J. A., Mielke, R. E., and Nadeau, J. L. (2005). Uptake of CdSe and CdSe/ZnS Quantum Dots into Bacteria via Purine-Dependent Mechanisms. *Applied and Environmental Microbiology* **71**(5), 2548-2557.

Kowshik, M., Ashtaputre, S., Kharrazi, S., Vogel, W., Urban, J., Kulkarni, S. K., and Paknikar, K. M. (2003). Extracellular synthesis of silver nanoparticles by a silver-tolerant yeast strain. MKY3. *Nanotechnology* **14**, 95–100.

Krishna, B. and Dan, G. V. (2009). Silver nanoparticles for printable electronics and biological applications. *Journal of Materials Research* **24**(9), 2828-2836.

Kroger, N., Deutzmann, R., and Sumper, M. (1999). Polycationic peptides from diatom biosilica that direct silica nanosphere formation. *Science* **286**, 1129–1132.

Kuber, C. B. and D'Souza, S. F. (2006). *Colloids Surf. B* **47**, 160–164.

Kumar, S. A., Abyaneh, M. K., Gosavi, S. W., Kulkarni, S. K., Pasricha, R., Ahmad, A., and Khan, M. I. (2007). Nitrate reductase-mediated synthesis of silver nanoparticles from AgNO$_3$. *Biotechnology Letters* **29**, 439-445.

Kuo, C. H. and Huang, M. H. (2005).Synthesis of Branched Gold Nanocrystals by a Seeding Growth Approach. *Langmuir* **21**, 2012-2016.

Kvitek Libor, Prucek Robert, Panacek Ales, Novotny Radko, Hrbác Jan, Zbořil, and Radek (2005). *Journal of Materials Chemistry* **15**, 1099.

Lara, H. H., Ayala-Nunez, N. V., Turrent, L. d. C. I., and Padilla, C. R. (2010). Bacterial effect of silver nanoparticles against multidrug-resistant bacteria. *World Journal of Microbiology. Biotechnology* **26**, 615-621.

Law, N., Saadia Ansari, Francis R. Livens, Joanna C. Renshaw, and Jonathan R. Lloyd (2008). Formation of Nanoscale Elemental Silver Particles via Enzymatic Reduction by Geobacter sulfurreducens. *Applied and Environmental Microbiology* **74**(22). 7090-7093.

Lee, G. J., Shin, S. I., Kim, Y. C., and Oh, S. G. (2004). Preparation of silver nanorods through the control of temperature and pH of reaction medium. *Materials Chemistry and Physics* **84**, 197–204.

Lee, H. J., Yeo, S. Y., and Jeong, S. H. (2003). Antibacterial effect of nanosized silver colloidal solution on textile fabrics. *Journal of Materials Science* **38**, 2199.

Leela, A. and Vivekanandan, M. (2008a). Tapping the unexploited plant resources for the synthesis of silver nanoparticles. *African Journal of Biotechnology* **7**, 3162-3165.

Leela, A. and Vivekanandan, M. (2008b). Tapping the unexploted plant resources for the synthesis of silver nanoparticles. *African Journal of Biotechnology* **7**(17), 3162-3165.

Lengke, M F., Michael E Fleet, and Gordon Southam (2007). Biosynthesis of silver nanoparticles by filamentous cyanobacteria from a silver (I) nitrate complex. *Lagmuir* **23**, 2694.

Li, Q., Mahendra, S., Lyon, D. Y., Brunet, L., Liga, M. V., Li D., and Alvarez, P. J. J. (2008). Antimicrobial Nanomaterials for Water Disinfection and Microbial Control: Potential Applications and Implications. *Water Research*, **42**(18), 4591-4602.

Li, S., Yuhua Shen, Anjian Xie, Xuerong Yu, Lingguang Qiu, Li Zhang, and Qingfeng Zhang. (2007). Green synthesis of silver nanoparticles using *Capsicum annuum* L. extract. *Green Chemistry* **9**, 852-858.

Li, Z., Lee, D., Sheng, X. X., Cohen, R. R., and Rubner, M. F.(2006). Two-Level Antibacterial Coating with Both Release-Killing and Contact-Killing Capabilities. *Langmuir* **22**, 9820-9823.

Linga Rao, M. and Savithramma, N. (2011). Biological synthesis of silver nanopartilces using *Svensonia hyderbadensis* Leaf extract and evaluation of their antimicrobial efficacy. *Journal of Pharmaceutical Sciences* **3**(3), 1117-1121.

Link, S., Wang, Z. L., and El-Sayed, M. A. (1999). Alloy Formation of Gold-Silver Nanoparticles and the Dependence of the Plasmon Absorption on their Composition. *The Journal of Physical Chemistry B* **103**, 3529.

Liu, S., Weiping Huang, Siguang Chen, Sigalit Avivi, and Aharon Gedanken (2001). Synthesis of X-ray amorphous silver nanoparticles by the pulse sonoelectrochemical method. *Journal of Non-Crystalline Solids* **283**(1-3), 231-236.

Liz-Marzán, L. M. and Philipse, A. P. (1995). Stable hydrosolo of metallic and bimetallic nanoparticles immobilized on imogolite fibers. *The Journal of Physical Chemistry* **99**(41), 15120-15128.

Long, D., Wu, G., and Chen, S. (2007). Preparation of oligochitosan stabilized silver nanoparticles by gamma irradiation. *Radiation Physics and Chemistry*, **76**, 1126-1131.

Luoma, S. N. (2008). Silver nanotechnologies and the environment: Old problems or new challenges? Project on Emerging Nanotechnologies, the Pew Charitable Trusts.

Maillard, M., Giorgio, S., and Pileni, M. P. (2002). Silver nanodisks. *Advanced Materials* **14**(15), 1084–1086.

Maliszewska, I. and Sadowski, Z. (2009). Synthesis and anti- bacterial activity of silver nanoparticles. J.of Phyc., Conference Series **146**,1-7.

Mallin, M. P. and Murphy, C. J. (2002). Solution-Phase Synthesis of Sub-10 nm Au−Ag Alloy Nanoparticles. *Nano Letters* **2**, 1235-1237.

Mandal, S., Arumugam, S. K., Pasricha, R., and Sastry, M. (2005). Silver nanoparticles of variable morphology synthesized in aqueous foams as novel templates. *Bulletin of Material Science* **28**, 503-510.

Manish, B., Seema, B., and Kushwah, B. S. (2009). Green synthesis of nanosilver particles from extract of *Eucalyptus hybrida* (Safeda) leaf. *Digest Journal of Nano materials and Biostructures* **4**(3), 537-543.

Mann, S. (1993). Molecular tectonics in biomineralization and biomimetic materials chemistry. *Nature* **365**, 499.

Mann, S, (Ed.) (1996). *BIomimetric Materials Chemistry*. VCH, Weinheim.

Matsumura, Y., Kuniaki Yoshikata, Shin-ichi Kunisaki., and Tetsuaki Tsuchido. (2003). Mode of Bactericidal Action of Silver Zeolite and Its Comparison with That of Silver Nitrate. *Applied and Environmental Microbiology* **69**(7), 4278-4281.

Maxwell, D. J., Taylor, J. R., and Nie, S. (2002). Self-Assembled nanoparticle probes for recognition and detection of biomolecules. *Journal of the American Chemical Society* **124**, 9606.

Mazur, M. (2004). Electrochemically prepared silver nanoflakes and nanowires. *Electrochemistry Communications* **6**, 400-403.

Mc Farland, A. D. and Richard P. Van Duyne (2003). Single Silver Nanoparticles as Real-Time Optical Sensors with Zeptomole Sensitivity. *Nano Letters* **3**(8), 1057–1062.

Medentsev, A. G and Akimenko, V. K. (1998). Naphthoquinone metabolites of the fungi. *Phytochemistry* **47**, 935-959.

Melaiye, A. Sun, Z., Hindi, K., Milsted, A., Ely, D., Reneker, D., Tessier, C., Youngs, W. (2005). Silver (I)-imidazole Cyclophane Gem-diol Complexes Encapsulated by Electrospun Tecophilic Nanofibers: Formation of Nanosilver Particles and Antimicrobial Activity. *Journal of the American Chemical Society* **127**, 2285-2291.

Miller, L. P. and McCallan, S. E. A. (1957). Toxic action of metal ions to fugus spores. *Journal of Agricultural and Food Chemistry* **5**, 116-122.

Mohanpuria, P., Rana, N. K., and Yadav, S. K. (2008). Biosynthesis of nanoparticles : Technological concepts and future applications. *Journal of Nanoparticle Research* **10**, 507-517.

Morones, J. R., Elechiguerra, J. L., Camacho, A., Holt, K., Kouri, J. B., Ramírez, J. T., and Yacaman, M. J. (2005). The bactericidal effect of silver nanoparticles. *Nanotechnology* **16**, 2346-2353.

Moyer, C. A, (1965). A treatment of burns. *Trans. Stud. Coll. Physicians Philadelphia* **33**, 53-103.

Mukherjee, P., Ahmad, A., Mandal, D., Senapati, S., Sainkar, S. R., Khan, M. I., Ramani, R., Parischa, R., Kumar, P. A. V., Alam, M., Sastry, M., and Kumar, R. (2001a). Bioreduction of AuCl(4) (-) Ions by the Fungus, *Verticillium* sp. and Surface Trapping of the Gold Nanoparticles Formed D.M. and S.S. thank the Council of Scientific and Industrial Research (CSIR), Government of India, for financial assistance. *Angew Chem. Int. Ed.* **40**, 3585–3588.

Mukherjee, P., Ahmad, A., Mandal, D., Senapati, S., Sainkar, S. R., Khan, M. I., Parischa, R., Ajayakumar, P. V., Alam, M., Kumar, R., and Sastry, M. (2001b). Fungus-Mediated Synthesis of Silver Nanoparticles and Their Immobilization in the Mycelial Matrix: A Novel Biological Approach to Nanoparticle Synthesis. *Nano Letters* **1**, 515–519.

Mukherjee, P., Roy, M., Mandal, B., Dey, G., Mukherjee, P., and Ghatak. (2008). J. Green synthesis of highly stabilized nanocrystalline silver particles by a non-pathogenic and agriculturally important fungus *T. asperellum. Nanotechnology* **19**,7510.

Mukherjee, P., Senapati, S., Mandal, D., Ahmad, A., Khan, M. I., Kumar, R., and Sastry, M. (2002). Extracellular synthesis of gold nanoparticles by the fungus *Fusarium oxysporum. Chemistry and Biochemistry* **3**, 461-463.

Nair, B. and Pradeep, T. (2002). Coalescence of nanoclusters and formation of submicron crystallites assisted by *Lactobacillus* strains. *Crystal Growth & Design* **2**, 293-298.

Nanda, A. and Saravanan, M. (2009). Biosynthesis of Silver-nanoparticles from *Staphylococcus aureus* and its antimicrobial activity against MRSA and MRSE. *Nanomedicine NBM* **5**, 453-457.

Navaladian, S., Viswanathan, B., Viswanath, R. P., and. Varadarajan, T. K. (2007). Thermal decomposition as route for silver nanoparticles. *Nanoscale Research Letters* **2**, 44-48.

Newman, D. K. and Kolter, R. (2000). A role for excreted quinones in extracellular electron transfer. *Nature* **405**, 94-97.

Nidhi, N., Santosh, K., Ghosh, T., and Dutta, P. K. (2009). Preparation of Chitosan-based silver nanocomposites by a facile method. International. Conference on Optics and Photonics. Chandigiah: CSIO.

Nikhil, S. S., Mahesh, B., Rahul, B., Rekha, S. S., George Szakacs, and Ashok Pandey (2009). Biosynthesis of silver nanoparticles using aqueous extract from the compactin producing fungal strain. *Process Biochemistry* **44**, 939-943.

Niu, H., Xu, X. S., and Wang, J. H. (1993). Removal of lead from Aqueous solutions of Pencillium biomass. *Biotechnology and Bioengineering* **42**, 785-787.

Oksanen, T., Pere, J., Paavilainen, L., Buchert, J., and Viikari, L. (2000). Treatment of recycled kraft pulps with *Trichoderma reesei* hemicellulases and cellulases. *Journal of Biotechnology* **78**(1), 39–44.

Oliveira, M. M., Ugarte, D., Zanchet, D., and Zarbin, A. J. G. (2005). Influence of synthetic parameters on the size, structure, and stability of dodecanethiol-stabilized silver nanoparticles. *Journal of Colloid and Interface Science* **292**(2), 429-435.

Pal, A., Shah, S., and Devi, S. (2007). Synthesis of Au, Ag and Au-Ag Alloy Nanoparticles in Aqueous Polymer Solution. *Colloids Surface A: Physicochemical and Engineering Aspects* **302**(1-3), 51-57.

Pal, T. and Maity, D. S. (1986). Silver(I)-gelatin interaction: Spectrophotometric determination of trace amounts of silver in water. *Analyst* **111**, 1413.

Panacek, A., Kolar, M., Vecerova, R. et al. (2009). Antifungal activity of silver nanoparticles against *Candida* spp. *Biomaterials* **30**, 6333-6340.

Panacek, A., Kvitek, L., Prucek, R., Kolar, M., Veerova, R., Pizurova, N., Sharma, V. K., Nevena, T., and Zboril, R. (2006). Silver colloid nanoparticles: Synthesis, characterization and their anti bacterial activity.*The Journal of Physical Chemistry B* **110**, 16248-16253.

Papp, S., Patakfalvi, R., and Dekany, I.(2008). Metal nanoparticle formation on layer silicate lamellae. *Colloid & Polymer Science* **286**, 3-14.

Parashar, V., Parashar, R., Sharma, B., and Pandey, A. C. (2009). Parthenium leaf extract mediated synthesis of silver nanoparticles: A novel approach towards weed utilization. *Digest Journal of Nanomaterials and Biostructures* **4**(1), 45-50.

Parikh, R. Y., Singh, S., Prasad, B. L. V., Patole, M. S., Sastry, M., and Schouche, Y. S. (2008). Extracellular synthesis of crystalline silver nanoparticles and molecular evidence of silver resistance from *Morganella* sp.: Towards understanding biochemical synthesis mechanism. *Chemistry and Biochemistry* **9**, 1415–1422.

Pastoriza-Santos and Liz-Marzán, L. M. (2002). Formation of PVP-Protected Metal Nanoparticles in DMF. *Langmuir* **18**, 2888-2894.

Patel, K., Kapoor, S., Dave, D. P., and Murherjee, T. (2005). *Journal of Chemical Sciences* **117**(1), 53-60.

Patel, K., Kapoor, S., Dave, D. P., and Murherjee, T. (2007). *Journal of Chemical Sciences* **117**(4), 311-315.

Patterson, T. F. (2007). Treatment and prevention of fungal infections. Focus on candidemia. Newyork: *Applied Clinical Education* **100**, p VII-VIII.

Petit, C., Lixon, P., and Pileni, M. P. (1993). *In situ* synthesis of silver nanocluster in AOT reverse micelles. *The Journal of Physical Chemistry* **97**, 12974-12983.

Phong, N T P., Ngo Hoang Minh, Ngo Vo Ke Thanh, and Dang Mau Chien (2009). Green synthesis of silver nanoparticles and silver colloidal solutions. *Journal of Physics*: *Conference Series* **187**, 012078 doi:10.1088/1742-6596/187/1/012078.

Pileni, M. P. (2001). Self-Assemblies of nanocrystals: Fabrication and Collective Properties. *Applied Surface Sciences* **171**, 1-14.

Pillai, Z. S. and Kamat, P. V. (2004). What Factors Control the Size and Shape of Silver Nanoparticles in the Citrate Ion Reduction Method? *Journal of Physical Chemistry B* **108**, 945.

Porter, A. E., Muller, K., Skepper, J., Midgley, P. and Welland, M. (2006) Uptake of C "6"0 by human monocyte macrophages, its localization and implications for toxicity: Studied by high resolution electron microscopy and electron tomography. *Acta Biomaterialia* **2**, 409-419.

Prabhu, N., Divya, T. R., Gowri, Y. K., Siddiqua, A. S., and Innocent, J. P. D. (2010). Synthesis of silver nanoparticles and their antibacterial efficacy. *Journal of Nanobiotechnology* **5**, 185-189.

Pugazhenthiran, N., Anandan, S., Kathiravan, G., and Udaya-Prakash, N. K. (2009). Microbial synthesis of silver nanoparticles by *Bacillus* sp. *Journal of Nanoparticle Research* **11**, 1811-1815.

Purwar, V. and Pokharkar, V. (2011). Green synthesis of silver nanoparticles using marine polysaccharide: Study of *in vitro* antibacterial activity. *Materials Letters* **65**, 999–1002.

Qourzal, S., Tamimi, M., Assabbane, A., Bouamrane, A., Nounah, A., Laanab, L., and Ait-Ichou, Y. (2006). Preparation of TiO_2 Photocatalyst Using $TiCl_4$ as a Precursor and its Photocatalytic Performance. *Journal of Applied Sciences* **6**(7), 1553-1559.

Rai, M., Yadav, A., and Gade, A. (2009). Silver nanoparticles: A novel antimicrobial agent. *Biotechnology Advances* **27**, 76-83.

Rajesh, R., Stringer, Sarah, J., Agarwal Gunjan, Jones Sharon, E., and Stone Morley, O. (2002). Diomimetis synthesis and patterning os silver nanoparticles. *Letters* 169-172.

Raveendran, P., Fu, J., and Wallen, S. L. (2003). Completely "green" synthesis and stabilization of metal nanoparticles. *Journal of the American Chemical Society* **125**, 13940-13941.

Rayman, M. K., Lo, T. C., and Sanwal, B. D. (Octuber 10, 1972). Transport of succinate in *Escherichia coli*. II. Characteristics of uptake and energy coupling with transport in membrane preparations. *The Journal of Biological Chemistry* **247**(19), 6332-6339.

Revathi, N. and Prabhu, N. (2009). Fungal silver nanoparticles: Preparation and its pH characterization. *Trends in Biotechnology* **8**, 27-29.

Rocio Balaguera-Gelves, M. (2006). Detection of nitroexplosives by surface enhanced Raman spectroscopy on colloidal metal nanoparticles. *Master thesis*. University of Puerto Rico, Mayaguez Campus.

Rodriguez-Sanchez, L., Blanco, M. C., and Lopez-Quintela, M. A. (2000). Electrochemical synthesis of silver nanoparticles. *Journal of Physical Chemistry B* **104**, 9683-9688.

Roe, D., Balu Karandikar, Nathan Bonn-Savage1, Bruce Gibbins, and Jean-Baptiste Roullet. (2008). Antimicrobial surface functionalization of plastic catheters by silver nanoparticles. *Journal of Antimicrobial Chemotherapy* **61**(4), 869-876.

Rosei, F. (2004). Nanostructured surfaces: Challenges and frontiers in nanotechnology. *Journal of Physics: Condensed Matter* **16**, S1373-1436.

Rosemary, M. J. and Pradeep, T. (2003). Solvothermal synthesis of silver nanoparticles from thiolates. *Colloids and Surfaces A* **268**, 81-84.

Rosi, N. L. and Mirkin, C. A. (2005). Nanostructures in biodiagnostics. *Chemical Reviews* **105**, 1547-1562.

Rouch, D. A., Lee, B. T. O., and Morby, A. P. (1995). Understanding cellular responses to toxic agents: A mechanism-choice in bacterial metal resistance. *Journal of Industrial Microbiology and Biotechnology* **14**, 132–141.

Roy, N. and Barik, A. (2010). Green synthesis of silver nanoparticles from the unexploited weed resources. *International journal of nanotechnology and applications* **4**, 95-101.

Roy, R., Hoover, M. R., Bhalla, A. S., Slaweekl, T., Dey, S., Cao, W., Li J., and Bhaskar, S. (2008). Ultradilute Ag-auasols with extraordinary bactericidal properties: Role of the system Ag-O-H$_2$O. *Materials Research Innovations* **11**, 3-18.

Russell, A. D. and Hugo, W. B. (1994). Antibacterial activity and action of silver. *Progress in Medicinal Chemistry* **31**, 351–370.

Saifuddin, N., Wong, C. W., and Nur Yasumira, A. A. (2009). Rapid Biosynthesis of Silver Nanoparticles Using Culture Supernatant of Bacteria with Microwave Irradiation. *E-Journal of Chemistry* **6**(1), 61-70.

Sakaguchi, T., Tsuji, T., Nakajima, A., and Horikoshi, T. (1979). Accumulation of cadmium by green micro algae. *European Journal of Applied Microbiology* **8**, 207-215.

Salata, O.V. (2004). Application of nanoparticles in biology and medicine. *Journal of Nanobiotechnology* 2:3, 3-6.

Salkar, R. A., Jeevanandam, P., Aruna, S. T., Yuri Koltypin, and Gedanken, A. (1999).The sonochemical preparation of amorphous silver nanoparticles. *Journal of Materials Chemistry* **9**, 1333-1335.

Saravanan, M. and Nanda, A. (2010) Extracellular synthesis of silver bionanoparticles from *Aspergillus clavatus* and its antimicrobial activity against MRSA and MRSE. *Colloids and Surfaces B: Biointerfaces* **77**, 214-218.

Sastry, M., Ahmad, A., Khan, M. I., and Kumar, R. (2003). Biosynthesis of metal nanoparticles using fungi and actinomycete. *Current Science* **85**, 162-170.

Sato, Y., Wang, J. J., Batchelder, D. N., and Smith, D. A. (2003). *Langmuir* **19**, 6857.

Sau, T. K. and Murphy, C. J. (2004). Room Temperature, High-Yield Synthesis of Multiple Shapes of Gold Nanoparticles in Aqueous Solution. *Journal of the American Chemical Society* **126**, 8648-8649.

Schreurs, W. J. and Rosenberg, H. (1982). Effect of silver ions on transport and retention of phosphate by *Escherichia coli. The Journal of Bacteriology* **152**, 7-13.

Senapati, S., Ahmad, A., Khan, M. I., Sastry, M., and Kumar, R. (2005). Extracellular Biosynthesis of Bimetallic Au-Ag Alloy Nanoparticles. *Small* **1**, 517-520.

Senapati, S., Mandal, D., Ahmad, A., Khan, M. I., Sastry, M., and Kumar, R. (2004). Fungus mediated synthesis of silver nanoparticles: A novel biological approach. *Indian Journal of Physics* **78A**, 101–105.

Setua, P., Chakraborty, A., Seth, D., Bhatta, U. M., Satyam, P. V., and Sarkar, N. (2007). Synthesis, optical properties, and surface enhanced Raman scattering of silver nanoparticles in nonaqueous methanol reverse micelles. *The Journal of Physical Chemistry C* **111**(10), 3901.

Shahverdi, A. R., Fakhimi, A., Shahverdi, H. R., and Sara, M. (2007). Synthesis and effect of silver nanoparticles on the antibacterial activity of different antibiotics against *Staphylococcus aureus* and *Escherichia coli. Nanomedicine: Nanotechnology, Biology and Medicine* **3**, 168-171.

Shankar, S. S., Rai, A., Ahmad, A., and Sastry, M. (2005). *Chemistry of Materials* **17**, 566.

Shankar, S. S., Rai, A., Ahmad, A., and Sastry. (2004). Rapid synthesis of Au, Ag, and bimetallic Au core-Ag shell nanoparticles using Neem (*Azadirachta indica*) leaf broth. *Journal of Colloid and Interface Science* **275**, 496–502.

Shiv Shankar, S., Ahmad, A. M., and Sastry, M. (2003). Geranium Leaf Assisted Biosynthesis of Silver Nanoparticles. *Biotechnology Progress* **19**, 1627-1631.

Shon, Y. S., Choo, H., and Chim, C. R. (2003). Organic Reactions of Monolayer-Protected Metal Nanoparticles. In *Dendrimers and Nanosciences*. D. Astruc (Ed.). *C. R. Chime,*Paris, **6**, 1009.

Shrivastava, S., Bera, T., Roy, A., Singh, G, Ramachandrarao, P., and Dash, D. (2007). Characterization of enhanced antibacterial effects of novel silver nanoparticles. *Nanotechnology* **18**, 225103.

Silver, S. (2003). Bacterial silver resistance: Molecular biology and uses and misuses of silver compounds. *FEMS Microbiology Reviews* **27**(2-3), 341–353.

Simi, C. K. and Abraham, T. E. (2007). Hydrophobic grafted and cross-linked starch nanoparticles for drug delivery. *Bioprocess and Biosystems Engineering* **30**, 173-180.

Singh, A., Jain, D., Upadhyay, M. K., Khandelwal, N., and Verma, H. N. (2010). Green synthesis of silver nanoparticles using Argemone *Mexicana* leaf extract and evaluation of their antimicrobial activities. *Digest Journal of Nanomaterials and Biostructures* **5**, 483-489.

Smetana, A. B., Klabunde, K. J., and Sorensen, C. M. (2005). Synthesis of spherical silver nanoparticles by digestive ripening, stabilization with various agents, and their 3-D and 2-D superlattice formation. *Journal of Colloid and Interface Science* **284**, 521–526.

Smith, A. M., Duan, H. W., Rhyner, M. N., Ruan, G., and Nie, S. (2006). A systematic examination of surface coatings on the optical and chemical properties of semi conductor quantum dots. *Physical Chemistry Chemical. Physics* **8**, 3895-3903.

Soroushian, B., Lampre, I., Belloni, J., and Mostafavi, M. (2005). Radiolysis of silver ion solutions in ethylene glycol. Solvated electron and radical scavenging yields. *Radiation, Physics and Chemistry* **72**, 111-118.

Souza, G. I. H., Marcato, P. D., Duran, N., and Esposito, E. (2004). Utilization of *Fusarium oxysporum* in the biosynthesis of silver nanoparticles and its antibacterial activities. In *IX National Meeting of Environmental Microbiology Curtiba*. pp. 25.

Sreeram, K. J., Nidhin, M., and Nair, B. U. (2008). Microwave assisted template synthesis of silver nanoparticles. *Bulletin of Materials Science* **31**(7), 937-942.

Starowicz, M., Stypula, B., and Banaœ, J. (2006). *Electrochemistry Communications* **8**, 227-230.

Stepanov, A. L., Khaibullin, I. B., Townsend, P. D., Hole, and Bukharaev, A. A., (2000). *RF Patent*, 2156490.

Sudeep, P. K. and Kamat, P. V. (2005). Photosensitized Growth of Silver Nanoparticles under Visible Light Irradiation: A Mechanistic Investigation. *Chemistry of Materials* **17**, 5404-5410.

Summers, A. O. and Silver, S. (1978). Microbial transformations of metals. *Annual Review of Microbiology*. **32**, 637–672.

Sun, Y. G. and Xia, Y. N. (2002). Shape-Controlled Synthesis of Gold and Silver Nanoparticles. *Science* **298**, 2176-2179.

Sun, Y. G., Mayers, B., Herricks, T., and Xia, Y. N. (2003). Polyol Synthesis of Uniform Silver Nanowires: A Plausible Growth Mechanism and the Supporting Evidence. *Nano Letters* **3**, 955-960.

Sun, Y. G., Yin, Y. D., Mayers, B. T., Herricks, T., and Xia, Y. N. (2002). Uniform silver nanowires can be synthesized by reducing $AgNO_3$ with ethylene glycol in the presence of seeds and poly (vinyl pyrrolidone). *Chemistry of Materials* **14**, 4736–4745.

Szłyk, E., Piszczek, P., Grodzicki, A., Chaberski, M., Goliński, A., Szatkowski, J., and Błaszczyk, T. (2001). CVD of Ag^I complexes with tertiary phosphines and perfluorinated carboxylates-A new class of silver precursors. *Advanced Materials, Chemical Vapour Deposition* 7, 111-116.

Taleb, A., Petit, C., and Pileni, M. P. (1997). Synthesis of Highly Monodisperse Silver Nanoparticles from AOT Reverse Micelles: A Way to 2D and 3D Self-Organization. *Chemistry of Materials* **9**, 950–959.

Tan, Y., Wang, Y., Jiang, L., and Daoben Zhu (2002).Thiosalicylic Acid-Functionalized Silver Nanoparticles Synthesized in One-Phase System. *Journal of Colloid and Interface Science* **249**, 336–345.

Tang, Z., Liu, S., Dong, S., and Wang, E. (2001). Electrochemical synthesis of Ag nanoparticles on functional carbon surfaces. *Journal of Electroanalytical Chemistry* **502**, 146-151.

Tessier, P. M., Velev, O. D., Kalambur, A. T., Rabolt, J. F., Lenhoff, A. M., and Kalar, E. W. (2000). Assembly of gold nanostructured films templated by colloidal crystals and used in surface enhanced Raman spectroscopy. *Journal of American chemical society* **122**(39), 9554-9555.

Toshima, N., Yonezawa, T., and Kushihashi, K. (1993). 2543Polymer-protected palladium–platinum bimetallic clusters: Preparation, catalytic properties and structural considerations. *Journal of the Chemical Society, Faraday Transactions* **89**, 2537-2543.

Townsend, P. T., Chandler, P. J., and Zhang, L. (1994). *Optical effects of ion implantation*. Cambridge Univ. Press, Cambridge.

Tripathi, A., Ashok, M. R., Chandrasekaran, N., Prathna, T. C. N., Prathna, T. C., and Mukherjee, A. (2010). Process variables in biomimetic synthesis of silver nanoparticles by aqueous extract of *Azadirachta indica* (Neem) leaves. *Journal of Nanoparticle Research* **12**, 237-246.

Tripathi, R. M., Antariksh Saxena, Nidhi Gupta, Harsh Kapoor, and Singh, R. P. (2010). High antibacterial activity of silver nanoballs against *E.coli* mtcc 1302, *S typhimurium* MTCC 1254, *B. subtilis* MTCC 1133 and *P. aeruginosa* MTCC 2295. *Digest journal of nanomaterials and Biostrucutres* **5**(2), 323-330.

Troupis, A., Hiskia, A., and Papaconstantinou, E. (2002). *Angewandte Chemie International Edition* **41**, 1911.

Vahabi, K., Ali Mansoori, G., and Sedighe Karimi (2011). Biosynthesis of Silver Nanoparticles by Fungus *Trichoderma reesei* (A Route for Large-Scale Production of AgNPs). *Insciences Journal* **1**(1), 65-79.

Vigneshwaran, N., Ashtaputrea, N. M., Varadarajana, P. V., Nachanea, R. P., Paralikara, K. M., and Balasubramanyaa, R. H. (2007). Biological Synthesis of Silver Nanoparticles using the Fungus *Aspergillus flavus*. *Materials Letters* **61**(6), 1413-1418.

Vigneshwaran, N., Kathe, A. A., Varadarajan, P. V., Nachane, R. P., and Balasubramanya, R. P. (2006). Biomimetics of silver nanoparticles by

white rot fungus, *Phaenerochaete chrysosporium. Colloids and Surfaces B: Biointerfaces* **53**, 55–59.

Vigneshwaran, N., Nachane, R. P., Balasubramanya, R. H., and Varadarajan, P. V. (2006). A novel one-pot "green" synthesis of stable silver nanoparticles using soluble starch. *Carbohydrate Research* **341**, 2012-2018.

Virender, S. K., Yngard Ria, A., and Lin Yekaterina. (2009). Silver nanoparticles: Green synthesis and their antimicrobial activities. *Colloid and Interface Science* **145**, 83-96.

Volesky, B. (Ed.) (1990). *Biosorption of Heavt metals*. pp. 139-172. Boca Raton, FL, CRC press.

Vorobyova, S. A., Lesnikovich, A. I., and Sobal, N. S. (1999). Preparation of silver nanoparticles by interphase reduction. *Colloids Surf. A* **152**, 375–379.

Vyom parashar, Rashmi parashara, Bechan Sharma, and Avinash Pandeyc. (2009). parthenium leaf extract mediated synthesis of silver nanoparticles: A novel approach towards weed utilization. *Digest Journal of Nanomaterials and Biostructures* **4**(1), 45-50.

Walter, E. C., Ng, K., Zach, M. P., Penner, R. M., and Favier, F. (2002). Electronic devices from electrodeposited metal nanowires. *Microelectronic Engineering* **61-62**, 555-561.

Wei, D. and Qian, W. (2008). Facile Synthesis of Ag and Au nanoparticles utilizing chitosan as a mediator agent. *Colloid Surface B* **62**, 136-142.

Weinstock, I. A. (1998). *Chemical Reviews* **98**,113.

Whitesides, G. M. (2003). The "right" size in nanobiotechnology. *Nature Biotechnology* **21**, 1161-1165.

Willems, and van den Wildenberg. (2005). *Roadmap report on nanoparticles*. Barcelona, Spain: W&W. Espana sl.

Windt, W. D. (2009), United States Patent Application Publication. *Methods for producing metal nanoparticles* (2009) US2009/0239280 A1.

Xie, Y., Ye, R., and Liu, H. (2006). Synthesis of silver nanoparticles in reverse micelles stabilized by natural biosurfactant. *Colloids and Surfaces A* **279**, 175-178.

Xiong, Y. J., Xie, Y., Du, G. O., Liu, X. M., and Tian, X. (2002). B.Ultra sound assisted self-regulated route to Ag nano rods. *Chemistry Letters* **1**, 98–99.

Yanagihara, N., Tanaka, Y., and Okamoto, H. (2001). Formation of silver nano particles in poly(methyl methacrylate) by UV irradiation. *Chemistry Letters* **8**, 796-797.

Yin Yadong, Li Zhi-Yuan, Zhong Ziyi, Gates Byron, and Venkateswaran Sagar (2002). Synthesis and characterization of stable aqueous dispersions of silver nanoparticles through the Tollens process. *Chemistry of Materials* **12**, 522-527.

Young-Ki Jo, Byung H. Kim, and Geunhwa Jung (2009). Antifungal activity of silver ions and nanoparticles on phytopathogenic fungi. *Plant Disease* **93**, 1037-1043.

Yu, D. and Yam, V. W. W. (2004). Controlled Synthesis of Monodisperse Silver Nanocubes in Water. *Journal of the American Chemical Society* **126**, 13200.

Yu, D. and Yam, V. W. W. (2005). Hydrothermal-Induced Assembly of Colloidal Silver Spheres into Various Nanoparticles on the Basis of HTAB-Modified Silver Mirror Reaction. *Journal of Physical Chemistry B*, **109**(12), 5497-5503.

Yu, D. G. (2007). Formation of colloidal silver nanoparticles stabilized by Na$^+$–poly(γ-glutamic acid)–silver nitrate complex via chemical reduction process. *Colloids Surf. B* **59**, 171-178.

Yu, Y. Y., Chang, S. S, Lee, C. L, and Wang, C. R. C. (1997). Gold nanorods: Electrochemical synthesis and optical properties. *Journal of Physical Chemistry B* 101, 6661-6664.

Zeng, F., Chao Hou, Shuizhu Wu, Xinxing Liu, Zhen Tong, and Shuning Yu. (2007). Silver nanoparticles directly formed on natural macroporous matrix and their anti-microbial activities. *Nanotechnology* **18**, 1-8.

Zhang, G., Keita, B., Dolbecq, A., Mialane, P., Secheresse, F., Miserque, F., and Nadjo, L. (2007). Green Chemistry-type One-Step Synthesis of Silver Nanostructures Based on MoV-MoVI Mixed Valence Polyoxometalate. *Journal of Materials Chemistry* **19**, 5821-5823.

Zhang, J. Z. (2009). *Optical properties and spectroscopy of nanomaterials*. World Scientific, Singapore, Vol. xvi, pp. 359-383.

Zhang, J., Chen, P., Sun, C., and Hu, X. (2004). Sonochemical synthesis of colloidal silver catalysts for reduction of complexing silver in DTR system. *Applied Catalysis A* **266**, 49.

Zhang, L., Yu, J. C., Yip, H. Y., Li, Q., Kwong, K. W., Xu, A.W. et al. (2003). *Langmuir* **19**, 10372

Zhou, Y., Yu, S. H., Cui, X. P., Wang, C. Y., and Chen, Z. Y. (1999). Formation of silver nanowires by a naovel solid-liquid phase arc discharge method. *Chemistry of materials* **11**, 545–546.

Zhu Jian, Zhu Xiang, and Wang Yongchang (2005). *Mictoelectronic Engineering* **77**, 58.

Zhu, J. J., Liao, X. H., Zhao, X. N., and Chen, H. Y. (2001). Preparation of silver nanorods by electrochemical methods. *Materials Letters* **49**(2), 91-95.

Zhu, J. J., Liu, S. W., Palchik, O., Koltypin, Y., and Gedanken, A. (2000). *Langmuir* **16**, 6396.

6

Aggarwal, B., Takata, Y., and Oommen, O, V, (2004). From chemoprevention to chemotherapy: Common targets and common goals. *Expert Opinion on Investigational Drugs* **13**(10), 1327-1338.

Arivazhagan, S., Velmurugan, B., Bhuvaneswari, V., and Nagini, S. (2004). Effects of aqueous extracts of garlic (*Allium sativum*) and neem (*Azadirachta indica*) leaf on hepatic and blood oxidant-antioxidant status during experimental gastric carcinogenesis. *Journal of Medicinal Food* **7**(3), 334-339.

Ashidi, J. S., Houghton, P. J., Hylands, P. J., and Efferth, T. (2010). Ethnobotanical survey and cytotoxicity testing of plants of South-western Nigeria used to treat cancer, with isolation of cytotoxic constituents from *Cajanus cajan Millsp.* leaves. *Journal of Ethnopharmacology* **128**(2), 501-512.

Bairwa, N. K., Sethiya, N. K., and Mishra, S. H. (2010). Protective effect of stem bark of *Ceiba pentandra* linn. against paracetamol-induced hepatotoxicity in rats. *Pharmacognosy Research* **2**, 26-30.

Bingfen, X., Zongchao, L., Qichao, P., Yongju, L., Xiurong, S., Likai, W., Runmei, Z., and Hongda, Z. (1994). The anticancer effect and anti-DNA topoisomerase II effect of extracts of *Camellia ptilophylla chang* and *camellia sinesis* Chinese *Journal of Cancer Research* 6(3), 184-190.

Bonham, M., Posakony, J., Coleman, I., Montgomery, B., Simon, J., and Nelson, P. S. (2005). Characterization of chemical constituents in *Scutellaria baicalensis* with antiandrogenic and growth-inhibitory activities toward prostate carcinoma. *Clinical Cancer Research* 11, 3905-3914.

Chao, A., Thun, M. J., and Connell, C. J. (2005). Meat consumption and risk of colorectal cancer. *The Journal of American Medical Association* 293(2), 172–182.

Choi, S. U., Ryu, S. Y., Yoon, S. K., Jung, N. P., Park, S. H., Kim, K. H., Choi, E. J., and Lee, C. O. (1999). Effects of flavonoids on the growth and cell cycle of cancer cells. *Anticancer Research* 19, 5229-5233.

Chung, C. P., Park, J. B., and Bae, K. H. (1995). Pharmacological effects of methanolic extract from the root of *Scutellaria baicalensis* and its flavonoids on human gingival fibroblast. *Planta Medica* 61, 150-153.

Costa-Lotufo L. V., Khan, M. T., Ather, A., Wilke, D. V., Jimenez, P. C., Pessoa, C., de Moraes, M. E., de Moraes, M. O. (2005). Studies of the anticancer potential of plants used in Bangladeshi folk medicine. *Journal of Ethnopharmacology* 99(1), 21–30.

Cragg, G. M., and Newman, D. J. (2004). A tale of two tumour targets: Topoisomerase I and tubulin. The Wall and Wani contribution to cancer chemotherapy. *Journal of Natural Products* 67, 232–244.

Dai, H. F., Zeng., Y. B.; Xiao, Q., Han, Z., Zhao, Y. X., and Mei, W. L. (2010). Caloxanthones O and P: Two New Prenylated Xanthones from *Calophyllum inophyllum*. *Molecules* 15, 606-612.

Das, U. N. (2002). A radical approach to cancer. *Medicinal Science Monitor* 8, 79–92.

Dhanamani, M., Devi, L., and Kannan, S. (2011). Ethnomedicinal plants for cancer therapy--A Review. Hygeia. *Journal of Drug and Medicine*.3(1), 1-10.

Dhanarasu, S., Masoud Al-hazimi, A., Sethuraman, P., and Selvam, M. (2010). Chemopreventive and Antilipdperoxidative Potential of *Thespesia populnea* (L.) on Experimental Buc-cal Pouch Carcinogenesis. Ibnosina. *Journal of Medicine and BS* 2(6), 269-277.

Fei, Y., Xui, L., Yi, J., Zhang, W., and Zhang, D. Y. (2002). Anticancer activity of *Scutellaria baicalensis* and its potential mechanism. *Journal of Alternative and Complementary Medicine* 8, 567-572.

Gálvez, M., Martín-Cordero, C., López-Lázaro, M., Cortés, F., and Ayuso, M. J. (2003). Cytotoxic effect of *Plantago* spp. on cancer cell lines. *Journal of Ethnopharmacology* 88(2-3), 125-130.

Heber, D. (2004). Vegetables, fruits and phytoestrogens in the prevention of diseases. *Journal of Postgraduate Medicine* 50(2), 145-149.

Hirano, T., Abe, K., Gotoh, M., and Oka, K. (1995). Citrus flavone tangeretin inhibits leukaemic HL-60 cell growth partially through induction of apoptosis with less cytotoxicity on normal lymphocytes. *British Journal of Cancer* 72(6), 1380-1388.

Hsu, S. D., Singh, B. B., Lewis, J. B., Borke, J. L., Dickinson, D. P., Drake, L., Caughman, G. B., and Schuster, G. S. (2002). Chemoprevention of oral cancer by green tea. *General Dentistry* 50(2), 140-146.

Jainu, M. and Shyamala Devi, C. S. (2003). Potent antiulcerogenic activity of *Cissus quadrangularis* on aspirin induced gastric ulcer by its antioxidative mechanism. *Journal of Clinical Biochemistry and Nutrition* 34, 43-47.

Janin, D., Pathak, N., Khan, S., Raghuram, G. V., Bhargava, A., Samarth, R., and Mishra, P. K. (2011). Evaluation of Cytotoxicity and Anticarcinogenic Potential of Mentha Leaf Extracts. *International Journal of Toxicology* 30(2), 225-236.

Joon Surh, Y. (2003). Cancer chemoprevention with dietary phytochemicals. *Nature* 3, 768-780.

Kathiresan, K., Sithranga Boopathy, N., and Kavitha, S. (2005). Coastal vegetation An underexplored source of anticancer drugs. *Natural Product Radiance* 5(2), 115-119.

Konczak, I, Okuno, S, Yoshimoto, M., and Yamakawa, O. (2004). Caffeoylquinic Acids Generated *In Vitro* in a High-Anthocyanin-Accumulating Sweet potato Cell Line. *Journal of Biomedicine and Biotechnology* 5, 287-292.

Konczak-Islam, I., Yoshimoto, M., Hou, D. X., Terahara, N., and Yamakawa, O. (2003). Potential chemopreventive properties of anthocyanin-rich aqueous extracts from *in vitro* produced tissue of sweetpotato (*Ipomoea batatas* L.). *Journal of Agricultural Food Chemistry* **51**(20), 5916-5922.

Kouidhi, B., Zmantar, T., and Bakhrouf, A. (2010). Anticariogenic and cytotoxic activity of clove essential oil (*Eugenia caryophyllata*) against a large number of oral pathogens. *Annals of Microbiology* **60**, 599–604.

Kumar, R. A., Sridevi, K., Kumar, N. V., Nanduri, S., and Rajagopal, S. (2004). Anticancer and immunostimulatory compounds from *Andrographis paniculata*. *Journal of Ethnopharmacology* **92**(2-3), 291-295.

Kyung-A. H., Yu-Jin, H., Dong-Sik, P., Jaehyun, K., and Ae-Son, O. (2011). *In vitro* investigation of antioxidant and anti-apoptotic activities of Korean wild edible vegetable extracts and their correlation with apoptotic gene expression in HepG2 cells. *Food Chemistry* **125**, 483–487.

Lee, C. K., Park, K. K., Lim, S. S., Park, J. H., and Chung, W. Y. (2007). Effects of the licorice extract against tumor growth and cisplatin-induced toxicity in a mouse xenograft model of colon cancer. *Biological and Pharmaceutical Bulletin* **30**(11), 2191-2195.

Liu, J. J., Huang, T. S., Cheng, W. F., and Lu, F. J. (2003). Baicalein and baicalin are potent inhibitors of angiogenesis: Inhibition of endothelial cell proliferation, migration and differentiation. *International Journal of Cancer* **106**, 559-565.

Lu, X., Yu, H., Ma, Q., Shen, S., and Das, U. N. (2010). Linoleic acid suppresses colorectal cancer cell growth by inducing oxidant stress and mitochondrial dysfunction. *Lipids in Health and Disease* **9**, 106.

Maloney, D. (1998). *The American Association of Oriental Medicine's Complete Guide to Chinese Herbal Medicine*. The Berkley Publishing Group, New York.

Markowitz, S. D. and Bertagnolli, M. M. (2009). Molecular basis of colorectal cancer. *The New England Journal of Medicine* **361**(25), 2449–2460.

Nanduri, S., Thunuguntla, S. S., Nyavanandi, V. K., Kasu, S., Kumar, P. M., Ram, P. S., Rajago-pal, S., Kumar, R. A., Deevi, D. S., Rajagopalan, R., Venkateswarlu, A. (2003). Biological investigation and structure-activity relationship studies on azadirone from *Azadirachta indica A. Juss*. *Bioorganic and Medicinal Chemistry Letters* **13**(22), 4111-4115.

Natesan, S., Badami, S., Dongre, S. H., and Godavarthi, A. (2007). Antitumor activity and antioxidant status of the methanol extract of *Careya arborea* bark against Dalton's lymphoma ascites induced ascetic and solid tumor in mice. *Journal of Pharmacological Sciences* **103**(1), 12-23.

Neto, C. C. (2007). Cranberry and its phytochemicals: A review of *in vitro* anticancer studies. *Journal of Nutrition* **137**, 186-193S.

Park, K. K., Chun, K. S., Lee, J. M., and Surh, Y. J. (1998). Inhibitory effects of [6]-gingerol, a major pungent principle of ginger, on phorbol ester-induced inflammation, epidermal ornithine decarboxylase activity and skin tumors promotion in ICR mice. *Cancer Letter* **129**, 139-144.

Pfisterer, P. H., Rollinger, J. M., Schyschka, L., Rudy, A., Vollmar, A. M., and Stuppner, H. (2010). Neoandrographolide from *Andrographis paniculata* as a potential natural chemosensitizer. *Planta Medica* **76**(15), 1698-1700.

Romero-Jimenez, M., Campos-Sanchez, J., Analla, M., Munoz-Serrano, A., and Alonso-Moraga, A. (2005). Genotoxicity and anti-genotoxicity of some traditional medicinal herbs. *Mutation Research* **585**, 147–155.

Sadava, D. and Winesburg, J. (2005). Contaminants of PC-SPES are not responsible for cytotoxicity in human small-cell lung carcinoma cells. *Cancer Letter* **220**, 171-175.

Sakarkar, D. M. and Deshmukh, V. N. (2011). Ethnopharmacological Review of Traditional Medicinal Plants for Anticancer Activity. *International Journal of PharmTech Research* **3**(1), 298-308.

Sakpakdeejaroen, I. and Itharat, A. (2009). Cytotoxic compounds against breast adenocarcinoma cells (MCF-7) from Pikutbenjakul. *Journal of Health Research* **23**(2), 71-76.

Seeram, N. P., Adams, L. S., Hardy, M. L., and Heber, D. (2004). Total cranberry extract versus its phytochemical constituents: Antiproliferative and synergistic effects against human tumor cell lines. *Journal of Agricultural and Food Chemistry* **52**(9), 2512-2517.

Sharma, V. A. (2011). Polyphenolic compound rottlerin demonstrates significant *in vitro* cytotoxicity against human cancer cell lines: Isolation and characterization from the fruits of *Mallotus philippinensis. Journal of Plant Biochemistry and Biotechnology* **20**(2), 190-195.

Singh, R. P., Banerjee, S., and Rao, A. R. (2001). Modulatory influence of *Andrographis paniculata* on mouse hepatic and extrahepatic carcinogen metabolizing enzymes and antioxidant status. *Phytotherapy Research* **15**(5), 382-390.

Subapriya, R., Bhuvaneswari, V., and Nagini, S. (2005). Ethanolic neem (*Azadirachta indica*) leaf extract induces apoptosis in the hamster buccal pouch carcinogenesis model by modulation of Bcl-2, Bim, caspase 8 and caspase 3. *Asian Pacific Journal of Cancer Prevention* **6**(4), 515-520.

Su, L. J. and Arab, L. (2002). Tea consumption and the reduced risk of colon cancer--results from a national prospective cohort study. *Public Health Nutrition* **5**(3), 419-425.

Sun, J. and Hai Liu, R. (2006). Cranberry phytochemical extracts induce cell cycle arrest and apoptosis in human MCF-7 breast cancer cells. *Cancer Letter* **241**(1), 124-134.

Tepsuwan, A., Kupradinun, P., and Kusamran, W. R. (2002). Chemopreventive Potential of Neem Flowers on Carcinogen-Induced Rat Mammary and Liver Carcinogenesis. *Asian Pacific Journal Cancer Prevention* **3**(3), 231-238.

Tyagi, S., Singh, G., Sharma, A., and Aggarwal, G. (2010). Phytochemical candidate therapeutics: An overview. *International Journal of Pharmaceutical Sciences* 53-55.

Uma Devi, P., Selvi, S., Devipriya, D., Murugan, S., and Suja, S. (2009). Antitumor and antimicrobial activities and inhibition of *in-vitro* lipid peroxidation by Dendrobium nobile. *African Journal of Biotechnology* **18**, 2289-2293.

Zhang, M., Binns, C. W., and Lee, A. H. (2002). Tea consumption and ovarian cancer risk: A case-control study in China. *Cancer Epidemiology, Biomarkers, and Prevention* **11**(8), 713-718.

7

Abu-Surrah, A. S., Al-Sa'doni, H. H., and Abdalla, M. Y. (2008). Palladium-based chemotherapeutic agents: Routes toward complexes with good antitumor activity. *Cancer Therapy* **6**, 1-10.

Ackrell, B. A. C., Armstrong, F. A., Cochran, B., Sucheta, A., and Yu, T. (1993). Classification of fumarate reductases and succinate dehydrogenases based upon their contrasting behavior in the reduced benzylviologen/fumarate. *Federation of European Biochemical Societies* **326**(1, 2, 3), 92-94.

Aggarwal, B. B. and Shishodia, S. (2006). Molecular targets of dietary agents for prevention and therapy of cancer. *Biochemical Pharmacology* **71**, 1397-1421.

Alberts, B., Bray, D., Lewis, J., Raff, M., Roberts, K., and Watson, J. D. (1989). *Molecular Biology of the Cell.* Garland Publishing Inc., New York.

Antonawich, F. J., Fiore, S. M., and Welicky, L. M. (2004). Regulation of ischemic cell death by the lipoic acid-palladium complex, Poly MVA, in gerbils. *Experimental Neurology* **189**, 10-15.

Bass, J and Takahashi, J. S. (2010). Circadian Integration of Metabolism and Energetics. *Science* **330**, 1349-1354.

Baumgartner, M. R., Schmalle, H., and Dubler, E. (1996). The Interaction of transition metals with the coenzyme α-lipoic acid: Synthesis, structure and characterization of copper and zinc complexes. *Inorg. Chim. Acta* **252**, 319-331.

Beattie, D. S. (2002). Bioenergetics and Oxidative Metabolism. In *Textbook of Biochemistry with Clinical Correlations.* T. M. Devlin (Ed.), 5th ed. Wiley-Liss, John Wiley & Sons, Inc., Publication, New York.

Berliner, L. J., Eaton, S. S., and Eaton, G. R. (Eds.) (2000). Distance Measurements in Biological Systems by EPR, Kluwer. In *Biological Magnetic Resonance*, vol 19. Academic Press/Plenum Publishers, New York.

Berrisford, J. M. and Sazanov, L., A. (2009). Structural Basis for the Mechanism of Respiratory Complex. *J. Biol. Che*, **284**, 29773-29783.

Biasutto, L., Dong, L. F., and Zoratti, M., and Neuzil, J. (2010). Mitochondrially targeted anticancer agents. *Mitochondrion* **10**(6), 670-681.

Bubber, P., Haroutunian, V., Fisch, G., Blass, J. P., and Gibson, G. E. (2005). Mitochondrial Abnormalities in Alzheimer Brain: Mechanistic Implications. *Ann. Neurol.* **57**, 695-703.

Buettner, G. R. (1993). The Pecking Order of Free Radicals and Antioxidants: Lipid Peroxidation, α-Tocopherol, and Ascorbate. *Arch. Biochem. Biophys* **300**, 535-543.

Caires, A. C. F. (2007). Recent Advances Involving Palladium(II) Complexes for the Cancer Therapy. *Anti-Cancer Agents In Medicinal Chemistry* **7**, 484-491.

Carew, J. S. and Huang, P. (2002). Mitochondrial defects in cancer. *Molecular Cancer* **1**, 9. http://www.molecular-cancer.com/content/1/1/9.

Carlson, D. A., Young, K. L., Fischer, S. J., and Ulrich, H. (2008). An Evaluation of the Stability and Pharmacokinetics of R-Lipoic Acid and R-Dihydrolipoic Acid Dosage Forms in Human Plasma from Healthy Subjects. In *Lipoic Acid: Energy Production, Antioxidant Activity and Health Effects*. M. S. Patel and L. Packer (Eds.). CRC press, Taylor & Francis Group, Florida, p. 255.

Castellani, R., Hirai, K., Aliev, G., Drew, K. L., Nunomura, A., Takeda, A., Cash, A. D., Obrenovich, M. E., Perry, G., and Smith, M. A. (2002). Role of mitochondrial dysfunction in Alzheimer's disease. *Journal of Neuroscience Research*, **70**(3), 357-360.

Chan, S. W., Chan, P. C., and Bielski, B. H. J. (1974). Studies on the lipoic acid free radical. *Biochim. Biophys. Acta, General Subjects* **338**, 213-223.

Chatterjee, A., Mambo, E., and Sidransky, A. (2006). Mitochondrial DNA mutations in human cancer. *Oncogene* **25**, 4663-4674.

Chen, G., Wang, F., Trachootham, D., and Huang, P. (2010). Preferential killing of cancer cells with mitochondrial dysfunction by natural compounds. *Mitochondrion* **10**(6), 614-625.

Corduneanu, O., Garnett, M., and Oliveira Brett, A. M. (2007). Anodic oxidation of α-lipoic acid at a glassy carbon electrode and its determination in dietary supplements. *Anal. Letters* **40**, 1763-1778.

Corduneanu, O., Paquim, A. M. C., Garnett, M., and Oliveira Brett, A. M. (2009). Lipoic acid-palladium complex interaction with DNA, voltammetric and AFM characterization. *Talanta* **77**, 1843-1853.

Cotton, F. A. and Wilkinson, G. (1972). *Advanced Inorganic Chemistry*, 3rd ed. Interscience Publishers, New York, p. 415.

Dabrowiak, J. C. (2009). *Metals in Medicine*. John Wiley & Sons Ltd., UK.

Dennery, P. A. (2010). Oxidative Stress in Development: Nature or nurture?. *Free radical Biology & Medicine* **49**, 1147-1151.

Dröge, W. (2006). Oxidative Stress in HIV Infection. In: *Oxidative Stress, Disease and Cancer*. K. K. Singh (Ed.). Imperial College Press, London, WC2H 9HE, pp. 885-895.

Elliott, S. J., Léger, C., Pershad, H. R., Hirst, J., Heffron, K., Ginet, N., Blasco, F., Rothery, R. A., Weine,r J. H., and Armstrong, F. A. (2002). Detection and interpretation of redox potential optima in the catalytic activity of enzymes. *Biochimica. Et. Biophysica. Acta (BBA) Bioenergetics* **1555**, 54-59.

Everhard, M. E., Gross, Jr. P. M., and Turner, J. W. (1962). Properties of Electrolytes in Hydrogen Peroxide-Water Solutions. 1. Solvation of Alkali Nitrates. *J. Phys. Chem.* **66**(5), 923-926.

Field, J. and Gyorgyi, L. (Eds.), (1993). In *Chaos in Chemistry and Biochemistry*. World Scientific Publishing Co., NJ 07661, USA.

Fink D. G. (Ed.). (1975). *Electronic Engineers Handbook*. McGraw Hill, New York.

Frezza, C. and Gottlieb, E. (2009). Mitochondria in cancer: Not just innocent bystanders. *Seminars in Cancer Biology* **19**, 4-11.

Fricker, S. P. (2007). Metal based drugs: From serendipity to design. *Dalton Trans* 4903-4917.

Fukushima, S., Nakanishi, S., Fukami, K., Sakai, S., Nagai, T., Tada, T., and Nakato, Y. (2005). Observation of synchronized spatiotemporal reaction waves in coupled electrochemical oscillations of an NDR type. *Electrochemistry Communications* **7**, 411-415.

Gao, E., Liu, C., Zhu, M., Lin, H., Wu, Q., and Liu, L. (2009). Current Development of Pd(II) Complexes as Potential Antitumor Agents. *Anti-*

cancer *Agents in Medicinal Chemistry* **9**(3), 356-368.

Galkin, A. and U. Brandt U. (2005). Superoxide Radical Formation by Pure Complex I (NADH:Ubiquinone Oxidoreductase) from Yarrowia lipolytica. *J. Biol. Chem.* **280**, 3019-10135.

Galluzzi, L., Larochette, N., Zamzami, N., and Kroemer, G. (2006). Mitochondria as therapeutic targets for cancer chemotherapy. *Oncogene* **25**, 4812-4830.

Garnett, M. (1995a). Synthetic DNA Reductase, Contents of 7th EBIC Conference Abstracts Issue, C 48. *J. Inorg. Biochem* **59**, 231.

Garnett, M. (October 31, 1995b). Palladium Complexes and Methods for Using Same in the Treatment of Tumors or Psoriasis, U.S.Patent, No. 5,463,093.

Garnett, M. (October 21, 1997). Palladium Complexes and Methods for Using same in the Treatment of Tumors, U.S.Patent, No. 5,679,697.

Garnett M. (July 7, 1998). Palladium Complexes and Methods for using same in the Treatment of Psoriasis, U.S.Patent, No. 5,776,973.

Genereux, J. C. and Barton, J. K (2010). Mechanisms for DNA Charge *Transport. Chem. Rev.* **110**, 1642-1662.

Gibson, G. E., Haroutunian, V., Zhang, H., Park, L. C. H., Shi, Q, Lesser, M., Mohs, R. C., Sheu, R. K. F., and Blass, J. P. (2000). Mitochondrial Damage in Alzheimer's Disease Varies with Apolipoprotein E Genotype. *Ann. Neurol.* 48, 297-303.

Gogvadze, V., Orrenius, S., and Zhivotovsky, B. (2008). Mitochondria in cancer cells: What is so special about them?. *Trends in Cell Biology* **18**(4), 165-173.

Gorin, M. H. (1935). The "Salting-in" of Hydrogen Peroxide by Electrolytes. *J. Am. Chem. Soc.* **57**, 1975-1978.

Greenamyre, J. T., MacKenzie, G., Peng T., and Stephans, S. E. (1999). Mitochondrial dysfunction in Parkinson's disease. *Biochem. Soc. Symp.* **66**, 85-97.

Gwyer, J. D., Richardson, D. J., and Butt, J. N. (2005). Diode or Tunnel-Diode Characteristics? Resolving the Catalytic Consequences of Proton Coupled Electron Transfer in a Multi-Centered

Oxidoreductase. *J. Am. Chem. Soc.* **127**(43), 14964-14965.

Hanahan, D. and Weinberg, R. A. (2000). The Hallmarks of Cancer. *Cell* 100, 57-70.

Heiden, M. G. V., Cantley, L. C., and Thompson, C. B. (2009). Understanding the Warburg Effect: The Metabolic Requirements of Cell Proliferation. *Science* **324**, 1029-1033.

Higuchi, M. (2007). Regulation of mitochondrial DNA content and cancer. *Mitochondrion* 7, 53-57.

Hoffman, M. Z. and Hayon, E. (1972). One-Electron Reduction of the Disulfide Linakge in Aqueous Solution. Formation, Protonation, and Decay Kinetics of RSSR⁻ Radical. *J. Am. Chem. Soc.* **94**, 795-797.

Hsu, P. P. and Sabatini, D. M. (2008). Cancer Cell Metabolism: Warburg and Beyond. *Cell* **134**, 703-707.

Hurst, J., Sucheta, A, Ackrell, B. A., and Armstrong, F. A. (1996). Electrocatalytic Voltammetry of Succinate Dehydrogenase: Direct Quantification of the Catalytic Properties of a Complex Electron Transport Enzyme. *J. Am. Chem. Soc.* **118**(21), 5031-5038.

Jaruga, P., Jaruga, B., Gackowski, D., Olczak, A., Halota, W., Pawlowska, M., and Olinski, R. (2002). Supplementation with antioxidant vitamins prevents oxidative modification of DNA in lymphocytes of HIV-infected patients. *Free Radical Biology & Medicine* **32**(5), 414-420.

Jones, S., Zhang, X., Parsons, D. W., Lin, J. C. H., Leary, R. J., Angenendt, P., Mankoo, P., Carter, H., Kamiyama, H., Jimeno, A., Hong, S. M., Fu, B., Lin, M. T., Calhoun, E. S., Kamiyama, M., Walter, K., Nikolskaya, T., Nikolsky, Y., Hartigan, J., Smith, D. R., Hidalgo, M., Leach, S. D., Klein, A. P., Jaffee, E. M., Goggins, M, Maitra, A., Donahue, C. L., Eshleman, J. R., Kern, S. E., Hruban, R. H., Karchin, R., Papadopoulos, N., Parmigiani, G., Vogelstein, B., Velculescu, V. E., and Kinzler, K. W. (2008). Core Signaling Pathways in Human Pancreatic Cancers Revealed by Global Genomic Analyses. *Science* **321**, 1801-1806.

Keasling, J. D. (2010) Manufacturing Molecules through Metabolic Engineering. *Science* **330**, 1355-1358.

Koper, M. T. M. (1996). Oscillations and Complex Dynamical Bifurcations in Electrochemical systems. In *Advances in Chemical Physics*. I. Prigogine and S. A. Rice, (Eds.). John Wiley & Sons, New York,vol 92, pp. 161-297.

Korkina, L. G., Afanas'ef, I. B., and Diplock, A. T. (1993). Antioxidant therapy in children affected by irradiation from the Chernobyl nuclear accident. *Biochemical Society Transactions* 314S, 21.

Krishnan, C. V. and Garnett, M. (2006). Liquid crystal behavior in solutions, electrode passivation, and impedance loci in four quadrants. In *Passivation of Metals and Semiconductors, and Properties of Thin Oxide Layers*. P. Marcus and V. Maurice, (Eds.). Elsevier, Amsterdam, pp. 389-394.

Krishnan, C. V., Garnett, M., and B., Chu (2007a). Spatiotemporal Oscillation in Peroxo-Molybdate Complexes in Acidic Solutions: 1. Impedance Measurements of $H_2Mo_2O_3(O-O)_4(H_2O)_2$. *Int. J. Electrochem Sci.* 2, 444-461.

Krishnan, C. V., Garnett, M., and Chu, B (2007b). Solute-Solvent Interactions from Admittance Measurements: Potential Induced and Water Structure-Enforced Ion-Pair Formation. *Int. J. Electrochem. Sci.* 2, 958-972.

Krishnan, C. V., Garnett, M., and Chu, B. (2008a). Solute-solvent interactions in biological molecules: L-Cysteine. *Int. J. Electrochem. Sci.* 3, 854-872.

Krishnan, C. V., Garnett, M., and Chu, B. (2008b). Spatiotemporal oscillations in biological molecules: Molybdate-L-Cysteine. *Int. J. Electrochem. Sci.* 3, 873-890.

Krishnan, C. V., Garnett, M., and Chu, B. (2008c). Oxidative Stress and Parkinson's Disease: Electrochemical Behavior of Hydrogen Peroxide in Aqueous Sodium Chloride. *Int. J. Electrochem. Sci.* 3, 1348-1363.

Krishnan, C. V., Garnett, M., and Chu, B. (2008d). Spatiotemporal oscillations in biological molecules: Hydrogen peroxide and Parkinson's disease. *Int. J. Electrochem. Sci.* 3, 1364-1385.

Krishnan, C. V., Garnett, M., Hsiao, B., and Chu, B. (2009a). Solute-Solvent Interactions from Impedance Measurements: 'π–way' Conduction and Water Structure-Enforced Ion Pair Forma-

tion in Aqueous Lidocaine Hydrochloride. *Int. J. Electrochem. Soc.* 4, 1085-1099.

Krishnan, C. V., Garnett, M., and Chu, B. (2009b). Admittance as a useful tool for investigation of solute-solvent interactions at the double layer. *Electrochem. Communications* 11, 2229-2232.

Kroemer, G. (2006). Mitochondria in cancer. *Oncogene* 25, 4630-4632.

Kroemer, G., Galluzzi, L., and Brenner, C. (2007). Mitochondrial Membrane Permeabilization in Cell Death. *Physiol. Rev.* 87, 99-163.

Kroemer, G. and Pouyssegur, J. (2008). Tumor Cell Metabolism: Cancer's Achilles Heel. *Cancer Cell* 13, 472-482.

Kussmaul, L. and Hirst, J. (2006). The mechanism of superoxide production by NADH: Ubiquinone oxidoreductase (complex I) from bovine heart mitochondria. *Proc. Natl. Acad. Sci.*, USA 103, 7607-7612.

Lasia, A. (1999). Electrochemical Impedance Spectroscopy and its Applications. In *Modern Aspects of Electrochemistry*. No 32, B. E. Conway, J. O'M. Bockris, and R. E. White (Eds.). Kluwer Academic/Plenum Publishers, New York.

Lázaro, M. L. (2007). Dual role of hydrogen peroxide in cancer: Possible relevance to cancer chemoprevention and therapy. *Cancer Letters* 252, 1-8.

Léger, C. and Bertrand, P. (2008). Direct Electrochemistry of Redox Enzymes as a Tool for Mechanistic Studies. *Chem. Rev.* 108, 2379-2438.

Levine, H and Jacob, E. B. (2004). Physical schemata underlying biological pattern formation-examples, issues and strategies. *Physical Biology* 1(1-2), P14-22.

Levine, A. J. and Puzio-Kuter, A. M. (2010). The Control of the Metabolic switch in Cancers by Oncogenes and Tumor Suppressor Genes. *Sceince* 330, 1340-1344.

Livingston, R. (1928). The Activity of Hydrogen Peroxide in Sodium Chloride and Sodium Sulfate Solutions. *J. Am. Chem. Soc.* 50, 3206.

Macdonald, J. R. and Johnson, W. B. (2005). Fundamentals of Impedance Spectroscopy. In *Impedance Spectroscopy: Theory, Experiment, and Applications*, 2nd ed. E. Barsoukov, J. R.

Macdonald (Eds.). Wiley Interscience, New Jersey.

Maloň, M., Trávníček, Z., Maryško, M., Zbořil, R., Mašláň, M., Marek, J., Doležal, K., Rolčík, J., Kryštof, V., and Strnad, M. (2001). Metal complexes as anticancer agents 2. Iron(III) and copper(II) bio-active complexes with N6-benzylaminopurine derivatives. *Inorg. Chim. Acta* **323**, 119-129.

Massey, V., Gibson, Q. H., and Veeger, C. (1960). Intermediates in the Catalytic Action of Lipoyl Dehydrogenase (Diaphorase). *Biochem. J.* **77**, 341-351.

Matesanz, A. I., Perez, J. M., Navarro, P., Moreno, J. M., Colacio, E., and Souza, P. (1999). Synthesis and characterization of novel palladium (II) complexes of bis (thiosemicarbazone). Structure, cytotoxic activity and DNA biding of Pd (II)-benzyl bis (thiosemicarbazonate). *J. Inorg. Biochem.* **76**, 29-37.

Mayevsky, A. (2009). Mitochondrial function and energy metabolism in cancer cells: Past Overview and future perspectives. *Mitochondrion* **9**, 165-179.

McKnight, S. L. (2010). On getting there from here. *Science* **330**, 1338-1339.

Mecocci, P., MacGarvey, U., and Beal, M. F. (1994). Oxidative Damage to mitochondrial DNA is increased in Alzheimer's disease. *Annals of Neurology* **36**(5), 747-751.

Menon, A., Krishnan, C. V., and Nair, C. K. K. (2009). Protection from gamma radiation insult to antioxidant defense and cellular DNA by POLY-MVA, a dietary supplement containing palladium lipoic acid formulation. *Int. J. Low Radiation* **6**, 248-262.

Mukouyama, Y., Nakanishi, S., Chiba, T., Murakoshi, K., and Nakato, Y. (2001). Mechanisms of Two Electrochemical Oscillations of Different Types, Observed for H_2O_2 Reduction on a Pt Electrode in the Presence of Small Amount of Halide Ions. *J. Phys. Chem. B* **105**, 7246-7253.

Mukouyama, Y., Hommura, H., Nakanishi, S., Nishimura, T., Konishi, H., and Nakato, Y. (1999). Mechanism and Simulation of Electrochemical Current Oscillations Observed in the H_2O_2-Reduction Reaction on Platinum Electrodes in Acidic Solutions. *Bull. Chem. Soc. Jpn.* **72**, 1247-1254.

Neustadt, J. and Pieczenik, S. R. (2008). Medication-induced mitochondrial damage and disease. *Mol. Nutr. Food Res.* **52**, 780-788.

Niki, E. and Noguchi, N. (2004). Dynamics of Antioxidant Action of Vitamin E. *Acc. Chem. Res.* **37**, 45-51.

Noodleman, L., Peng, C. Y., Case, D. A., and Mouesca, J.-M. (1995). Orbital interactions, electron delocalization and spin coupling in iron-sulfur clusters. *Coord. Chem. Rev.* **144**, 199-244.

Nualart, F., Rivas, C., Montecinos, V., Godoy, A., Guaiquil, V., Golde, D., and Vera, J. (2003). Recycling of vitamin C by a bystander effect. *J. Bio. Chem.* **278**(12), 10128-10133.

Ogilvie, G. K. and Moore, A. S. (2000). Tumors of Bone. In *Managing the Canine Cancer Patient: A practical Guide to Compassionate Care*. R. A. Henry and P. A Yardley, (Eds.) Veterinary Learning Systems, pp. 565-589.

Ohnishi, T. (1998). Iron-sulfur clusters/semiquinones in Complex I. *Biochim. Biophys. Acta* **1364**, 186-206.

Olanow, C. W and Lieberman, A. N. (Eds.) (1992). In *The Scientific Basis for the Treatment of Parkinson's Disease*. The Parthenon Publishing Group, New Jersey, 07656, USA.

Packer, L., Witt, E. H., and Tritschler, H. J. (1995). Alpha Lipoic Acid as a Biological Antioxidant. *Free Radical Biology and Medicine* **19**(2), 227-250.

Parker, Jr. W. D., Boyson, S. J., and Parks, J. K. (1989). Abnormalities of the Electron Transport Chain in Idiopathic Parkinson's Disease. *Ann. Neurol* **26**, 719-723.

Parsons, D. W., Jones, S., Zhang, X., Lin, J. C. H., Leary, R. J., Angenendt, P., Mankoo, P., Carter, H., Siu, I. M., Gallia, G. L., Olivi, A., McLendon, R., Rasheed, B. A., Keir, S., Nikolskaya, T., Nikolsky, Y., Busam, D. A., Tekleab, H., Diaz, Jr. L. A., Hartigan, J., Smith, D. R., Strausberg, R. L., Marie, S. K. N., Shinjo, S. M. O., Yan, H., Riggins, G. J., Bigner, D. D., Karchin, R., Papadopoulos, N., Parmigiani, G., Vogelstein, B., Velculescu, V. E., and K. W. Kinzler, K. W. (2008). An Integrated Genomic Analysis of Human Glioblastoma Multiforme. *Science* **321**, 1807-1812.

Patel, M. S. and Packer, L. (Eds.), (2008). *Lipoic Acid: Energy Production, Antioxidant Activity and Health Effects.* CRC Press, Taylor & Francis Group, New York.

Pershad, H. R., Hirst, J., Cochran, B., Ackrell, B. A. C., and Armstrong, F. A. (1999). Voltammetric studies of bidirectional catalytic electron transport in *Escherichia coli* succinate dehydrogenase: comparison with the enzyme from beef heart mitochondria. *Biochimica et Biophysica Acta (BBA)–Bioenergetics* **1412**(3), 262-272.

Portakal, O., Özkaya, O., Inal, M. E., Bozan, B., Koşan, M., and Sayek, I. (2000). Coenzyme Q10 concentrations and antioxidant status in tissues of breast cancer patients. *Clinical Biochemistry* **33**(4), 279-284.

Principal, S. G., Quiles, J. L., Tortosa, C. L. R., Rovira, P. S., and Tortosa, M. R. (2010). New advances in molecular mechanisms and the prevention of Adriamycin toxicity by antioxidant nutrients. *Food and Chemical Toxicology* **48**, 1425-1438.

Punnonen, K., Ahotupa, M., Asaishi, K., Hyöty, M., Kudo, R., and Punnonen, R. (1994). Antioxidant enzyme activities and oxidative stress in human breast cancer. *Journal of cancer Research and Clinical Oncology* **120**(6), 374-377.

Rabinowitz, J. D and White, E. (2010). Autophagy and Metabolism. *Science* **330**, 1344-1348.

Ramachandran, L., Krishnan, C. V., and Nair, C. K. K. (2010). Radioprotection by α-Lipoic Acid Palladium Complex Formulation (POLY-MVA) in Mice. *Cancer Biotherapy and Radiopharmaceuticals* **25**(4), 395-399.

Ramakrishnan, N., Wolfe, W. W., and Catravas, G. N. (1992). Radioprotection of Hematopoietic Tissues in Mice by Lipoic Acid. *Radiation Research* **130**, 360-365.

Rajneesh, C. P., Manimaran, A., Sasikala, K. R., and Adaikappan, P. (2008). Lipid peroxidation and antioxidant status in patients with breast cancer. *Singapore Med. J.* **49**(8), 640-643.

Rau, T., Alsfasser, R., Zahl, A., and van Eldik, R. (1998). Structural and Kinetic Studies on the Formation of Platinum(II) and Palladium(II) Complexes with L-Cysteine-Derived Ligands. *Inorg. Chem.* **37**, 4223-4230.

Roscoe, S. G. (1996). Electrochemical Investigations of the Interfacial Behavior of Proteins. In *Modern Aspects of Electrochemistry.* B. E. Con-

way and J. O'M. Bockris (Eds.). Plenum Press, New York, vol 29, pp. 319-399.

Rouach, N., Calvo, C., Duquennoy, H., Glowinski, J., and Giaume, C. (2004). Hydrogen Peroxide Increases Gap Junctional Communication and Induces Astrocyte Toxicity: Regulation by Brain Macrophages. *Glia* **45**, 28-38.

Saad, E. I., Gowilly, S. M. E., Sherhaa, M. O., and Bistawroos, A. E. (2010). Role of oxidative stress and nitric oxide in the protective effects of α-lipoic acid and aminoguanidine against isoniazid-rifampicin-induced hepatotoxicity in rats. *Food and Chemical Toxicology* **48**, 1869-1875.

Sandhya, B., Manoharan, S., Lavanya, G. S., and Manmohan, Ch. R. (2010). Lipid peroxidation and antioxidant status in prostate cancer patients. *Indian Journal of Science and Technology* **3**(1) 83-86.

Sarkar, F. H., Li, Y., Wang, Z., and Kong, D. (2009). Cellular signaling perturbation by natural products. *Cellular Signaling* **21**, 1541-1547.

Schapira, A. H. V. (2004). Mitochondrial dysfunction in Parkinson's disease. *Cell Death and Differentiation* **14**, 1261-1266.

Senthil, K., Aranganathan, S., and Nalini, N. (2004). Evidence of oxidative stress in the circulation of ovarian cancer patients. *Clinica Chimica Acta* **339**, 27-32.

Sherman, S. E. and Lippard, S. J. (1987). Structural Aspects of Platinum Anticancer Drug Interactions with DNA. *Chem. Rev.* **87**, 1153-1181.

Simonnet, H., Alazard, N., Pfeiffer, K., Gallour, C., Béroud, C., Demont, J., Bouvier, R., Schägger, H., and Godinot, C. (2002). Low mitochondrial respiratory chain content correlates with tumor aggressiveness in renal cell carcinoma. *Carcinogenesis* **23**, 759-768.

Singh, K. K. (Ed.) (2006). In *Oxidative Stress, Disease and Cancer.* Imperial College Press, London, WC2H 9HE.

Sinha, R. J., Singh, R., Mehrotra, S., and Singh, R. K. (2009). Implications of free radicals and antioxidant levels in carcinoma of the breast: A never-ending battle for survival. *Indian Journal of Cancer* **46**(2), 146-150.

Strasdeit, H., von Dollen, A., and Duhme, A. K. (1995). Metal Complexes of the Drug and Coenzyme α-Lipoic acid and Related Ligands. Contents of 7th EBIC Conference Abstracts Issue, C 45. *J. Inorg. Biochem* **59**, 228.

Sudheesh, N. P., Ajith, T. A., Janardhanan, K. K., and Krishnan, C. V. (2009). Palladium α-lipoic acid complex formulation enhances activities of Krebs cycle dehydrogenases and respiratory complexes I-IV in the heart of aged rats. *Food and Chemical Toxicology* **47**, 2124-2128.

Sudheesh, N. P., Ajith, T. A., Janardhanan, K. K., and Krishnan, C. V. (2010). Effect of POLY-MVA, a palladium α-lipoic acid complex formulation against declined mitochondrial antioxidant status in the myocardium of aged rats. *Food and Chemical Toxicology* **48**, 1858-1862.

Sucheta, A., Ackrell, B. A. C., Cochran, B., and Armstrong, F. A. (1992). Diode-like behavior of a mitochondrial electron transport enzyme. *Nature* **356**, 361-362.

Tabassum, H., Parvez, S., Pasha, S. T., Banerjee, B. D., and Raisuddin, S. (2010). Protective effect of lipoic acid against methotrexate-induced oxidative stress in liver mitochondria. *Food and Chemical Toxicology* **48**, 1973-1979.

Tanriverdi, T., Hanimoglu, H., Kacira, T., Sanus, G. Z., Kemerdere, R., Atukeren, P., Gumustas, K., Canbaz, B., and Kaynar, M. Y. (2007). Glutathione peroxidase, glutathione reductase and protein oxidation in patients with glioblastoma multiforme and transitional meningioma. *J. Cancer Res Clin Oncol.* **133**, 627-633.

Thomas, D. K. and Maass, O. (1958). Electrolytic Conductance in Hydrogen Peroxide-Water Mixtures. *Can. J. Chem.* **36**, 449-455.

Van Hellemond, J. J., Klockiewicz, M., Gaasenbeek, C. P. H., Roos, M. H., and Tielens, A. G. M. (1995). Rhodoquinone and Complex II of the Electron Transport Chain in Anaerobically Functioning Eukaryotes. *Journal of Biological Chemistry* **270**, 31065-31070.

Vazquez, A, Liu, J, Zhou, Y., and Oltvai, Z. N. (2010) Catabolic efficiency of aerobic glycolysis: The Warburg effect revisited. *BMC Systems Biology* **4**, 58, doi 1752-0509/4/58.

Voet, D. and Voet, J. G. (1995). *Biochemistry*, 2nd ed. John Wiley & Sons, Inc., New York.

Wallace, D. C. and Fan W. (2010). Energetics, epigenetics, mitochondrial genetics. *Mitochondrion* **10**, 12-31.

Warburg, O. (1956). On the Origin of Cancer Cells. *Science* **123**, 309-314.

Weiner, W. J., Shulman, L. M., and Lang, A. E. (2007). *Parkinson's Disease*, 2nd ed. The John Hopkins University, Maryland, USA.

Winklhofer, K. F and Haass, C. (2010). Mitochondrial dysfunction in Parkinson's disease. *Biochim Bipophys Acta (BBA) Molecular Basis of Disease* **1802**, 29-44.

Wood, Z. A., Poole, L. B., and Karplus, P. A. (2003). Peroxoredoxin Evolution and the Regulation of Hydrogen Peroxide. *Science* **300**, 650-653.

8

Adamekova, E., Markova, M., Kubatka, P., Bojkova, B., Ahlers, I., and Ahlersova, E. (2003). NMU-induced mammary carcinogenesis in female rats is influenced by repeated psychoemotional stress. *Neoplasma* **50**, 428-432

Anokhin, P. K. (1970). The theory of a functional system. *Uspekhi Matematicheskikh Nauk* **1**, 19-54.

Bekhterev, V. M. (1998). *Suggestion and its role in social life*. Transaction Publishers, New Brunswick, New Jersy.

Bernstein, N. A. (1967). *The coordination and regulation of movements*. Pergamon Press, Oxford.

Dimsdale, J. E. (2008). Psychological stress and cardiovascular disease. *Journal of the American College of Cardiology* **51**, 1237-1246.

Gidron, Y., Russ, K., Tissarchondou, H., and Warner, J. (2006). The relation between psychological factors and DNA-damage: A critical review. *Biological Psychology* **72**, 291-304.

Grossardt, B. R., Bower, J. H., Geda, Y. E., Colligan, R. C., and Rocca, W. A. (2009). Pessimistic, anxious, and depressive personality traits predict all-cause mortality: The mayo clinic cohort study of personality and aging. *Psychosomatic Medicine* **71**, 491-500.

Jemal, A., Siegel, R., Ward, E., Hao, Y., Xu, J., Murray, T., and Thun, M. J. (2008). Cancer Statistics. *Cancer Journal for Clinicians* **58**, 71-96.

Knox, S. S. (2001). Psychosocial stress and the physiology of atherosclerosis. *Advances in Psychosomatic Medicine* **22**, 139-151.

Leont'ev, A. N. (1978). *Activity, consciousness, and personality*. Englewood Cliffs, New Jersy, Prentice-Hall.

Lester, D. (2009). Voodoo death. *Omega* (Westport) **59**, 1-18.

Levav, I., Kohn, R., Iscovich, J., Abramson, J. H., Tsai, W. Y., and Vigdorovich, D. (2000). Cancer incidence and survival following bereavement. *American Journal of Public Health* **90**, 1601-1607.

Li, J., Johansen, C., Brønnum–Hansen, H., Stenager, E., Koch-Henriksen, N., and Olsen, J. (2004). The risk of multiple sclerosis in bereaved parents: A nationwide cohort study in Denmark. *Neurology* **62**, 726-729.

Lloyd-Williams, M., Shiels, C., Taylor, F., and Dennis, M. (2009). Depression–an independent predictor of early death in patients with advanced cancer. *Journal of Affective Disorders* **113**, 127-132.

Luria, A. R. (1970). The functional organization of the brain. *Scientific American* **222**, 66-78.

Maslow, A. H. (1943). A theory of human motivation. *Psychological Review* **50**, 370-396.

McEwen, B. S. (2007). Physiology and neurobiology of stress and adaptation: Central role of the brain. *Physiological Reviews* **87**, 873-904.

Mravec, B., Gidron, Y., and Hulin, I. (2008). Neurobiology of cancer: Interactions between nervous, endocrine and immune systems as a base for monitoring and modulating the tumorogenesis by the brain. *Seminars in Cancer Biology* **18**, 150-163.

Nemeroff, C. B. (2008). Recent findings in the pathophysiology of depression. *Focus* **6**, 3-14.

Ostrander, M. M., Ulrich-Lai, Y. M., Choi, D. C., Richtand, N. M., and Herman, J. P. (2006). Hypoactivity of the hypothalamo-pituitary-adrenocortical axis during recovery from chronic variable stress. *Endocrinology* **147**, 2008-2017.

Perelman, Ya. (2008). *Physics for entertainment*, Book two. Hyperion, New York.

Reiche, E. M., Morimoto, H. K., and Nunes, S. M. (2005). Stress and depression-induced immune dysfunction: Implications for the development and progression of cancer. *International Review of Psychiatry* **17**, 515-527.

Rodin, G., Lo, C., Mikulincer, M., Donner, A., Gagliese, L., and Zimmermann, C. (2009). Pathways to distress: The multiple determinants of depression, hopelessness, and the desire for hastened death in metastatic cancer patients. *Social Science and Medicine* **68**, 562-569.

Rotenberg, V. S. and Arshavsky, V. V. (1984). *Search activity and adaptation*. Nauka, Moscow.

Rotenberg, V. S. (2009). Search activity concept: Relationship between behavior, health and brain functions. *Activitas Nervosa Superior* **51**, 12-44.

Roy-Byrne, P. P., Davidson, K. W., Kessler, R. C., Asmundson, G. J. G., Goodwin, R. D., Kubzansky, L., Lydiard, R. B., Massie, M. J., Katon, W., Laden, S. K., and Stein, M. B. (2008). Anxiety disorders and comorbid medical illness. *Focus* **6**, 467-485.

Seymour, J. and Benning, T. B. (2009). Depression, cardiac mortality and all-cause mortality. *Advances in Psychiatric Treatment* **15**, 107-113.

Shpagina, L. A., Ermakova, M. A., Volkova, E. A., and Iakovleva, S. A. (2008). Clinical, functional and biochemical characteristics of arterial hypertension in military men under chronic stress. *Meditsina Truda i Promyshlennaia Ekologiia* **7**, 24-29.

Simon, N. M., Smoller, J. W., McNamara, K. L., Maser, R. S., Zalta, A. K., Pollack, M. H., Nierenberg, A. A., Fava, M., and Wong, K. K. (2006). Telomere shortening and mood disorders: Preliminary support for a chronic stress model of accelerated aging. *Biological Psychiatry* **60**, 432-435.

Spinelli, S., Chefer, S., Suomi, S. J., Higley, J. Dee., Barr, C. S., and Stein, E. (2009). Early-life stress induces long-term morphologic changes in primate brain. *Archives of General Psychiatry* **66**, 658-665.

Surtees, P. G., Wainwright, N. W. J., Luben, R. N., Wareham, N. J., Bingham, S. A., and Khaw, K. T. (2008). Depression and ischemic heart disease mortality: Evidence from the EPIC-Norfolk United Kingdom prospective cohort study. *American Journal of Psychiatry* **165**, 515-523.

Ukhtomsky, A. A. (1927). The dominant as a working principle of nervous centers. *Russkii Fiziologicheskii Zhurnal* **6**.

Ukhtomsky, A. A. (1966). *The Dominant*. Nauka, Moscou.

Uznadze D. N. (1997). *The theory of installation*. Metsniereba, Tbilisi.

Yousef, N. (2008). From the wild side. *History Workshop* **65**, 213-220.

9

Anbuselvam, C., Vijayavel, K., and Balasubramaniam, M. P. (2007). Protective effect of *Operculina turpethum* against 7,12-dimethylbenz(a) anthracene induced oxidative stress with reference to breast cancer in experimental rats. *Chem. Biol. Interact.* **168**, 229-236.

Barros, A. C. S. D., Muranaka, E. N. K., and Mori, L. J. (2004). Induction of experimental mammary carcinogenesis in rats with 7, 12-dimethylbenz(a)anthracene. *Cancer Pharma.* **21**, 257-261.

Bryle, P., Leon, M. E., and Maisonneuve, P. (2003). Cancer control in women. *Int. J. Gynacecol. Obes.* **83**, 179-202

Comporti, M. (1989). Three models of free-radicals induced cell injury. *Chem. Biol. Intract.* **72**, 1–56.

Deb, L., Dubey, S. K., Jain, A., Pandian, G. S., and Rout, S. P. (2007). Antidiarrhoel activity of *Thuja occidentalis Linn* ethanol extract on experimental animal. *Ind. Drug* **44**, 319-321.

DeSantis, C, Center, M. M, Sighel, R., and Jemal, A. (2009-2010). *Breast cancer facts and figures*. American Cancer Society, Department of Surveillance and Health Policy Research, Atlanta, Georgia 1-40.

Dubey, S. K and Batra, A. (2008). Hepatoprotective activity from ethanol fraction of *Thuja occidentalis Linn*. *Asian J. Chem. Res.* **1**, 32-35.

Frieauff, W., Hartmann, A., and Suter, W. (2001). Automatic analysis of slides processed in the Comet assay. *Mutagenesis* **16**(2), 133-137.

Ghumare, S. S. and Cunningham, J. E. (2007). Breast cancer trends in Indian residents and emigrants portend an emerging epidemic for India. *Asian Pac. J. Cancer Prev.* **8**, 507-512.

Gupta, G. (2002). *In-vitro* Antimycotic potential of *Thuja occidentalis* against Curvularia-lunata

causing Phaeoyphomycosis in humans. *Nat. J. Homeopath.* **4**, 1-3.

Halliwell, B., Gutteridge, J. M. C., and Cross, C. E. (1992). Free radicals, antioxidants and human disease: Where are we now? *J. Lab. Clin. Med.* **119**(6), 598–620.

In vivo cancer model (1976-1982). Developmental therapeutic programme, Division of Cancer Treatment, National Cancer Institute, NIH Publication No. 84–2695, Pg no. 25, Protocol No. 3MBH2, 1984.

Kanekar, S. A. (1962). *Biological study of breast cancer in the albino strain of mouse inbred at the ICRC. M.Sc. thesis*. University of Bombay.

Khoobchandani, M, Ojeswi, B. K., Hazra, D. K., and Srivastava, M. M. (2009). *Brassica oleracea* extracts: Potential for antioxidative and anticancer activities for B16F10 & B16F1 mice melanoma cell lines. *Nat. Acad. Sci. Let.* **32**(9, 10), 297-302.

Khoobchandani, M, Ojeswi, B. K., Sharma, B, and Srivastava, M. M. (2009). Chenopodium album preventive progression of cell growth and enhancement in cell toxicity in human breast cancer cell lines. *Oxi. Med. Cellular Longivity* **2**(3), 160-165.

Kun-Young, K., Jae, H., Sun, Y. K., and Chi, H. C. (2003). Cadmiun induced acute lung injury and tunel expression of apoptosis in respiratory cells. *J. Korean Med. Sci.* **18**, 655-662.

Lee, S. E., Ju, E. M., and Kim, J. H. (2002). Antioxidant activity of extracts from Euryale ferox seed. *Exp. Mol. Med.* **34**(2), 100-106.

Millspaugh, C. F. (1974). *American Medicinal Plant-Thuja occidentalis*. Dover Publications, New York.

Nam, S. H and Kang, M. Y. (2008). Antioxidant activity of medicinal plants. *Pharma Biotech* **42**, 409-415.

Naser, B, Bodinet, C, Tegtmeier, M., and Lindequest, V. (2009). *Thuja occidentalis* (Arborvitae): A review of its pharmaceutical, pharmacological and clinical properties. *Adv. Access. Publ.* **2**, 69-78.

Ojeswi, B. K, Khoobchandani, M., and Srivastava, M. M. (2009). Green Chemicals: Prospects and Future in designing new drugs for cancer. *Int. J. Waste Wat. Treat. Green Chem.* **1**(1), 17-21.

Ojeswi, B. K., Khoobchandani, M., Hazra, D. K., and Srivastava, M. M. (2010). Protective effect of *Thuja occidentalis* against DMBA induced breast cancer with reference to oxidative stress. *Human Exp. Toxi.* **29**(5), 369-375.

Ojeswi, B. K., Khoobchandani, M., Hazra, D. K., and Srivastava, M. M. (2009). *In vitro* antibreast cancer efficacy of two indigenous plants on human cancer cell line MCF-7. *National Academy Science Letter* **32** (3, 4), 105-109.

Savage, J. R. K. (1993). Update on target theory as applied to chromosomal aberrations. *Env. Mol. Mutagen.* **22**, 198-202.

Shimada, K., Fujikawa, K., Yahara, K., and Nakamura, T. (1992). Antioxidative properties of xanthin on autoxidation of soybean oil in cyclodextrin emulsion. *J. Agric. Food Chem.* **40**, 945-948.

Sunde, R. A. and Hoekstra, W. G. (1980). Structure, synthesis and function of glutathione peroxidase. *Nutr. Rev.* **6**, 265-273.

Werneke, U, Ladenheim, D., and McCarthy, T. (2004). Complementary alternative medicine for cancer: A review of effectiveness and safety. *Cancer Therapy* **2**, 475-500.

Yao, M., Song, D. H., Rana, B., and Wolfe, M. M. (2002). COX-2 selective inhibition reverses the tropic properties of gastrin in colorectal cancer. *Brit. J. Can.* **87**, 574–579.

10

Block, K. I. (2004). Antioxidants and Cancer Therapy: Furthering the Debate. *Integrative Cancer Therapy* **3**, 342348.

Borek, C. (2004). Dietary antioxidants and human cancer. *Integrative Cancer Therapy* **3**, 333341.

Carmia, B. (2004). Dietary Antioxidants and Human Cancer. *Integrative Cancer Therapy* **3**, 333.

Chinery, R., Brockman, J. A., Peeler, M. O., Shyr, Y., Beauchamp, R. D., and Coffey, R. J. (1997). Antioxidants enhance the cytotoxicity of chemotherapeutic agents in colorectal cancer: A p53-independent induction of p21$^{WAF1/CIP1}$ via C/EBP β. *Nature Medicine* **3**, 1233–1241.

Duthie, S. J., Ma, A., Ross, M. A., and Collins, A. R. (1996). Antioxidant supplementation decreases oxidative damage in human lymphocytes. *Cancer Research* **56**, 12911295.

Hogan, F. S., Krishnegowda, N. K., Mikhailova, M., and Kahlenberg, M. S. (2007). Flavonoid, Silibinin, Inhibits Proliferation and Promotes Cell-Cycle Arrest of Human Colon Cancer. *Journal of Surgical Research* **143**, 58–65.

Kaur, M. and Agarwal, R. (2007). Silymarin and epithelial cancer chemoprevention: How close we are to bedside? *Toxicology and Applied Pharmacology* **224**, 350–359.

Kedar, N., Prasad, K. N., Kumar, A., Kochupillai, V., and Cole, W. C. (1999). High Doses of Multiple Antioxidant Vitamins: Essential Ingredients in Improving the Efficacy of Standard Cancer Therapy. *Journal of American College of Nutrition* **18**(1), 1325.

Labriola, D. and Livingston, R. (1999). Possible interactions between dietary antioxidants and chemotherapy. *Oncology* **13**, 10031012.

Lamm, D. L., Riggs, D., Shriver, J., VanGilder, P., Rach, J., and DeHaven, J. (1994). Megadose vitamins in bladder cancer. A double-blind clinical trial. *Journal of Urology* **151**, 2126.

Lamson, D. W. and Brignall, M. S. (1999). Antioxidants in cancer therapy: their actions and interactions with oncologic therapies. *Alternative Medicine Review* **4**, 304329.

Lamson, D. W. and Brignall, M. S. (2000) Antioxidants and cancer therapy II: Quick reference guide. *Alternative Medicine Review* **5**, 152163.

Lee, I. M., Cook, N. R., and Manson, J. E. (1999). Beta-carotene supplementation and incidence of cancer and cardiovascular disease: Women's Health Study. *Journal of National Cancer Institute* **91**, 2102–2106.

Liu, Q. Y. and Tan, B. K. H. (2002). Dietary Fish Oil and Vitamin E Enhance Doxorubicin. Effects in P388 Tumor-Bearing Mice. *Lipids* **37**, 549–556.

Prasad, K. N. (2004). Multiple dietary antioxidants enhance the efficacy of standard and experimental cancer therapies and decrease their toxicity. *Integrative Cancer Therapy* **3**, 10322.

Sangeetha, P., Das, U. N., Koratkar, R., and Suryaprabha, P. (1990). Increase in free radical generation and lipid peroxidation following chemotherapy in patients with cancer. *Free Radical Biology Medicine* **8**, 1519.

Saxena, A., Saxena, A. K., Singh, J., and Bhushan, S. (2010). Natural antioxidants synergistically enhance the anticancer potential of AP9-cd, a novel lignan composition from *Cedrus deodara* in human leukemia HL-60 cells. *Chemico. Biological Interactions* **188**, 580590.

Singh, S. K., Shanmugavel, M., Kampasi, H., Singh, R., Mondhe, D. M., Rao, J. M., Adwankar, M. K., Saxena, A. K., and Qazi, G. N. (2007) Chemically standardized isolates from *Cedrus deodara* stem wood having anticancer activity. *Planta Medical* **73**, 519526.

Weij, N. I., Hopman, G. D., Wipkink-Bakker, A., Lentjes, E. G. W. M., Berger, H. M., Cleton1, F. J., and Osanto, S. (1998). Cisplatin combination chemotherapy induces a fall in plasma antioxidants of cancer patients. *Annals of Oncology* **9**, 13311337.

Whelan, R. L., Horvath, K. D., Gleason, N. R., Forde, K. A., Treat, M. D., Teitelbaum, S. L., Bertram, A., and Neugut, A. I. (1999). Vitamin and calcium supplement use is associated with decreased adenoma recurrence in patients with a previous history of neoplasia. *Dis. Colon Rectum* **42**, 212217.

11

Altekruse, S. F., Kosary, C. L., Krapcho, M., Neyman, N., Aminou, R., Waldron, W., Ruhl, J., Howlader, N., Tatalovich, Z., Cho, H., Mariotto, A., Eisner, M. P., Lewis, D. R., Cronin, K., Chen, H. S., Feuer, E. J., Stinchcomb, D. G., and Edwards, B. K. (2010). SEER Cancer Statistics Review, 1975–2007, National Cancer Institute. M. D. Bethesda, http://seer.cancer.gov/csr /1975_2007/, based on November 2009 SEER data submission, posted to the SEER web site.

Auerbach, C. (1962). *Mutation: An introduction to research on mutagenesis Part I: Methods*. Oliver and Boyed, Edinburgh, pp. 422–428.

Balch, C. M. (1992). Cutaneous melanoma: Prognosis and treatment results worldwide, Semin. *Surgical Oncology* **8**, 400–414.

Balch, C. M., Soong, S. J., Gershenwald, J. E., Thompson, J. F., Reintgen, D. S., Cascinelli N., Urist, M., McMasters, K. M., Ross, M. I., Kirkwood, J. M., Atkins, M. B., Thompson, J. A., Coit, D. G., Byrd, D., Desmond, R., Zhang, Y., Liu, P. Y., Lyman, G. H., and Morabito, A.

(2001). Prognostic factors analysis of 17,600 melanoma patients: validation of the American Joint Committee on Cancer melanoma staging system. *Journal of Clinical Oncology* **19**(16), 3622–3634.

Barnhill, R. L., Piepkorn, M. W., Cochran, A. J., Flynn, E., Karaoli, T., and Folkman, J. (1998). Tumor vascularity, proliferation, and apoptosis in human melanoma micrometastases and macrometastases. *Archive Dermatology* **134**(8), 991–994.

Bianco, V. (1995). Rocket, an ancient underutilized Vegetable crop and its potential. *Rocket Genetic Resources Network*. S. Paludosi (compiler). IPGRI, Rome, pp. 35–58.

Cassileth, B. (2009). *Mediterranean diet. Oncology* **23**(14), 1315.

Chen, S. and Andreasson, E. (2001). Update on glucosinolate metabolism and transport. *Plant Physiology and Biochemistry* **39**, 743–758.

Comporti, M. (1989). Three models of free-radicals induced cell injury. *Chemico Biological Interaction*, **72**, 1–56.

Diepgen, T. L. and Mahler, V. (2002). The epidemiology of skin cancer. *The British Journal of Dermatology* **146**(61), 1–6.

Fahey, J. W., Zhang, Y., and Talalay, P. (1997). Broccoli sprouts: An exceptionally rich source of inducers of enzymes that protect against chemical carcinogens. *Proceeding of Natural Academic Science USA* **89**, 10367–10372.

Frieauff, W., Hartmann, A., and Suter, W. (2001). Automatic analysis of slides processed in the Comet assay. *Mutagenesis* **16**(2), 133–137.

Greenlee, R. T., Hill-Harmon, M. B., Murray, T., and Thun, M. (2001). Cancer statistics. *CA Cancer Journal of Clinical* **51**, 15–36.

Guerrero, R. F., Garcia-Parrilla, M. C., Puertas, B., and Cantos-Villar, E. (2009). Wine, resveratrol and health: A review. *Natural Products Communication* **4**(5), 635–658.

Halliwell, B., Gutteridge, J. M. C., and Cross, C. E. (1992). Free radicals, antioxidants and human disease: Where are we now? *Journal of Laboratory Clinical Medicine* **119**(6), 598–620.

Higdon, V., Delage, B., Williams, D. E., and Dashwood, R. H. (2007). Cruciferous vegetables and human cancer risk: Epidemiologic evidence and mechanistic basis. *Pharmacological Research* **55**, 224–236.

Hoey, S. H. E., Devereux, C. E. J., and Murray, L. (2007). Skin cancer trends in Northern Ireland and consequences for provision of dermatology services. *The British Journal of Dermatology* **156**, 1301–1307.

Jeffery, E. H. and Jarrell, V. (2001). Cruciferous vegetables and cancer prevention. *In Handbook of Nutraceuticals and Functional Foods*. R. E. C. Wildman, (Ed.). CRC Press LLC, Boca, Raton, FL, pp. 169–192.

Khoobchandani, M., Ojeswi, B. K., Ganesh, N., Srivastava, M. M., Gabbanini, S., Matera, R., Iori, R., and Valgimigli, L. (2010). Antimicrobial properties and analytical profile of traditional *Eruca sativa* seed oil. Comparison with various aerial and root plant extracts. *Food Chemistry* **120** (1), 217–224.

Khoobchandani, M., Ojeswi, B. K., Hazra, D. K., and Srivastava, M. M. (2009). *Brassica oleracea* extracts: Potential for antioxidant and anticancer activities for B16F10 & B16F1 mice melanoma cell lines. *National Academy Science Letter* **32** (9, 10), 297–302.

Kun-Young, K., Jae, H., Sun, Y. K., and Chi, H. C. (2003). Cadmiun induced acute lung injury and tunel expression of apoptosis in respiratory cells. *Journal of Korean Medical Science* **18**, 655–662.

Lee, W. R., Shen, S. C., Lin, H. Y., Hou, W. C., Yang, L. L., and Chen, Y. C. (2002). Wogonin and fisetin induce apoptosis in human promyeloleukemic cells, accompanied by a decrease of reactive oxygen species, and activation of caspase 3 and Ca(2þ)-dependent endonuclease. *Biochemical Pharmacology* **63**, 225–236.

Melchini, A., Costa, C., Traka, M., Miceli, N., Mithen, R., De Pasquale, R., and Trovato, A. (2009). Erucin, a new promising cancer chemopreventive agent from rocket salads, shows antiproliferative activity on human lung carcinoma A549 cells. *Food Chemical and Toxicology* **47**(7), 1430–1436.

Nam, S. H. and Kang, M. Y. (2008). Antioxidant activity of medicinal plants. *Pharmaceutical Biotechnology* **42**, 409–415.

Nascimento, N. C. D., Fragoso, V., Moura, D. J., Silva, A. C. R., Fett-Neto, A. G., and Saffi, J. (2007). Antioxidant and Antimutagenic effects of the Crude Foliar Extract and the Alkaloid Brachycerine of *Psychotria brachyceras*. *Environmental and Molecular Mutagenesis* **48**, 728–734.

Ojeswi, B. K., Khoobchandani, M., and Srivastava, M. M. (2009). Green Chemicals: Prospects and Future in designing new drugs for cancer. *International Journal of Waste Water Treatment and Green Chemistry* **1**(1), 17–21.

Pauwels, E. K. J. and Covas, M. I. (2009). The Mediterranean diet, part I: The anticancer effect of olive oil. *Drugs Future* **34**(4), 307–313.

Poppel, V. G., Verhoeven, D. T., Terhagen, H., and Goldbohm, R. A. (1999). *Brassica* vegetables and cancer prevention. Epidemiology and mechanisms. *Advance Experimental Medicinal Biology* **472**, 159–168.

Savage, J. R. K. (1993). Update on target theory as applied to chromosomal aberrations. *Environmental and Molecular Mutagenesis* **22**, 198–207.

Schmid, W. (1975). The micronucleus test. *Mutation Research* **31**, 9–12.

Shimada, K., Fujikawa, K., Yahara, K., and Nakamura, T. (1992). Antioxidative properties of xanthin on autoxidation of soybean oil in cyclodextrin emulsion. *Journal of Agricultural and Food Chemistry* **40**, 945–948.

Shureiqi, I., Reddy, P., and Brenner, D. E. (2000). Chemoprevention: General perspective. *Critical reviews in oncology/hematology* **33**, 157–167.

Tang, F. Y., Cho, H. J., Pai, M. H., and Chen, Y. H. (2009). Concomitant supplementation of lycopene and eicosapentaenoic acid inhibits the proliferation of human colon cancer cells. *Journal of Nutrition Biochemistry* **20**(6), 426–434.

Tseng, M., Sellers Thomas, A., Vierkant Robert, A., Kushi Lawrence, H., and Vachon Celine, M. (2008). Mediterranean diet and breast density in the Minnesota Breast Cancer Family Study. *Nutrition Cancer* **60**(6), 703–709.

Verhoeven, D. T., Goldbohm, R. A., Van Poppel, G., Verhagen, H., and Brandt van den, P. A. (1996). Epidemiological studies on *Brassica* vegetables and cancer risk. *Cancer Epidemiology, Biomarkers and Prevention* **5**, 733–748.

Warwick, S. I. (1994). Guide to the wild germplasm of *Brassica* and allied crops. Part V. Life History and Geographical Data for wild species in the tribe Brassicaceae (Cruciferae). *Agricultural Canadian Technical Bulletin* **2E**, 61.

Zeven, A. C. and de Wet, J. M. J. (1982). *Dictionary of cultivated plants and their regions of diversity,* 2nd ed. Centre for Agricultural Publishing and Documentation, Wageningen, p. 107.

Zhang, Y., Talalay, P., Cho, C., and Posner, G. H. (1992). A Major Inducer of Anticarcinogenic Protective Enzymes from Broccoli: Isolation and Elucidation of Structure. *Proceedings of the National Academy of Sciences* **89**, 2399–2403.

12

Albers, B. J., Schwendemann, T. C., Baykara, M. Z., Pilet, N., Liebmann, M., Altman, E. I., and Schwarz, U. D. (2009). Three-dimensional imaging of short-range chemical forces with picometre resolution. *Nat. Nanotechnol.* **4**, 307.

Albrecht, T. R., Grütter, P., Horne, D., and Rugar, D. (1991). *J. Appl. Phys.* **69**, 668.

Andreeva, N., Ferrini, G., Bassi, D., Cappa, F., Cocconcelli, P. S., Prato, S., Troian, B., and Parmigiani, F. (2009). Preliminary results of combined scanning near-field optical microscopy and atomic force microscopy applied to a model biological system: Clostridium tyrobutyricum spores. *Boll. Geof. Teor. Appl.* **50**, 396.

Andreeva, N., Bassi, D., Cappa, F., Cocconcelli, P. S., Parmigiani, F., and Ferrini, G. (2010). Nanomechanical analysis of Clostridium tyrobutyricum spores. *Micron* **41**, 945.

Auld, B. (1990). *Acoustic Fields and Waves in Solids.* Krieger, Malabar FL.

Banfi, F., Pressacco, F., Revaz, B., Giannetti, C., Nardi, D., Ferrini, G., and Parmigiani, F. (2010). Abinitio thermodynamics calculation of all-optical time-resolved calorimetry of nanosize systems: Evidence of nanosecond decoupling of electron and phonon temperatures. *Phys. Rev. B* **81**, 155-426.

Bartels, A., Dekorsy, T., and Kurz, H. (1999). Coherent zone-folded longitudinal acoustic phonons in semiconductor superlattices: Excitation and detection. *Phys. Rev. Lett.* **82**, 1044–1047.

Bartels, A., Cerna, R., Kistner, C., Thoma, A., Hudert, F., Janke, C., and Dekorsy, T. (2007). Ultrafast time-domain spectroscopy based on high-speed asynchronous optical sampling. *Rev. Sci. Instrum.* **78**, 035-107.

Butt, H. J., Cappella, B., and Kappl, M. (2005). Force measurements with the atomic force microscope: technique, interpretation and applications. *Surf. Sci. Rep.* **59**, 1–152.

Cecchini, M., Piazza, V., Simoni, G. D., Beltram, F., Beere, H. E., and Ritchie, D. A. (2006). Acoustic charge transport in a n-i-n three terminal device. *Appl. Phys. Lett.* **88**, 212101.

Chao, W., Harteneck, B. D., Liddle, J. A., Anderson, E. H., and Attwood, D. T. (2005). Soft X-ray microscopy at a spatial resolution better than 15 nm. *Nature* **435**, 1210–1213.

Cilento, F., Giannetti, C., Ferrini, G., Dal Conte, S., Sala, T., Coslovich, G., Rini, M., Cavalleri, A., and Parmigiani, F. (2010). Ultrafast insulator-to-metal phase transition as a switch to measure the spectrogram of a supercontinuum light pulse. *Appl. Phys. Lett.* **96**, 021-102.

Cross, S. E., Jin, Y. S., Rao, J., and Gimzewski, J. K. (2007). Nanomechanical analysis of cells from cancer patients. *Nat. Nanotechnol.* **2**, 780–783.

de Lima, M. M., Hey, R., Santos, P. V., and Cantarero, A. (2005). Phonon-induced optical superlattice. *Phys. Rev. Lett.* **94**, 126-805.

Ferrini, G., De Carlo, L., Giannetti, C., and Parmigiani, F. (2009). Evanescent wave spectroscopy of methylene blue solutions at surfaces using a continuum generated by a nonlinear fiber. *Optics and Spectroscopy* **107**, 464; ОПТИКА И СПЕКТРОСКОПИЯ 107, 490.

Fukuma, T., Higgins, M. J., and Jarvis, S. P. (2007). Direct Imaging of Lipid-Ion Network Formation under Physiological Conditions by Frequency Modulation Atomic Force Microscopy. *Phys. Rev. Lett.* **98**, 106101.

Garcia, R. and Perez, R. (2002). Dynamic atomic force microscopy methods. *Surf. Sci. Rep.* **47**, 197.

Giannetti, C., Revaz, B., Banfi, F., Montagnese, M., Ferrini, G., Cilento, F., Maccalli, S., Vavassori, P., Oliviero, G., Bontempi, E., Depero, L. E., Metlushko, V., and Parmigiani, F. (2007). Thermomechanical behavior of surface acoustic waves in ordered arrays of nanodisks studied by near-infrared pump-probe diffraction experiments. *Phys. Rev. B* **76**, 125-413.

Giannetti, C., Banfi, F., Nardi, D., Ferrini, G., and Parmigiani, F. (2009). Ultrafast Laser Pulses to Detect and Generate Fast Thermomechanical Transients in Matter. *IEEE Photonics Journal* **1**, 21.

Giessibl, F. J. (2003). Advances in atomic force microscopy. *Rev. Mod. Phys.* **75**, 949.

Gross, L., Mohn, F., Moll, N., Liljeroth, P., and Meyer, G. (2009). The Chemical Structure of a Molecule Resolved by Atomic Force Microscopy. *Science* **325**, 1110.

Gundrum, B. C., Cahill, D. G., and Averback, R. S. (2005). Thermal conductance of metal–metal interfaces. *Phys. Rev. B* **72**, 245-426.

von Gutfeld, R. J. and Nethercot, A. H. (1966). Temperature dependence of heat-pulse propagation in sapphire. *Phys. Rev. Lett.* **17**, 868–871.

Harrick, N. J. and du Pré, F. K. (1966). Effective Thickness of Bulk Materials and of Thin Films for Internal Reflection Spectroscopy. *Appl. Optics* **11**, 17-39.

Highland, M., Gundrum, B. C., Koh, Y. K., Averback, R. S., Cahill, D. G., Elarde, V. C., Coleman, J. J., Walko, D. A., and Landahl, E. C. (2007). Ballistic-phonon heat conduction at the nanoscale as revealed by time-resolved X-ray diffraction and time-domain thermoreflectance. *Phys. Rev. B* **76**, 075-337.

Hurley, D. H., Wright, O. B., Matsuda, O., Suzuki, T., Tamura, S., and Sugawara, Y. (2006). Time-resolved surface acoustic wave propagation across a single grain boundary. *Phys. Rev. B* **73**, 125-403.

Hurley, D. H., Lewis, R., Wright, O. B., and Matsuda, O. (2008). Coherent control of gigahertz surface acoustic and bulk phonons using ultrafast optical pulses. *Appl. Phys. Lett.* **93**, 113101.

Juvé, V., Scardamaglia, M, Maioli, P., Crut, A., Merabia, S., Joly, L., Del Fatti, N., and Vallée, F. (2009). Cooling dynamics and thermal interface resistance of glass-embedded metal nanoparticles. *Phys. Rev. B* **80**, 195-406.

Knoll, W. (1998). Interfaces and thin films as seen by bound electromagnetic waves. *Annu. Rev. Phys. Chem.* **49**, 569–638.

Landau, L. D., Pitaevskii, L. P., Kosevich, A. M., and Lifshitz, E. M. (1959). *Theory of Elasticity.* Pergamon Press Ltd., Oxford, U.K.

Landau, L. D. and Lifshitz, E. M. (1986). *Theory of Elasticity.* Butterworth-Heinemann, Oxford, U.K.

Lantz, M. A., Hug, H. J., Hoffmann, R., van Schendel, P. J. A., Kappenberger, P., Martin, S., Baratoff, A., and Güntherodt, H. J. (2001). Quantitative Measurement of Short-Range Chemical Bonding Forces. *Science* **291**, 25-80.

Lin, H. Y., Maris, H. J., Freund, L. B., Lee, K. Y., Luhn, H., and Kern, D. P. (1993). Study of vibrational modes of gold nanostructures by picosecond ultrasonics. *J. Appl. Phys.* **73**, 37.

Lyeo, H. K. and Cahill, D. G. (2006). Thermal conductance of interfaces between highly dissimilar materials. *Phys. Rev. B* **73**, 144-301.

Mallat, S. G. (1999). *A Wavelet Tour of Signal Processing.* Academic Press, New York.

Malegori, G. and Ferrini, G. (2010a). Tip-sample interactions on graphite studied in the thermal oscillation regime. *J. Vac. Sci. Technol. B* **28**, C4B18.

Malegori, G. and Ferrini, G. (2010b). Tip-sample interactions on graphite studied using the wavelet transform. *Beilstein J. Nanotechnol* **1**, 172.

Malegori, G. and Ferrini, G. (2011a). Wavelet transforms to probe long- and short-range forces by thermally excited dynamic force spectroscopy. *Nanotechnology* **22**, 195-702.

Malegori, G. and Ferrini, G. (2011b). Wavelet Transforms to Probe the Torsional Modes of a Thermally Excited Cantilever across the Jump-to-Contact Transition: Preliminary Results. *J. Surf. Sci. Nanotech* **9**, 228.

Maris, H. (1998). Picosecond ultrasonics. *Sci. Amer* **278**, 86.

Maznev, A. A. (2009). Laser-generated surface acoustic waves in a ring-shaped waveguide resonator. *Ultrasonics* **49**, 1–3.

Morita, S., Wiesendanger, R., and Meyer, E. (Eds.) (2002). *Noncontact Atomic Force Microscopy.* Springer, Berlin.

Nardi, D., Banfi, F., Giannetti, C., Revaz, B., Ferrini, G., and Parmigiani, F. (2009). Pseudo-surface acoustic waves in hypersonic surface phononic crystals. *Phys. Rev. B* **80**, 104-119.

Ohline, S. M., Lee, S., Williams, S., and Chang, C. (2001).*Chem. Phys. Lett.* **346**, 9.

Perrin, B., Péronne, E., and Belliard, L. (2006). Generation and detection of incoherent phonons in picosecond ultrasonics. *Ultrasonics* **44**, e1277–e1281.

Profunser, D. M., Wright, O. B., and Matsuda, O. (2006). Imaging ripples on phononic crystals reveals acoustic band structure and Bloch harmonics. *Phys. Rev. Lett.* **97**, 055-502.

Radmacher, M., Fritz, M., Kacher, C. M., Cleveland, J. P., and Hansma, P. K. (1996). Measuring the viscoelastic properties of human platelets with the atomic force microscope. *Biophys. J.* **70**, 556–567.

Robillard, J. F., Devos, A., and Roch-Jeune, I. (2007). Time-resolved vibrations of two-dimensional hypersonic phononic crystals. *Phys. Rev. B* **76**, 092-301.

Rosenbluth, M. J., Lam, W. A., and Fletcher, D. A. (2006). Force microscopy of nonadherent cells: a comparison of leukemia cell deformability. *Biophys. J.* **90**, 2994–3003.

Schirmeisen, A. (2010). Surfing on graphite waves. *Nat. Mat.* **9**, 615.

Siemens, M. E., Li, Q., Murnane, M. M., Kapteyn, H. C., Yang, R., Anderson, E. H., and Nelson, K. A. (2009). High-frequency surface acoustic wave propagation in nanostructures characterized by coherent extreme ultraviolet beams. *Appl. Phys. Lett.* **94**, 093-103.

Siemens, M. E., Li, Q., Yang, R., Nelson, K. A., Anderson, E. H., Murnane, M. M., and Kapteyn, H. C. (2010). *Nature Materials* **9**, 26.

Stoner, R. J. and Maris, H. (1993). Kapitza conductance and heat flow between solids at temperatures from 50 to 300 K. *Phys. Rev. B* **48**, 16373–16387.

Sugawara, Y., Wright, O. B., Matsuda, O., Takigahira, M., Tanaka, Y., Tamura, S., and Gusev, V. E. (2002). Watching ripples on crystals. *Phys. Rev. Lett.* **88**, 185-504.

Sugimoto, Y., Pou, P., Abe, M., Jelinek, P., Pérez, R., Morita, S., and Custance O. (2007). Chemical identification of individual surface atoms by atomic force microscopy. *Nature* **446**, 64.

Tobey, R. I., Gershgoren, E. H., Siemens, M. E., Murnane, M. M., Kapteyn, H. C., Feurer T., and Nelson K. A. (2004). *Appl. Phys. Lett.* **85**, 564.

Voisin, C., Del Fatti, N., Christofilos, D., and Vallée, F. (2000). Time resolved investigation of the vibrational dynamics of metal nanoparticles. *Appl. Surf. Sci.* **164**, 131–139.

Wilson, M. (2007). Ultrafast laser spectroscopy measures heat flow through molecular chains. *Physics Today* **60**, 20-23.

13

Apóstolo, J. L. A., Batista ,A. C., Macedo, C. M. R., and Pereira, E. M. R. (2006). Suffering and comfort in patients who undergo chemotherapy. *Referência* **2**ª Série (3), 55–64.

Apóstolo, J. L. A., Cunha, S. R. P., Cristo, J. M. F., and Lacerda, R. P. P. (2004). Experience of the patients' relatives with oncological illness terminal condition in a center of palliative care. *Revista Investigação Enfermagem* **10**, 28–37.

Barbosa, A. (2006). Sofrimento (Suffering). In *Manual de cuidados paliativos (Manual of palliative care)*, A. Barbosa and I. Neto (Eds.), Fundação Calouste Gulbenkian, Lisboa, Portugal, pp. 397–417.

Capela, R. (2010). O sofrimento de doentes oncológicos em cuidados paliativos (Suffering of oncological patients in palliative care). Master Dissertation, *Universidade Católica Portuguesa, Porto, Portugal.*

Cassell, E. J. (1991). Recognizing suffering. *Hastings Center Report* **21**(3), 24–31.

Cassell, E. J. (1999). Diagnosing suffering: A perspective. *Annals of Internal Medicine* **131**(7), 531–534.

Fleming, M. (2003). Dor sem nome: Pensar o sofrimento (Pain without a name: The thinking of suffering). Afrontamento, Porto, Portugal.

Ferreira, F. L. (2009). Suffering of women having chemotherapy after mastectomy. *Referência* **2**ᵃSérie(10), 65–76.

Frankl, V. (2004). *El hombre en busca de sentido (Man's search for meaning).* Herder, Barcelona.

Gameiro, M. G. H. (2000). IESSD: Um instrumento para a abordagem do sofrimento na doença (ISSEI: An instrument to approach suffering in illness), *Referência* **4**, 57–66.

Instituto de Lexicologia e Lexicografia da Academia das Ciências de Lisboa (Institute of Lexicology and Lexicography of the Lisbon Academy of Sciences) (2001). Dicionário da língua portuguesa contemporânea (Dictionary of contemporary Portuguese language). Editorial Verbo, Lisboa, Portugal.

Kolcaba, K. Y. (1991). A taxonomic structure for the concept comfort. *Image: Journal of Nursing Scholarship* **23**(4), 237–240.

Kolcaba, K. Y. (2003). Comfort theory and practice. *A vision for holistic health care and research*. Springer Publishing Company, New York.

Kolcaba, K. Y. and Kolcaba, R. J. (1991). An analysis of the concept of comfort. *Journal of Advanced Nursing* **16**(11), 1301–1310.

Mcintyre, T. M. (2004). Perda e sofrimento na doença: Contributo da psicologia da saúde (Loss and suffering during illness: Contributions from health psychology), *Psychologica* **35**, 167–179.

Neto, I. (2004). Para além dos sintomas: A dignidade e o sentido da vida na prática dos cuidados paliativos. In *A dignidade e o sentido da vida: uma reflexão sobre a nossa existência (Beyond symptoms: dignity and purpose of life in the practice of palliative care. In Dignity and purpose of life: a reflection on our existence).* I. Neto, H. Aitken, and T. Paldrön (Eds.), Pergaminho, Cascais, Portugal, pp. 13–40.

Index

A

Adenosine triphosphate (ATP), 76
Angiogenesis
  breast cancer, 3
  Down's syndrome, 3
  factors
    angiopoetins, 5
    angiostatin, 6
    CXC-chemokines, 6
    endostatin, 6–7
    fibroblast growth, 5
    integrins, 4–5
    thrombospondin-1, 6
    transforming growth, 5
    vascular endothelial growth, 5
  malignant metastatic cancer, 2–3
  mechanism, 2–4
  modulators of, 4
  physiological conditions, 2
  switch, 3
  tumor progression
    angiogenic switch, 4
    EPCs, 4
    vasculogenesis and lymphangiogenesis, 4
    VEGF expression, 4
  types, 4
  VEGF, 3
Angiogenic factors of angiogenesis
  angiopoetins, 5
  CXC-chemokines, 6
  fibroblast growth, 5
  integrins, 4–5
  transforming growth, 5
  vascular endothelial growth, 5
Angiostatic factors of angiogenesis
  angiostatin, 6
  endostatin, 6–7
  thrombospondin-1, 6
Antibacterial therapy and diagnosis
  AMPs
    biocidal efficiency, 37

clinical applications, 36–37
    DS polypeptide chains, 37
    EPR effect, 37
    immobilization of, 37
    leishmanicidal activity, 37
    magnetic nanoparticles, 37–38
    P. oreades and *P. hypochondrialis,* 37
  antibacterial activity of lysozyme, 33
  Bacillus anthracis, 31
  bacteriophage drug-carrying platforms, 35
  bioactive glasses, 34
  biopolymers, 34–35
  carbon nanotubes and fullerenes, 32
  mechanism of action, 32–33
  micellar nanocarriers, 36
  multifunctional nanoplatforms
    biofilm infections, 36
    mechanism of action, 36
    MRI, 36
  nanoemulsion
    Burkholderia cepacia, 35–36
    cystic fibrosis, 35
    systemic toxicity, 36
  nanomedicines, 31
  therapeutic and diagnostic applications, 31
Antimicrobial peptides (AMPs)
  biocidal efficiency, 37
  clinical applications, 36–37
  DS polypeptide chains, 37
  EPR effect, 37
  immobilization of, 37
  leishmanicidal activity, 37
  magnetic nanoparticles, 37–38
  P. oreades and *P. hypochondrialis,* 37
Antioxidants and combinatorial therapies
in cancer treatment
  anticancer potential
    Cedrus deodar, 158
    curcumin, 158
    cytotoxic and apoptotic, 158

lignan, 158
anti-neoplastic leads, 157
chemotherapeutic agents, 157
cisplatin-induced oxidative damage,
158–159
cytotoxic potential of chemotherapeutic
in colorectal cancer, 159
enhancement effect of doxorubicin, 159
heated debates
    cancer therapeutic agents, 160
    chemotherapy protocols, 161
    growth-inhibitory effects, 160
    growth promoting agents, 160–161
modulating effects, 157
Silymarin
    cancer protective effects, 160
    liver treatment, 160
    polyphenolic, 160
    silibinin's mechanism of action, 160
therapeutic effects, 158
Apoptosis
cell death, 2
chromalolysis, 2
combinational therapy, 2
disastrous effects, 2
mechanisms, 2
Applications of chitosan nanoparticles
anti-fungal delivery, 47
anti-microbial agents, 48–49
articular joint therapy, 51
brain delivery, 52
buccal and sublingual delivery system,
51
gene delivery system, 47–48
hepatitis treatment, 48
for hyperglycemia, 46
molecular imaging, 45
ocular delivery system, 51–52
protein delivery, 45
tumor targeting, 49–50
as vaccination, 45–46
via nasal route, 46–47
Aptamers
advantage, 10
oligonucleic acid/peptide molecules, 10
riboswitches, 10
therapeutic application, 10

Atomic force microscopy (AFM)
Brownian motion, 185
cantilever's dynamical parameters, 183
cell stiffness, 182
chemical specificity, 186
force measurements, 182
Fourier transform (FT), 183–184
frequency shift, 185
Heisenberg box, 185
Hooke's law, 182
linear elasticity theory, 182
mechanical properties, 182
quantitative analysis, 186
temporal oscillations of cantilever, 183
time–frequency representation, 183
Wavelet coefficients, 185
Wavelet transform (WT), 183–184
Young modulus, 182–183
ATP. *See* Adenosine triphosphate (ATP)

B

Brain tumours
anaplasia and pleomorphism, 20
astrocytic, 19
auto fluorescence spectroscopy, 21
catalytic nanomedicine, 21
chemotherapeutic agents, 21
fluorescence characteristics, 22
hemorrhage and necrosis, 19
histological characteristics, 19
infiltration pattern, 20
molar absorptivity and fluorescence
quantum, 21
necrotic regions, 20
optical spectroscopic methods, 21
radiation and chemotherapy, 20
Temozolomide, 20–21
Breast cancer
antioxidant levels, 88
antioxidant status, 86
D-loop region, 86
MDA, 87
superoxide dismutase and catalase
levels, 87–88
Brownian motion
AFM, 185
Burkholderia cepacia, 35–36

C

Caenorhabditis elegans, 16
Cancer disease in LPD
  disease dominant, 142
  iceberg psychosomatics, 142
  malignant tumors diseases, 141
  psychogenic
    carcinogenesis, 141
    component, 141–142
Chitosan nanoparticles
  applications of
    anti-fungal delivery, 47
    anti-microbial agents, 48–49
    articular joint therapy, 51
    brain delivery, 52
    buccal and sublingual delivery
      system, 51
    gene delivery system, 47–48
    hepatitis treatment, 48
    for hyperglycemia, 46
    molecular imaging, 45
    ocular delivery system, 51 52
    protein delivery, 45
    tumor targeting, 49–50
    as vaccination, 45–46
    via nasal route, 46–47
  biomedical material, 42
  drug delivery system, 41
  hydrophilic drug entrapment, 41
  ionic gelation and complex coacerva-
    tion, 41–42
  mechanism of transport, 52
  paracellular transport, 52–53
  pharmaceutical applications, 41
  preparation methods
    complex coacervation, 44
    covalent cross-links, 44
    desolvation, 44
    emulsion-droplet coalescence, 45
    ionic cross linking/ionic gelation,
      43–44
    reverse micellar, 45
    schematic representation of, 43
  solubility, 41
  structure of, 42
  therapeutic uses, 41
  transcellular transport

non-specific uptake, 53
specific uptake, 53–54
Chronic lymphoid leukemia (CLL), 8

D

Diseases in LPD
  pathological condition, 135
  psychogenic component, 135–136
  subdominants of, 135
Doctrine of dominant in LPD
  brain and spinal marrow, 132
  cortical, 133
  features, 132
  spiritual anatomy, 133
  topographic center, 132
  vital functions, 133
Down's syndrome, 3

E

Endothelial progenitor cells (EPCs), 4
Eruca sativa inhibits melanoma growth
  antimutagenic activity
    chromosomal aberration, 166–167
    histopathology study, 168–169
    micronuclei formation, 168
    micronucleus assay, 166, 168
    MPCE and MNCE, 167–168
    mutation effect, 168
  antitumor activity, 165–166
  cruciferous family, 166–164
  effect of seed oil, 166
  free radical scavenging, 164–165
  hydroxyl and DPPH radicals, 164–165
  isothiocyanates, 164
  mediterranean diet, 163
  seed oil, chemistry profile
    chemical structure of isothiocya-
      nates, 169
    chromatograms, 169–170
    epidemiological studies, 171
    isothiocyanate formation, 170
    mechanism depicting isothiocya-
      nates, 171
    taramira plant, 169–170

F

Fourier transform (FT), 183–184

G

Gene-based therapy in mitochondrial dysfunction and cancer
  Herculean challenge, 80
  isocitrate dehydrogenase 1 (IDH1), 80
  pharmacogenomics, 80
  SNPs, 80
Glioblastoma multiformes (GBM)
  biopsies, 25
  brain tissue fluorescence, 26
  brain tumours (*see* Brain tumours)
  cavity size, 26
  diffuse reflectance spectra, 27
  fluorescence measurements, 22, 25–26
  Hematoxyline-Eosine (H-E), 22–23
  histopathology
    anaplasia, 29
    bacterial-onslaught phase, 28
    coagulative necrosis, 28
    focal bacterial/fungal infections, 28
    malignant tissue, 29
    necrotic tissue, 28
    neoplasm of astrocytes, 29
    NPt treatment, 29
    vascularization, 29
  and Masson methods, 22–23
  microsurgical techniques, 24
  morphological change, 23
  MRI studies, 24
  nanostructured biocatalysts, 22
  optical spectra emissions, 25
  spectrofluorometer, 23–24
  tumor removal and surgical repair, 24
  and type I meningioma, 86
  WHO, 19
Glutathione (GSH), 146–147

H

Heisenberg box, 184
Histopathology for GBM
  anaplasia, 29
  bacterial-onslaught phase, 28
  coagulative necrosis, 28
  focal bacterial/fungal infections, 28
  malignant tissue, 29
  necrotic tissue, 28
  neoplasm of astrocytes, 29

  NPt treatment, 29
  vascularization, 29
Hooke's law, 182
Human concept in LPD
  basic integrated functional conditions, 136
  central nervous system, 133
  and current subdominants, 134
  dynamics of integrated condition, 137–139
  Homo ferus, 133
  iceberg psychosomatics, 137–138
  mental and somatic processes, 133
  occurrence and loss of, 135
  organs and systems, 133
  self-destruction dominant, 138–139

K

Kolcaba's conceptual framework, 192
Kretchmann configuration, 175

L

Life purpose dominant (LPD)
  in animal, 134
  cancer disease
    disease dominant, 141
    iceberg psychosomatics, 141
    malignant tumors diseases, 140
    psychogenic carcinogenesis, 140
    psychogenic component, 140–141
  chronic disease formation, 131–132
  concept implications, 142
  diseases
    pathological condition, 135
    psychogenic component, 135–136
    subdominants of, 135
  doctrine of dominant
    brain and spinal marrow, 132
    cortical, 133
    features, 132
    spiritual anatomy, 133
    topographic center, 132
    vital functions, 133
  in human
    basic integrated functional conditions, 136
    central nervous system, 133

and current subdominants, 134
dynamics of integrated condition,
    137–139
Homo ferus, 133
iceberg psychosomatics, 137–138
mental and somatic processes, 133
occurrence and loss, 135
organs and systems, 133
self-destruction dominant, 138–139
nervous centers and vital functions, 133
Pavlov's doctrine, 133
sole correct scientific idea, 133

M

Malondialdehyde (MDA)
    in breast cancer, 87
Medicinal plants
    anticancer agents, 70
    baikal skullcap (Scutellaria baicalen-
        sis), 70
    blocking agents, 73
    carcinogenesis, 73
    cytotoxic activity, 72
    kinase enzymes, 73
    phytochemicals, 70–73
    Plantago sp., 71
    potential bioactive compounds, 70
    suppressing agents, 73
Mendelian rules
    for mitochondrial dysfunction and
        cancer, 83
Methylene Blue (MB), 175
    molar absorbance spectra of, 176
Micro ribonucleic acids (miRNAs), 1
    breast carcinomas, 8
    CLL patients, 8
    downstream effecter molecules, 9
    genetic analysis, 8
    hypoxia, 9
    messenger RNAs, 7
    potential anticancer drugs, 9
    protein coding genes, 7
    stem loop structures, 7
    tumor necrosis factor alpha (TNF-α), 8
miRNAs. See Micro ribonucleic acids
    (miRNAs)
Mitochondrial dysfunction and cancer

alpha lipoic acid, 97–99
Alzheimer's disease, 97
apoptosis/programmed cell death, 83
ascorbic acid, 93–94
ATP
    turnover rates, 76
breast cancer, 86–88
catabolic processes, 82–83
chain reactions and free radical produc-
    tion, 92–93
defects, 77
depletion and deletion, 85
diameter and length, 81
drug induced toxicity, amelioration, 128
effects, 75–76
electron
    transfer, 78
    transport chain complexes, subunits
        of, 84
electronic properties, 84, 118
    admittance comparison of, 116
    current oscillations, 115
energy-converting organelles, 76
enzymatic composition, 82
Faradaic impedance, 115
free radicals and antioxidants
    capacitation process, 90
    chain reactions, 90
    enzymes, 91
    hydroxyl and superoxide, 89
    phagocytosis, 90
    physiologic reducing agents, 90
    reduction potentials, 91–92
    therapeutic applications, 92
function of, 83
GBM and type I meningioma, 86
gene-based therapy
    Herculean challenge, 80
    isocitrate dehydrogenase 1 (IDH1),
        80
    pharmacogenomics, 80
    SNPs, 80
glutathione, 95
glycolysis, 76–77
hallmarks of, 80–81
heteroplasmy and homoplasmy, 85
HIV infection, oxidative stress in, 128

holistic medicine, 75
hydrogen peroxide, 95–97
impedance spectroscopy, 113–114
Krebs cycle, enzymatic reactions, 77
matrix, 76
Mendelian rules, 83
mutated genes in different cancers, 84–85
mutations, 84, 86
natural compounds, 76
NDR, 116
neuron degeneration, 117
Nyquist plot, 115
ovarian cancer, 88
oxidative damage, 84
palladium α-lipoic acid complex, 99–112, 125–126
    formulation, 77–78
Parkinson's disease, 97
platinum(II) and palladium(II) complexes
    adenocarcinoma MCF7, 79–80
    biological action, 79
    cisplatin, 79
    gastrointestinal toxicity, 78
    hydrolysis, 79
    ovarian cancer treatment, 78
    palladium-based drugs, 80
    solid tumor chemotherapy, 78
powerhouse of cell, 81
production of ATP, 84
prostate cancer, 88–89
pyruvate dehydrogenase, 77
Raoult's law, 117
regulation of calcium homeostasis, 81
ROS, 78
SDH and shapes, 81
simple molecules, electronic properties of
    electrochemical impedance technique, 118
    enzyme activity, 118
    FAD, 121, 122
    impedance data, 122–123
    impedance spectra, 120
    L-lysine, 121
    neurotransmitter histamine, 124

Nyquist plot, 118–119, 122, 124
    transition metals, 118
    tunnel diode characteristics, 125
specific cytotoxic drugs, 75
spin coupling in electron transfer
    cytochromes, 126–127
    electron donor, 127
    EPR and ESR measurement, 126
    free radical reaction mechanism, 127
    iron-sulfur clusters, 126
    pulse radiolysis studies, 127
    semiquinone radicals, 126
    vectorial translocation, 126
tumorogenesis, 86
tunnel-diode behavior, 112–113
vitamin E, 94–95
Warburg effect/aerobic glycolysis, 85–86
Multifunctional nanoplatforms
    of antibacterial therapy and diagnosis
        biofilm infections, 36
        mechanism of action, 36
        MRI, 36

N

Nanoemulsion of antibacterial therapy and diagnosis
    Burkholderia cepacia, 35–36
    cystic fibrosis, 35
    systemic toxicity, 36
Nanostructures, optical and mechanical investigations
    AFM
        Brownian motion, 185
        cantilever's dynamical parameters, 183
        cell stiffness, 182
        chemical specificity, 186
        force measurements, 182
        Fourier transform (FT), 185–184
        frequency shift, 185
        Heisenberg box, 185
        Hooke's law, 182
        linear elasticity theory, 182
        mechanical properties, 182
        quantitative analysis, 187

temporal oscillations of cantilever, 183

time–frequency representation, 183

Wavelet coefficients, 185

Wavelet transform (WT), 183–184

Young modulus, 182–183

ligand-receptor complexes, 173

molecular detection at surfaces

  aggregation states, 175

  angle of incidence, 174

  application, 177

  evanescent wave, 173

  evanescent wave optics, 175

  Kretchmann configuration, 175

  Methylene Blue (MB), 175–176

  PCF, 174

  pump and probe techniques, 177

  refraction indexes, 174

molecular interactions, 173

single theoretical model, 173

study

  applications, 181–182

  energy density, 181

  energy radiation, 179

  features, 179

  gigahertz–terahertz frequency range, 177

  light penetration depth, 181

  oscillation dynamic, 181

  PEM, 180

  phononic crystal properties, 181

  pseudo-surface acoustic waves, 181

  pump and probe experiment, 178–179

  refractive index, 178

  relative intensity, 180

  SAWs, 178

  thermal conductance, 178

  thermal gradients, 177, 181

  thermoelastic stress, 178

  time-resolved measurements, 180

techniques, 173

Nanotechnological based systems for cancer

angiogenesis, 1, 2–7

anti-angiogenic drugs, 1

apoptosis, 2

aptamers, 10

carcinogenesis, 1

delivering anti-angiogenic/anticancer molecules, 11–12

gene delivery to target cells, 16

lactoferrin, 11

micro RNAS in, 7–9

miRNAs, 1

RNA interference (RNAi)

  Caenorhabditis elegans, 16

  endocytotic pathway, 17

  gene therapy, 16

  mechanism of, 16

  non-viral carriers, 17

  therapeutic applications, 16

tumor

  invasion and metastasis, 1

  suppressor genes, 1

uses of nano particles

  bioactive glass, 13–15

  calcium phosphate ceramics, 13

  doxorubicin and taxol loaded ACNC-NPs, 15

  lodamin, 12

  paciltaxil and ceramide, 12

  tumor vasculature, 12

VHL disease, 10–11

Negative differential resistance (NDR), 116

Nyquist plot, 115, 118–119, 122, 124

O

Ovarian cancer, 88

P

Palladium α-lipoic acid complex

antioxidant activity and prophylactic effects, 110–112

clinical human studies, 105–106

clinical veterinary studies, 103–104

effect of, 901

glioblastoma tumor volume, 102–103

mitochondrial studies

  antitumor activity, 108

  effect of, 106, 108

  enzyme activities, 106–107

  influence of, 109

Krebs cycle, 106
lactate dehydrogenase and pyruvate dehydrogenase, 110
lipid peroxidation and GSH level, 108
phosphorylation, 110
succinate dehydrogenase, 109
therapeutic effect, 107
open label veterinary oncology study, 104
oxygen radical absorbance capacity, 100
phase microscopy pictures, 125
protection from radiation, 110
self-assembly of, 125–126
synthesis of, 99
transient ischemia studies with gerbils, 104–105
in vitro cell line studies, 100–102
in vivo studies, 102–103
voltammetric studies, 100
Parkinson's disease
in mitochondrial dysfunction and cancer, 97
PCF. *See* Photonic-crystal fibers (PCF)
Photoelastic modulator (PEM), 180
Photonic-crystal fibers (PCF), 174
P. hypochondrialis, 37
Phytosynthesis in silver nanoparticles
Capsicum annum, 60
green chemistry methods, 59
mechanisms, 60
Menthapiperita leaf extract, 60
plant materials choice, 60–61
protocols and materials, 59
spectrometric analysis, 60
vascular plants leaf extracts, 60
P. oreades, 37
Portuguese cancer patients
comfort
ease and peaceful contentment, 191
health and well-being component, 191
Kolcaba's conceptual framework, 192
predict phenomena, 191
relief, 191–192

strengthen greatly, 192
comfort and suffering, 193–196
concept of suffering
dimensions, 189
existential and Socio-relational, 190
human experience, 189
human potential, 190
physical and psychological, 190
profile of suffering, 194
Prostate cancer, 88–89

R

Raoult's law, 117
Reactive oxygen species (ROS), 78
Recent advances in cancer therapy
causes, 69
chemotherapeutic agents, 69
dietary supplements, 70
medicinal plants
anticancer agents, 70
baikal skullcap *(Scutellaria ba-icalensis),* 70
blocking agents, 73
carcinogenesis, 73
cytotoxic activity, 71
kinase enzymes, 73
phytochemicals, 70–73
Plantago sp., 71
potential bioactive compounds, 70
suppressing agents, 73
natural products, 69
phytochemicals, 69–70
Taxol (paclitaxel), 69
RNA interference (RNAi)
Caenorhabditis elegans, 16
endocytotic pathway, 17
gene therapy, 16
mechanism of, 16
non-viral carriers, 17
therapeutic applications, 16
ROS. *See* Reactive oxygen species (ROS)

S

SAWs. *See* Surface acoustic waves (SAWs)
SDH. *See* Succinate dehydrogenase (SDH)
Silver nanoparticles

applications, 55
biomedical applications
    antibacterial effect, 65
    anti-infective topical medicine, 64
    antimicrobial activity, 64
    bactericidal effect, 64–65
    dimorphic transition, 66
    as disinfectant, 64
    fungicidal effect, 66
    hygienic and healing purposes, 64
    inhibitory and lethal effect, 65
    ulcer treatment, 64
biomemetric synthesis, 62
biosynthetic methods, 56–57
chemical synthesis
    chemical reductants, 62
    reducing agent, 61
    stabilizing agents, 62
    surfactants, 62
    wet chemical reduction, 61
classical chemical method, 56
intracellular magnetite/greigite nano
crystals, 57
microbial synthesis
    antimicrobial activity, 57–58
    bacterial strains, 59
    bactericidal effects, 57
    fungal strains used for biosynthesis,
    58–59
    Fusarium oxysporium and *Verticil-
    lium* sp, 57
    Fusarium semitectum, 57
    mechanism for, 58
physical synthesis procedures, 56
phytosynthesis
    Capsicum annum, 60
    green chemistry methods, 59
    mechanisms, 60
    Menthapiperita leaf extract, 60
    plant materials choice, 60–61
    protocols and materials, 59
    spectrometric analysis, 60
    vascular plants leaf extracts, 60
polyoxometalates method, 62
properties, 55
radiation chemical method, 56
synthesis from saccharides

irradiation method, 63
reducing and capping agent, 63
Tollen's method, 63
top-down approach, 56
Silymarin
    cancer protective effects, 160
    liver treatment, 160
    polyphenolic, 160
    silibinin's mechanism of action, 160
Single nucleotide polymorphisms (SNPs),
80
Succinate dehydrogenase (SDH)
    mitochondrial dysfunction and cancer,
    81
Surface acoustic waves (SAWs), 178
Synthesis from saccharides in silver
nanoparticles
    irradiation method, 63
    reducing and capping agent, 63
    Tollen's method, 63

T

Thuja occidentalis and breast cancer che-
    moprevention
    antibreast cancer activity
        bioassay of EtOAc fractions, 155
        doxorubicin drug, 151
        EtOAc and MeOH extracts effect,
        151–152
        growth inhibitory activity, 148–150
        TBE and MTT bioassays, 148
        tumor volume and body weight,
        150–151
    antimutagenic activity, 153–154
    carcinogenesis, 143
    cases of, 143
    chromosomal aberration in bone mar-
    row, 153–154
    coniferous pyramidal features, 143
    cupressaceae, 143
    ethyl acetate extract, chromatographic
    fractionation, 154–155
    experiments and protocol, 144–145
    folk medicine, 143
    free radical scavenging activity
        antioxidant, 145
        DMBA toxicity, 147

effect of solvent extracts, 146
EtOAc extract, effect of, 147
glutathione (GSH), 146–147
order of potency, 145
solvent extracts, 145
haematoxylin and eosin stained slides, 152
histopathological study, 152
morbidity and mortality, 143
phytochemical prevention, 143
therapies, 143
Tollen's method
for silver nanoparticles, 63
Transcellular transport of chitosan nanoparticles
non-specific uptake, 53
specific uptake, 53–54
Tumor necrosis factor alpha (TNF-α)

in micro RNAS, 8
Tumor progression for angiogenesis
angiogenic switch, 4
EPCs, 4
vasculogenesis and lymphangiogenesis, 4
VEGF expression, 4

V

Vascular endothelial growth factor (VEGF), 3
VEGF. *See* Vascular endothelial growth factor (VEGF)

W

Wavelet transform (WT), 183–184